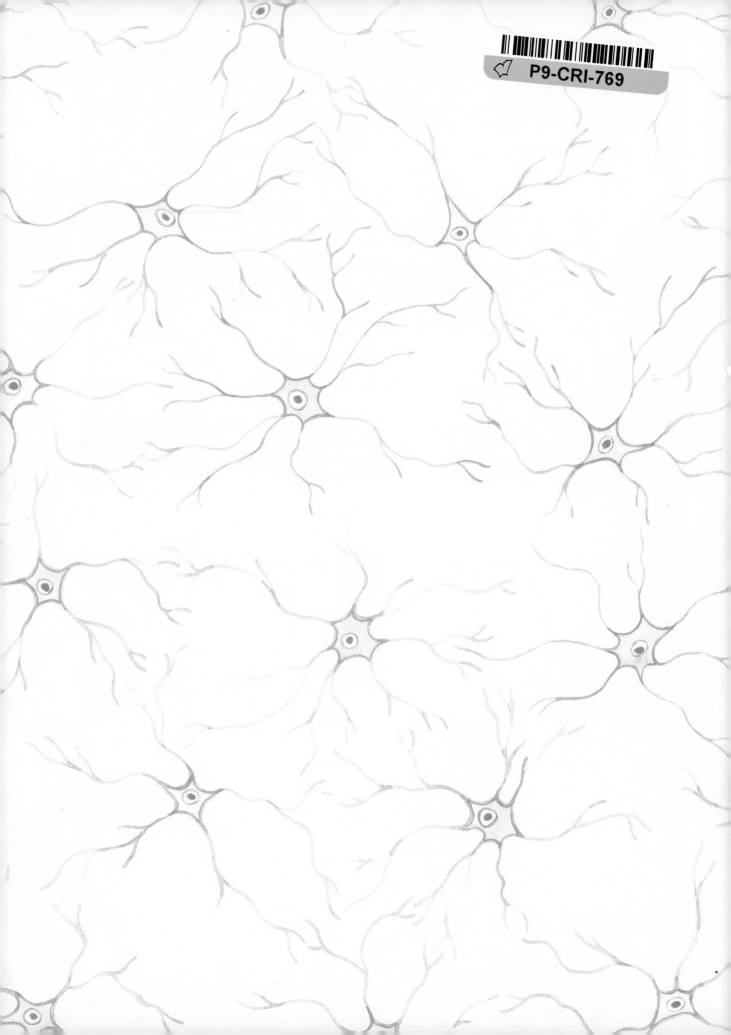

NURSE'S CLINICAL LIBRARY™

NEUROLOGIC DISORDERS

NURSING84 BOOKS™
SPRINGHOUSE CORPORATION
Springhouse, Pennsylvania

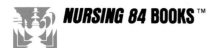

NURSING 84 BOOKS™

Nurse's Clinical Library™
Other volumes in this series:
Cardiovascular Disorders
Respiratory Disorders
Endocrine Disorders
Renal and Urologic Disorders
Gastrointestinal Disorders
Neoplastic Disorders

Nurse's Reference Library®
Diseases
Diagnostics
Drugs
Assessment
Procedures
Definitions
Practices
Emergencies

New Nursing Skillbook™ series
Giving Emergency Care
  Competently
Monitoring Fluid and
  Electrolytes Precisely
Assessing Vital Functions
  Accurately
Coping with Neurologic
  Problems Proficiently
Reading EKGs Correctly
Combatting Cardiovascular
  Diseases Skillfully
Nursing Critically Ill Patients
  Confidently
Dealing with Death and Dying

Nursing Photobook™ series
Providing Respiratory Care
Managing I.V. Therapy
Dealing with Emergencies
Giving Medications
Assessing Your Patients
Using Monitors
Providing Early Mobility
Giving Cardiac Care
Performing GI Procedures
Implementing Urologic
  Procedures
Controlling Infection
Ensuring Intensive Care
Coping with Neurologic
  Disorders
Caring for Surgical Patients
Working with Orthopedic
  Patients
Nursing Pediatric Patients
Helping Geriatric Patients
Attending Ob/Gyn Patients
Aiding Ambulatory Patients
Carrying Out Special
  Procedures

Nursing Now™ series
Shock
Hypertension
Drug Interactions
Cardiac Crises
Respiratory Emergencies
Pain

Nursing84 Drug Handbook™

Nurse's Clinical Library™

Editorial Director
Helen Klusek Hamilton

Clinical Director
Minnie Bowen Rose, RN, BSN, MEd

Art Director
Sonja E. Douglas

Clinical staff
Clinical Editors
Joanne Patzek DaCunha, RN;
Carole Arlene Pyle, RN, BSN, MA, CCRN

Drug Information Manager
Larry Neil Gever, RPh, PharmD

Contributing Clinical Editors
Sandra Ludwig Nettina, RN, BSN;
Jo-Ann Hopkins Olmstead, RN, BS

Acquisitions
Thomas J. Leibrandt, Susan H.
Brunt, Bernadette M. Glenn

Editorial staff
Managing Editor
Matthew Cahill

Associate Editors
Lisa Z. Cohen, H. Nancy Holmes,
Patricia Minard Shinehouse

Contributing Editors
Laura Albert, Barbara Hodgson,
Joan Twisdom-Harty, Marylou
Webster

Copy Supervisor
David R. Moreau

Copy Editors
Dale A. Brueggemann, Diane M.
Labus

Contributing Copy Editors
Laura Dabundo, Reni Fetterolf, Max
Fogel, Linda Johnson, Jane Paluda,
Doris Weinstock, William Wright

Production Coordinator
Sally Johnson

Editorial Assistants
Mary Ann Bowes, Maree DeRosa

Researchers
Vonda Heller, Elaine Shelly

Design staff
Senior Designer
Linda Jovinelly Franklin

Contributing Designers
Virginia Sloss, Mary Wise

Illustrators
Michael Adams, Dimitrios Bastas,
Maryanne Buschini, David
Christiana, Design Management,
Jean Gardner, William Haney, Tom
Herbert, Robert Jackson, Robert
Jones, Adam Mathews, Robert
Phillips, Eileen Rudnick, Dennis
Schofield

Production staff
Art Production
Robert Perry (manager), Diane Fox,
Donald Knauss, Robert Miele,
Sandy Sanders, Craig T. Siman,
Louise Stamper, Robert Wieder

Typography
David C. Kosten (manager), Ethel
Halle, Diane Paluba, Nancy Wirs

Senior Production Manager
Deborah C. Meiris

Production Manager
Wilbur D. Davidson

Production Assistant
Tim A. Landis

Library of Congress Cataloging in Publication Data
Main entry under title:
Neurologic disorders.
    (Nurse's clinical library)
    "Nursing84 Books."
    Bibliography: p.
    Includes index.
1. Neurological nursing.   I. Series.
[DNLM: 1. Neurology—nurses'
instruction. WY 160 N493]
RC350.5.N48 1984   610.73'68   84-5504
ISBN 0-916730-72-7

Cover: Color-enhanced cerebral angiogram. Photograph by Howard Sochurek.
Inside front and back covers: Neurons.

CONTENTS

CONTRIBUTORS AND CLINICAL CONSULTANTS

Contributors

At the time of publication, the contributors held the following positions:

Maryann C. Banko, RN, BSN, Project Coordinator, Stroke Data Bank, University of Maryland Medical System, Baltimore

Joan B. Davis, RN, CCRN, CNRN, Instructor, Pacific Northwest Inservice Specialists, Seattle

Carol A. Eggleston, RN, BSN, Neurosurgical Nurse Clinician, St. Louis University Hospital

Ann Fagerness, RN, BSN, CNRN, CCRN, Instructor, Pacific Northwest Inservice Specialists, Seattle

Lester J. Gardina, RN, BS, Head Nurse, Barrows Neurological Institute, Phoenix, Ariz.

Susan Hann, RN, MS, MSN, Neurosensory Nursing Instructor, Chester County Hospital School of Nursing, West Chester, Pa.

Marilynn S. Mitchell, RN, MSN, CNRN, Head Nurse, Neurologic Intensive Care and Intermediate Units, Denver General Hospital

Judith A. Rich, RN, MSN, Nurse Manager, Perioperative Unit, St. Mary's Hospital, West Palm Beach, Fla.

Therese S. Richmond, RN, MSN, CCRN, CN IV–Clinical Specialist, Neurosensory Intensive Care Unit, Thomas Jefferson University Hospital, Philadelphia

Amy Perrin Ross, RN, MSN, CNRN, Clinical Nurse Specialist, Neuroscience, Loyola University Medical Center, Maywood, Ill.

Cheryl Goldberg Sklar, RN, MSN, formerly Educational Coordinator, Hines (Ill.) Veterans Administration Hospital

Katherine Small, RN, MS, Nurse Supervisor, University of Maryland Hospital, Baltimore

Christina M. Stewart, RN, MSN, CCRN, CNRN, Neuroscience Clinical Nurse Specialist, St. Margaret Hospital, Hammond, Ind.

Connie A. Walleck, RN, MS, CNRN, Director of Nursing, Maryland Institute of Emergency Medical Services Systems, Baltimore

Joseph Warren, RN, BSN, Nurse Clinician, Head Injury Clinical Center, Medical College of Virginia, Richmond

Clinical Consultants

At the time of publication, the clinical consultants held the following positions:

John M. Bertoni, MD, PhD, Associate Professor of Neurology, Thomas Jefferson University, Philadelphia

Mimi Callanan, RN, MSN, CNRN, Epilepsy Clinical Specialist, Graduate Hospital, Philadelphia

Richard A. Chambers, MD, Professor of Neurology, Thomas Jefferson University Hospital, Philadelphia

Joanne Kirik Condi, RN, MN, Assistant Administrator, Neurology Division, Shadyside Hospital, Pittsburgh

John P. Conomy, MD, Chairman, Department of Neurology, Cleveland Clinic Foundation

Laura Johnson Farling, RN, CCRN, CNRN, Clinical Instructor, Neurosurgical Intensive Care Unit, Cleveland Clinic Hospital

Leon I. Gilner, MD, Assistant Professor of Surgery, Division of Neurosurgery, Medical College of Pennsylvania, Philadelphia

Lynn Joseph, RN, Head Nurse, Neurology Unit, Ottawa Civic Hospital

Joyce A. Kunkel, RN, BSN, CNRN, Neurology Nurse Associate, Miami Valley Neurosurgery, Inc., Dayton, Ohio

Cynthia J. Lange, RN, BSN, Assistant Director of Nursing, Laconia (N.H.) State School and Training Center

Kathleen M. Lupica, RN, CNRN, Assistant Head Nurse, Neurosurgical Intensive Care Unit, Cleveland Clinic Foundation

Roger M. Morrell, MD, PhD, FACP, Chief, Neurology Service, Veterans Administration Medical Center, Allen Park, Mich.; Professor of Neurology and Immunology/Microbiology, Wayne State University, Detroit

Patricio F. Reyes, MD, Assistant Professor of Neurology and Pathology, Thomas Jefferson University, Philadelphia; Consultant, Veterans Administration Hospitals, Coatesville, Pa. and Wilmington, Del.

Gizell Maria Rossetti, MD, Clinical Instructor in Neurology, Medical College of Pennsylvania, Philadelphia

William L. Shopp, RN, BSN, CNRN, Head Nurse, Neurosurgical Intensive Care Unit, Cleveland Clinic Hospital

Connie A. Walleck, RN, MS, CNRN, Director of Nursing, Maryland Institute of Emergency Medical Services Systems, Baltimore

FOREWORD

I f you find caring for patients with neurologic disorders unsettling, you're not alone. Providing meaningful care, emotional support, and adequate instruction for these patients has always been difficult. Why? Probably because we know comparatively little about this complex system and its control over all the others. Because too often, as after stroke or head injury, the patient may die within the first few hours or days regardless of the quality or immediacy of care. Because that care involves intricate, acute measures and persistent long-term rehabilitation, most patients sustain some permanent mental or physical impairment, and many face unrelenting decline. For others, such as those with brain tumor or Alzheimer's disease, the prognosis is similarly grim.

As nurses, our dilemma has long been how to give optimum and optimistic care in the face of limited knowledge and hope. Now, scientific advances have begun to supply more answers, creating new options for the patient—and new responsibilities for the nurse. New knowledge of neurologic anatomy and pathophysiology has led to improved medical and surgical treatments and has shifted neurologic care into the critical-care arena. In the last decade, the introduction of CT scan, the ability to identify and measure chemical neurotransmitters, and the use of intracranial pressure (ICP) monitoring have made diagnosis faster and more precise; patient care more timely and hopeful.

These advances have spawned new nursing protocols. No longer simply watching and waiting for problems to appear, we're now closely monitoring and constantly assessing patient status to anticipate problems and offset secondary damage. Current protocols emphasize early diagnosis and precautions, ongoing assessment, and quick recognition of potential complications. This approach to neurologic care challenges us to sharpen our assessment skills and to deepen our understanding of the nervous system and the devastating effects of its dysfunction.

NEUROLOGIC DISORDERS, the fourth volume in the Nurse's Clinical Library, combines theory and practice to help nurses at every level meet the challenge of neurologic care. Its introductory chapters lay firm ground for later discussions of individual disorders. Chapter 1 reviews the normal structures and functions of the nervous system in light of recent discoveries and explains the dynamics of nerve transmission and general pathophysiologic mechanisms. Chapter 2 takes us step-by-step through a careful neurologic assessment, so critical to our care planning. It acknowledges our expanded assessment role by covering new areas, such as cranial and peripheral nerve assessment. Chapter 3 describes current diagnostic tools, including ICP monitoring and advanced imaging techniques.

The subsequent 11 chapters explore the etiology and management of specific neurologic disorders in detail. Each chapter's three-part organization quickly locates needed information. *Pathophysiology* discusses each disorder's causes, identifying signs and symptoms, specific dysfunctional mechanisms, and systemic toll. *Medical management* summarizes important diagnostic tests, their results, and current medical and surgical treatments and introduces some of the experimental therapies under investigation. *Nursing management* follows each disorder through the nursing process from comprehensive nursing history through crucial assessment findings to the nursing diagnoses they suggest. For each diagnosis, this section details pertinent nursing goals, appropriate interventions, and guidelines for evaluating results.

Heavily illustrating this volume, you'll find anatomic drawings, physiologic diagrams, charts, tables, and sidebars of related material to clarify and augment the text. The appendix lists the most common neurologic drugs.

The information explosion and our expanded role compel us to keep current with neurologic nursing. With the comprehensive information in this volume, we can manage the neurologic patient more confidently.

CONNIE A. WALLECK, RN, MS, CNRN
Director of Nursing
Maryland Institute of Emergency Medical Services Systems
Baltimore

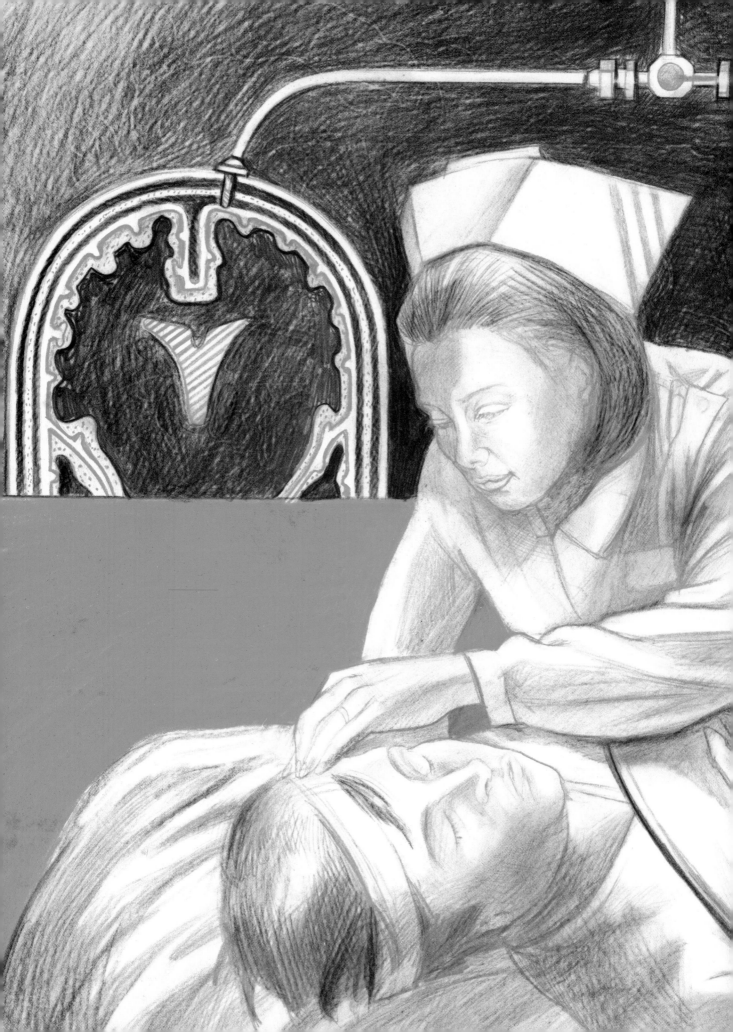

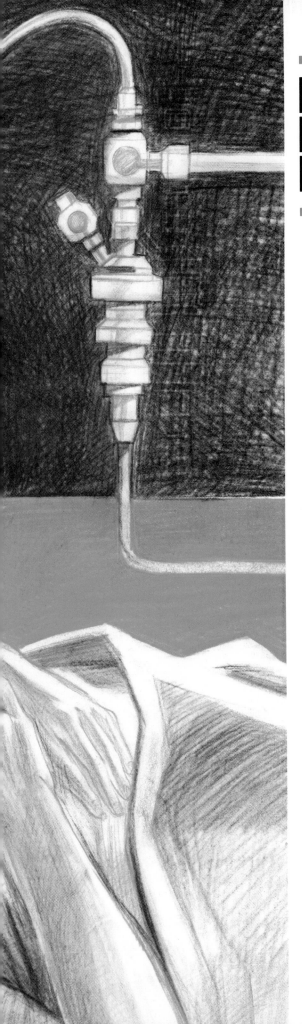

FUNDAMENTAL
NEUROLOGIC
FACTS

1 REVIEWING BASIC PRINCIPLES

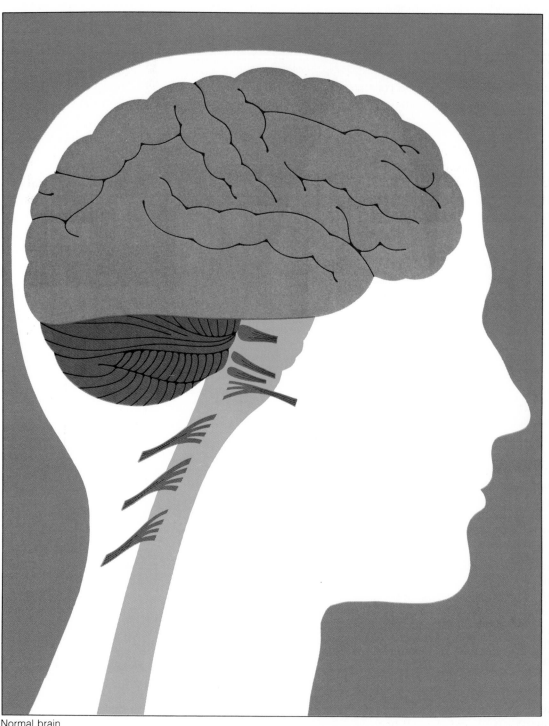

Normal brain

The discovery of two brain chemicals called enkephalins in 1975 heralded major advances in the study of brain structure and function. Researchers have identified more than 30 brain chemicals that are thought to act as neurotransmitters and have elucidated the architecture of the neuron, the nervous system's basic structural and functional unit.

Keeping current with this rapidly expanding body of knowledge is an important part of your nursing responsibilities. After all, an improved understanding of neurologic function and dysfunction directly affects the quality of your patient care. It allows you to give your patient a clear understanding of his disorder and its treatment, to refine your assessment skills, and to develop sound nursing interventions that promote rehabilitation.

NEUROGLIA AND NEURONS

The nervous system directs every body system and cell, governing all movement, sensation, thought, and emotion. Two types of cells make up the nervous system: neuroglial (or glial) cells and neurons. Neuroglial cells differ in type, function, and location in the nervous system. (See *Functions of neuroglial cells.*)

The neuron typically consists of a cell body and two types of appendage—one long, stalk-like axon and one or more shorter dendrites. Cell bodies form the gray matter in the brain, brain stem, and spinal cord.

The *axon* transmits impulses from the cell body to other neurons and, according to current theory, also transports substances needed by the cell back to the cell body. At its tip lie multiple tiny branches, each ending in a small swelling—the synaptic knob or presynaptic terminal—that transmits impulses to an adjoining neuron. Axons form the white matter in the brain, brain stem, and spinal cord. Groups of axons with a common origin, termination, and function, and projecting in the same direction within the central nervous system (CNS), constitute a tract. These axons are protected by the oligodendroglia; axons outside the CNS are protected by a segmented myelin covering generated by Schwann's cells, with each myelin segment extending between two nodes of Ranvier. Peripheral axons are further protected by a thin outer sheath of neurilemma, which plays an important role in peripheral nerve regeneration.

Dendrites are short, branched fibers that receive impulses from nearby cells and conduct them toward the cell body. In the simple, unipolar neuron, axon and dendrite appear at opposite ends of the neuron's single branch.

Neurons perform one of three roles in transmitting impulses: reception of sensory stimuli, transmission of motor responses, or integration of activities and coordination of communication between body parts. *Sensory* (afferent) *neurons* carry stimuli from a peripheral sensory organ, such as the skin, to the spinal cord and brain. *Motor* (efferent) *neurons* carry impulses from the brain and spinal cord back to remote tissues and organs. *Interneurons* (intercalary, or association neurons) relay impulses within the CNS.

All operations of mind and body rely on impulses passing from neuron to neuron. This transmission of impulses (neurotransmission) occurs across a synapse, the contact point between two neurons (see *Understanding neurotransmission,* pages 16 and 17).

Two anatomic divisions

The nervous system is composed of central and peripheral divisions. The CNS serves as the control center. The peripheral nervous system (PNS) links the CNS with the rest of the body and includes the autonomic nervous system (ANS), which regulates involuntary functions of internal organs.

CENTRAL NERVOUS SYSTEM

Consisting of the brain, brain stem, and spinal cord, the CNS is surrounded and protected by three meningeal membranes: the dura mater, the arachnoid membrane, and the pia mater. (See *Structures of the brain and spinal cord,* pages 10 and 11, and *Protecting the central nervous system,* page 12.)

Brain

The center of the nervous system, the brain is made up of the cerebrum, diencephalon, cerebellum, and brain stem and incorporates the ventricular system.

Cerebrum. Two matched hemispheres make up the cerebrum, the largest portion of the brain. Each hemisphere contains four major lobes named for the skull bones that lie over them: frontal, parietal, temporal, and occipital. Many fissures (sulci) divide the cerebral surface. A deep longitudinal fissure completely separates the two hemispheres. A lateral fissure (fissure of Sylvius) separates the frontal and temporal lobes. A central sulcus (fissure of Rolando) separates the frontal and parietal lobes. Portions of the cerebrum lying between fissures are called *gyri* or *convolutions.*

Functions of neuroglial cells

Neuroglial cells include four specialized types: astroglia, ependymal cells, microglia, and oligodendroglia.

Astroglia, or astrocytes, appear throughout the nervous system and form part of the blood-brain barrier. They supply nutrients to the neuron and help maintain its electrical potential.

Ependymal cells, lining the brain's four ventricles and the choroid plexuses, help produce cerebrospinal fluid.

Microglia, deployed throughout the nervous system, phagocytize waste products from injured neurons.

Oligodendroglia form the protective myelin sheaths for axons of central nervous system neurons, supporting and electrically insulating them.

Structures of the brain and spinal cord

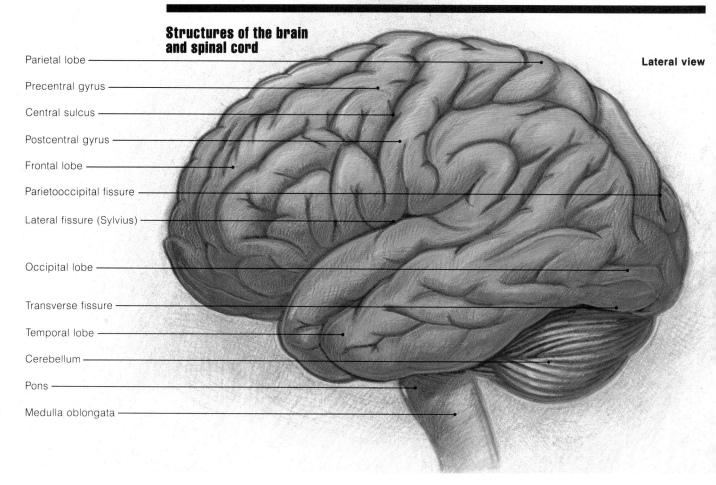

Lateral view

Parietal lobe

Precentral gyrus

Central sulcus

Postcentral gyrus

Frontal lobe

Parietooccipital fissure

Lateral fissure (Sylvius)

Occipital lobe

Transverse fissure

Temporal lobe

Cerebellum

Pons

Medulla oblongata

The cerebrum performs motor, sensory, associative, and mental functions in specialized areas of the hemispheres (see *Sites of cerebral function,* page 15). For example, on either side of the central sulcus lie areas controlling motor and sensory function. Along the precentral gyrus (frontal lobe) is the motor area (motor cortex), and in the neighboring area on the posterior side of the central sulcus is the sensory area (sensory cortex). The prefrontal area is associated with abstract thought, mature judgment, social inhibition, intellectual function, and storage of sensory information. The parietal lobe has functional areas for sensory discrimination and body image. The temporal lobe controls hearing, olfaction, sensory speech (Wernicke's area), and short-term memory. The occipital lobe integrates visual reception.

Current theory allots special functions to each hemisphere: the left is oriented to analytic and verbal skills, the right to spatial and pattern perception and to artistic forms of intelligence. From an equal potential at birth, one hemisphere (usually the left) develops more highly than the other and becomes dominant. Damage to the dominant hemisphere before age 6 may spur development of

its functions in the other hemisphere. For example, damage to the left hemisphere usually causes language function to develop in the right hemisphere. After age 6, however, such damage causes severe and permanent intellectual impairment.

Each hemisphere consists of gray matter (neuron cell bodies in the cortex and basal ganglia) and white matter (axon tracts). The corpus callosum, a mass of nerve fibers deep in the center of the longitudinal fissure, allows each area of one hemisphere to communicate with its corresponding area in the other hemisphere. Association fibers link different sections of the cortex within a single hemisphere. Projection fibers, tracts of axons that fan out from the brain stem, link the cortex with the subcortical areas, the brain stem, and the spinal cord.

The basal ganglia, groups of subcortical gray matter that surround the brain's lateral ventricles, are important in modulating voluntary body movements, especially of the hands and legs. Their major structures include the caudate nucleus, the putamen, the globus pallidus, the claustrum, and the amygdala.

Diencephalon. This major division of the brain includes the hypothalamus and thala-

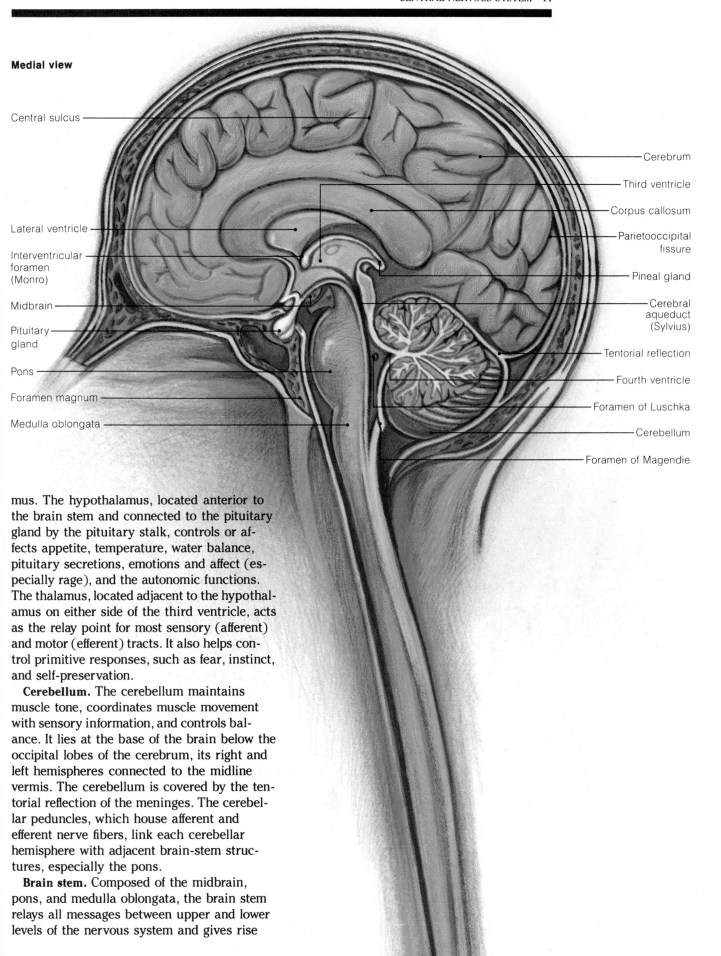

Medial view

Central sulcus

Lateral ventricle

Interventricular foramen (Monro)

Midbrain

Pituitary gland

Pons

Foramen magnum

Medulla oblongata

Cerebrum

Third ventricle

Corpus callosum

Parietooccipital fissure

Pineal gland

Cerebral aqueduct (Sylvius)

Tentorial reflection

Fourth ventricle

Foramen of Luschka

Cerebellum

Foramen of Magendie

mus. The hypothalamus, located anterior to the brain stem and connected to the pituitary gland by the pituitary stalk, controls or affects appetite, temperature, water balance, pituitary secretions, emotions and affect (especially rage), and the autonomic functions. The thalamus, located adjacent to the hypothalamus on either side of the third ventricle, acts as the relay point for most sensory (afferent) and motor (efferent) tracts. It also helps control primitive responses, such as fear, instinct, and self-preservation.

Cerebellum. The cerebellum maintains muscle tone, coordinates muscle movement with sensory information, and controls balance. It lies at the base of the brain below the occipital lobes of the cerebrum, its right and left hemispheres connected to the midline vermis. The cerebellum is covered by the tentorial reflection of the meninges. The cerebellar peduncles, which house afferent and efferent nerve fibers, link each cerebellar hemisphere with adjacent brain-stem structures, especially the pons.

Brain stem. Composed of the midbrain, pons, and medulla oblongata, the brain stem relays all messages between upper and lower levels of the nervous system and gives rise

Protecting the central nervous system

The bones of the skull and the vertebrae help protect the central nervous system from shock and infection, along with three membranes (meninges).

The dura mater, a fibrous membrane, lines the skull and forms folds (reflections) that descend into the brain's fissures and provide stability. These dural folds include the falx cerebri (which lies in the longitudinal fissure and separates the hemispheres of the cerebrum), the tentorium cerebelli (separating cerebrum from cerebellum), and the falx cerebelli (separating the two cerebellar lobes). The arachnoid villi, projections of the dura mater into the superior sagittal and transverse sinuses, serve as the exit points for cerebrospinal fluid drainage into venous circulation.

The arachnoid membrane, a fragile, fibrous layer with moderate vascularity, lies between the dura and pia mater. Injury to its blood vessels during lumbar or cisternal puncture may cause hemorrhage.

The pia mater, a very thin and highly vascular membrane, closely covers the brain's surface and extends into its fissures. Its intimate invaginations

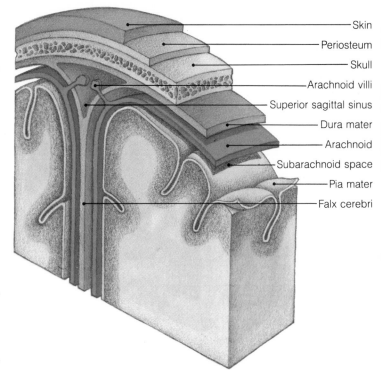

- Skin
- Periosteum
- Skull
- Arachnoid villi
- Superior sagittal sinus
- Dura mater
- Arachnoid
- Subarachnoid space
- Pia mater
- Falx cerebri

help form the choroid plexuses of the brain's ventricular system.

Three layers of space further cushion the brain and spinal cord against injury. The epidural space—actually, a potential space—lies over the dura mater. The subdural space lies between the dura mater and

arachnoid membrane. A closed area, which is often the site of hemorrhage after head trauma, it offers no escape route for hemorrhagic accumulations. The subarachnoid space, which is filled with cerebrospinal fluid, lies between the arachnoid membrane and the pia mater.

to cranial nerves III through XII. Along with the thalamus and hypothalamus, it constitutes the reticular formation, a nerve network that supplies constant muscle stimulation to counteract the force of gravity on the body. The reticular formation also forms part of the reticular activating system (RAS), which relays impulses to the rest of the brain to control consciousness, the sleep-wake cycle, and mental concentration. Damage to the RAS results in loss of consciousness. In fact, the most critical signs of coma—unconsciousness, pupillary and ocular reflex abnormalities, and respiratory irregularities—usually derive from pressure or other disruption of tissue in the brain stem.

The brain stem's three divisions are continuous structures. The midbrain, the top structure, connects to the cerebrum via the dien-

cephalon. The pons, the middle structure, connects to the cerebellum and contains the apneustic and pneumotaxic respiratory centers. The medulla oblongata, the bottom structure, connects to the spinal cord; it contains the vital centers for cardiac, respiratory, vasomotor, and rhythmicity functions and the center for initiating protective pharyngeal reflexes, such as sneezing, swallowing, coughing, gagging, and vomiting. The site of contralateral crossing (decussation) for most motor nerve tracts descending from the cerebrum is called the pyramids of the medulla.

Ventricles. The ventricular system, located in the center of the brain, contains four communicating compartments: two lateral ventricles and a third and fourth ventricle. The lateral ventricles communicate with the third ventricle through the dual interventricular foramina (foramina of Monro). The third and fourth ventricles communicate through the cerebral aqueduct (aqueduct of Sylvius).

Folds of pia and arachnoid mater invaginated into the ventricles and covered with ependymal cells form the choroid plexuses, which produce cerebrospinal fluid (CSF).

Spinal cord

Besides serving as a communication pathway between the brain and the PNS, the spinal cord mediates the reflex arc—the neural pathway used in a reflex action. It joins the brain stem at the level of the foramen magnum and terminates near the second lumbar vertebra as the conus medullaris.

A cross section of the spinal cord shows a central H-shaped mass of gray matter (neuron cell bodies) divided into dorsal (posterior) and ventral (anterior) horns. Cell bodies in the dorsal horn relay sensory (afferent) impulses; those in the ventral horn relay motor (efferent) impulses. White matter surrounding these horns consists of myelinated axons of sensory and motor nerves grouped in ascending and descending tracts. (See *Spinal cross section*.) These fibers cross to the contralateral side so that nerves in one hemisphere control or respond to impulses on the body's opposite side. This crossing (decussation) occurs in the spinal cord or brain stem.

Ascending tracts carry sensory impulses from the spinal cord to the brain. Impulses enter the cord at the dorsal (sensory) horn and eventually reach the contralateral postcentral gyrus (primary somatosensory cortex) for processing. The primary ascending tracts include the anterior and posterior spinocerebellar tracts (which govern unconscious proprioception); the fasciculus gracilis and cuneatus (conscious proprioception and vibratory and tactile stimuli from the legs and arms); the anterior spinothalamic tract (tactile sensations, especially light touch); and the lateral spinothalamic tract (pain and temperature sensations).

Descending tracts carry motor impulses from the spinal cord to the PNS. These impulses travel from the precentral gyrus to muscles, exiting the spinal cord at the ventral (motor) horn. Major descending tracts are the lateral and anterior corticospinal and the rubrospinal tracts.

PERIPHERAL NERVOUS SYSTEM

The cranial and spinal nerves, which form the PNS, carry sensory messages from organs and tissues to the brain and motor instructions from the brain to these outlying areas.

Cranial nerves

The 12 pairs of cranial nerves, numbered CN I through CN XII, serve the sensory and motor needs mainly of the head but also of the neck, chest, and abdomen. CN I (olfactory nerve) and CN II (optic nerve) are integrated in the brain, while CN III through CN XII originate in the brain stem. (See *Guide to cranial nerve assessment,* pages 30 and 31.)

Spinal nerves

The 31 pairs of spinal nerves originate in the spinal cord, each pair numbered for its level of origin among the cord's 31 segments. The

Spinal cross section

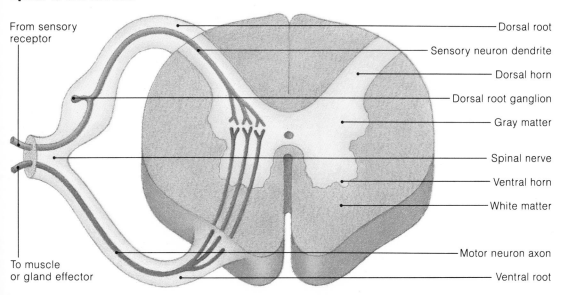

From sensory receptor

To muscle or gland effector

- Dorsal root
- Sensory neuron dendrite
- Dorsal horn
- Dorsal root ganglion
- Gray matter
- Spinal nerve
- Ventral horn
- White matter
- Motor neuron axon
- Ventral root

nerves include 8 pairs of cervical nerves, 12 thoracic, 5 lumbar, 5 sacral, and 1 coccygeal nerve and extend to outlying body areas through the intervertebral foramina. Nerves of the cervical enlargement (cervical 3 to thoracic 2) supply the upper extremities; those of the lumbar enlargement (thoracic 9 through 12) supply the lower extremities (see *Mapping sensory function by dermatomes,* page 33).

CEREBROVASCULAR DYNAMICS
An intact cerebrovascular system is crucial for sufficient cerebral blood flow to supply brain tissue with oxygen and glucose. Otherwise, impaired blood flow will eventually reduce production of adenosine triphosphate (ATP), the intracellular energy source. When ATP levels drop, brain tissue may suffer irreversible damage.

Cerebrovascular structures
The paired carotid and vertebral arteries, which arise from the aorta, provide the brain with its needed blood supply. The internal carotids, which supply about 80% of the total cerebral flow, provide blood to the anterior and middle parts of the cerebral hemispheres. The two vertebral arteries, which supply the remaining 20% of the total cerebral flow, join to form the basilar artery, which provides blood to the posterior parts of the cerebral hemispheres, the cerebellum, brain stem, and part of the spinal cord. At the base of the brain, surrounding the pituitary stalk, these arterial structures connect via communicating arteries to form the circle of Willis. When one or more of the four chief supplying arteries becomes occluded, the circle of Willis promotes collateral circulation to all cerebral structures (see Chapter 12). However, its structure, which is not a perfect circle but contains angles that deflect blood flow, may predispose to cerebral aneurysms; the pressure of high-velocity blood flow may locally weaken vessel walls and cause ballooning.

Cerebrovascular perfusion
The brain receives about 20% of the entire cardiac output, or 750 to 850 ml/minute. Cerebral circulation, however, must remain constant because the rigid skull and fragile brain tissue allow little room for safe expansion. Consequently, any increase in arterial flow, as results from arterial dilation, must be balanced by a corresponding increase in venous flow to avoid increases in intracranial pressure (ICP).

Cerebral circulation responds to the same factors that influence systemic blood pressure. For example, hypoxia and hypercapnia cause vasodilation and thus increase cerebral blood flow. Elevated carotid sinus pressure, arteriovenous malformation, and reduced CSF pressure also increase cerebral blood flow. In contrast, reduced carbon dioxide and increased oxygen levels lead to vasoconstriction and decrease cerebral blood flow. Arteriosclerotic changes and elevated CSF pressure also decrease blood flow.

To support normal brain function, cerebral circulation must maintain cerebral perfusion pressure (CPP) at no less than 50 mm Hg. To maintain this pressure, mean arterial blood pressure (MABP) normally must exceed 70 mm Hg. Since the difference between MABP and ICP determines CPP, brain tissue becomes ischemic if MABP plummets or rises rapidly. If autoregulatory mechanisms, which maintain normal blood flow, fail to compensate for changing physical or chemical factors, cerebral edema or further ischemic damage may occur.

CEREBROSPINAL FLUID DYNAMICS
Normally, CSF is clear, colorless, and odorless, with a specific gravity of 1.007 and a pH of 7.35. It's produced by the choroid plexuses of the ventricular system. Any fluctuations in cerebral metabolism that alter cerebral blood flow and blood osmotic pressure cause corresponding fluctuations in CSF production, which averages about 840 ml daily.

CSF circulates from the lateral ventricles into the third ventricle and through the aqueduct of Sylvius into the fourth ventricle. From there, it enters the subarachnoid space and diffuses over the brain and the spinal cord.

CSF reabsorption into venous blood occurs mainly in the arachnoid villi, highly permeable tufts of arachnoid membrane that project into the venous sinuses, predominantly the superior sagittal sinus. When CSF pressure exceeds venous pressure, CSF diffuses into the blood. Reabsorption maintains circulating CSF volume at 135 to 150 ml.

CSF: Constant volume, constant pressure
Despite fluctuations in CSF production, a constant volume of CSF flows at constant pressure (10 to 12 mm Hg) as long as CSF reabsorption offsets production. In this closed system, factors that elevate CSF volume also elevate CSF pressure. For example, increased cerebral blood flow or arterial pressure in-

Sites of cerebral function

Lateral view

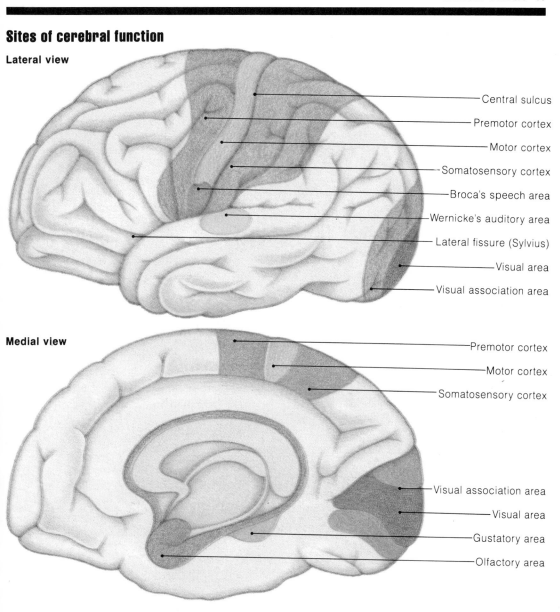

Central sulcus
Premotor cortex
Motor cortex
Somatosensory cortex
Broca's speech area
Wernicke's auditory area
Lateral fissure (Sylvius)
Visual area
Visual association area

Medial view

Premotor cortex
Motor cortex
Somatosensory cortex

Visual association area
Visual area
Gustatory area
Olfactory area

creases CSF production and pressure. Venous occlusion impedes reabsorption of CSF, raising both volume and pressure. Carbon dioxide retention, respiratory obstruction, Valsalva's maneuver, occlusion of venous outflow (as with head turning), and space-occupying intracranial lesions (such as hematoma, abscess, or tumor) also increase CSF pressure.

Four functional divisions
Functionally, the nervous system subdivides into four components: the sensory, motor, and autonomic systems, and the RAS.

SENSORY SYSTEM
This system converts sensory stimuli into neurochemical action potentials, which travel to the spinal cord and brain, where they're interpreted and acted upon. This system consists of sensory receptors and nerves, ascend-

ing sensory tracts, thalamic nuclei, and somatosensory strip of the cerebral cortex.

Sensory stimulus
Sensation may be characterized as superficial, deep, or combined. Superficial sensation includes touch, temperature, pain, and two-point discrimination. Deep sensation relates to muscle and joint position sense (proprioception), deep muscle pain, and vibration sense (pallesthesia). Combined superficial and deep sensation includes recognizing and naming familiar items held in the hand (stereognosis) and localizing cutaneous stimuli (topognosis). A complex process integrating receptive and interpretive functions with memory, combined sensation requires cerebrocortical integrity.

Five types of sensory receptors detect and respond to specific environmental changes. *(continued on page 18)*

Understanding neurotransmission

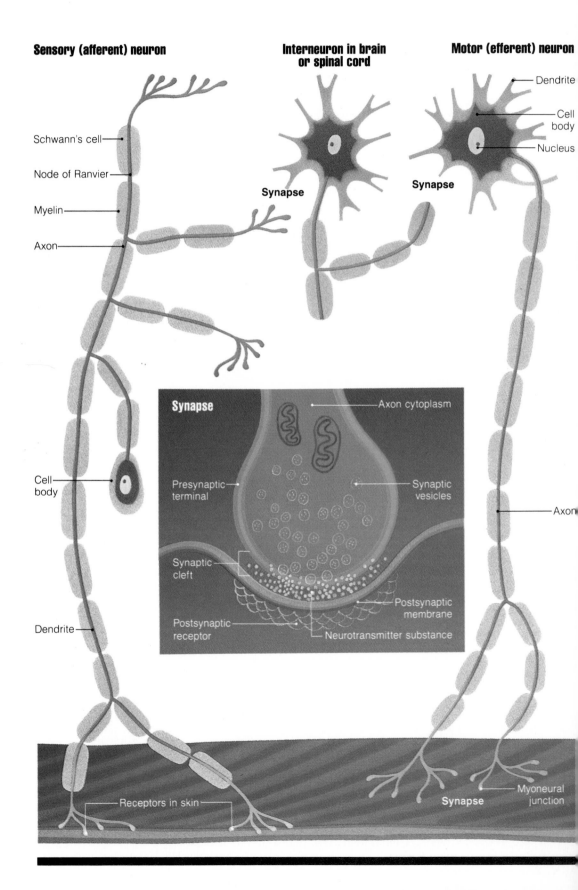

Sensory (afferent) neuron

Interneuron in brain or spinal cord

Motor (efferent) neuron

Dendrite

Cell body

Nucleus

Schwann's cell

Node of Ranvier

Myelin

Axon

Synapse

Synapse

Synapse

Axon cytoplasm

Presynaptic terminal

Synaptic vesicles

Cell body

Axon

Synaptic cleft

Postsynaptic membrane

Postsynaptic receptor

Neurotransmitter substance

Dendrite

Receptors in skin

Synapse

Myoneural junction

Impulse transmission at the synapse involves the transmitter neuron's presynaptic terminal, the target receptor neuron (postsynaptic receptor), and the narrow synaptic cleft between the two neurons.

Numerous presynaptic terminals branch from the tips of axons. These terminals contain synaptic vesicles, which, when stimulated, release neurotransmitter substances into the synaptic cleft to excite or inhibit the target receptor neuron. The excitatory or inhibitory effect of these chemical neurotransmitters depends not only on their composition but also on the target neuron's surface receptors, which may be excitatory or inhibitory for a specific neurotransmitter. Of more than 30 known neurotransmitters, acetylcholine, glutamic acid, and substance P usually produce excitatory effects. In contrast, dopamine, gamma-aminobutyric acid, glycine, norepinephrine, and serotonin usually produce inhibitory effects.

Because the vesicles exhaust their chemical stores after 3 minutes of peak synaptic activity, mitochondria within the presynaptic terminals produce adenosine triphosphate, which promotes rapid synthesis of both excitatory and inhibitory chemicals.

Ions: Their critical role

Changes in the concentrations of sodium, potassium, chloride, and calcium ions in intra- and extracellular fluids account for chemical propagation of nerve impulses. Sodium is the major extracellular cation, driven from the cell by a powerful sodium pump. Potassium is the major intracellular cation, but its pump is weaker than that of sodium. Thus, while both sodium and potassium ions carry a positive charge, more positive ions are pumped out of the cell than into it. Also, under resting conditions, the cell membrane prevents sodium diffusion inward but easily allows potassium to diffuse outward. Chloride, predominantly an extracellular ion, increases neuron excitability and regulates the duration and intensity of nerve transmission, but the mechanism is poorly understood. Calcium is required for vesicle release of neurotransmitters.

Removal of sodium cations from the cell leaves behind many nondiffusible anions, thus creating a negative intracellular charge and a positive extracellular charge *(resting potential)*. Nerve stimulation reverses these charges by changing cell membrane permeability. Sodium diffuses rapidly back into the cell, depolarizing the interior and shifting the normally negative charge to positive *(reversal potential)*. To correct this sudden electrical imbalance, membrane permeability swiftly ceases to sodium and increases to potassium. Rapid outward diffusion of potassium repolarizes the cell body to its negative resting potential. These two stages of depolarization and repolarization form the cell's *action potential,* which moves in a wave along the cell membrane as electrical reversals stimulate adjacent sites.

As the action potential reaches the cell's presynaptic terminals, terminal membrane permeability increases to extracellular calcium. Calcium ions leak into the terminals and stimulate the vesicles to release their excitatory or inhibitory chemicals into the synaptic cleft. These chemicals cross the cleft and bind with specialized protein receptors in the postsynaptic membrane, selectively increasing receptor membrane permeability. If the vesicles release excitatory chemicals, receptor membrane permeability increases to sodium. If the vesicles release inhibitory chemicals, receptor membrane permeability increases to potassium and chloride. These changes in permeability respectively promote or block extension of an action potential in the postsynaptic receptor, depending on the sum effect of other nearby synapses.

Excitability

After initiation of an impulse, the neuron can't be stimulated for 1 to 2 milliseconds (*absolute refractory period*) as ion concentrations equilibrate. A *relative refractory period* follows, during which the nerve responds only to an exceptionally strong stimulus. However, the nerve is capable of almost continuous transmission, because the total action potential cycle lasts only milliseconds.

Conduction velocity

The diameter of the nerve fiber carrying an impulse determines impulse velocity—the larger the diameter, the faster the conduction rate. Type A fibers, large-diameter myelinated fibers of the spinal nerves, possess rapid conduction properties. These fibers quickly transmit muscle position sense, sharp pain, temperature, and deep pressure and touch sensations that require immediate recognition. Type A fibers subdivide into alpha, beta, delta, and gamma fibers, with successively smaller diameters and decreasing conduction rates. Type C fibers, small-diameter nonmyelinated fibers that make up most peripheral and all autonomic nerves, conduct impulses very slowly. They transmit itch, temperature, crude touch, and protracted pain sensations that don't require quick recognition. In addition, the fatty myelin sheath surrounding many axons provides insulation that may slightly boost nerve stimulus.

In general, the conduction velocity for a nerve impulse doesn't depend on stimulus strength. A stimulus that's strong enough to initiate an action potential produces a maximum response regardless of the force of the original stimulus.

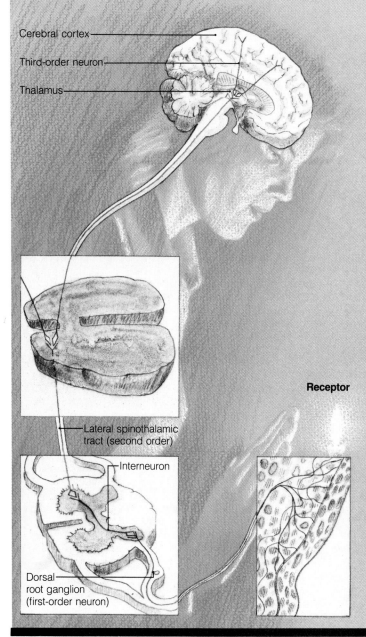

Sensory pathway for pain and temperature

Cerebral cortex

Third-order neuron

Thalamus

Lateral spinothalamic
tract (second order)

Interneuron

Receptor

Dorsal
root ganglion
(first-order neuron)

Sensory pathways are three-neuron chains. In the characteristic pain/temperature pathway, the first-order neuron is a unipolar cell. Its body lies in the dorsal root ganglion, and its free (nonencapsulated) nerve endings extend locally to the epidermis. Since pain and temperature represent important danger signals, the first-order neuron responds to the stimulus *nature* rather than *quality*, so that the body can rapidly take any necessary evasive action.

A sensory stimulus follows this neuron to the spinal cord, enters through the dorsal root, and travels along an interneuron to the contralateral ascending pain pathway, the lateral spinothalamic tract (LST). This interneuron lies in the gray matter of the dorsal horn. Its axon crosses the midline and joins the LST at the same level as, but contralateral to, the sensation's point of entry to the spinal cord.

The second-order neuron, part of the LST, ascends from the spine through the brain stem to the thalamus.

The third-order neuron, a thalamocortical neuron, lies in the thalamus, with its axon projecting to the postcentral gyrus (primary somatosensory cortex). While pain and temperature are perceived at the thalamic level, stimuli must reach the cerebral cortex to be localized.

Chemoreceptors detect and respond to changes in osmolality and in oxygen and carbon dioxide levels; *mechanoreceptors,* to mechanical changes as occur with the hearing process; *nocioreceptors,* to tissue damage; *thermoreceptors,* to temperature changes; and *light receptors,* to light on the retina.

Three-neuron pathway
The typical sensory pathway, such as the pain-temperature pathway, is a three-neuron chain from receptor to cortex. Specific struc-

tures and points of decussation may vary with the type of sensory stimulus that each tract carries, and tracts through the spinal cord may receive impulses along the length of the nerve bundle. However, each path has only three neurons. (See *Sensory pathway for pain and temperature.*)

The sensory pathway for pain, temperature, and touch for face and head includes the trigeminal nerve (mixed sensory/motor) as the first-order neuron, the contralateral medial lemniscus ascending to the thalamus as the

The reflex arc

The reflex arc is the simplest neural relay cycle for quick motor response to a harmful sensory stimulus.

Here's how it works: Sharp or painful stimulation of a sensory organ or subcutaneous end organ initiates an afferent impulse. This impulse travels along the dorsal sensory root to the spinal cord, where two synaptic transmissions occur simultaneously. One synapse continues the impulse along a sensory neuron to the brain for processing. The other doesn't wait for this processing but immediately relays the impulse to an interneuron (intercalary, or association, neuron), which passes it to a motor (efferent) neuron. The motor neuron delivers the impulse to a muscle or gland, producing an immediate response.

The prototypical reflex arc is the hand's recoil from a hot object. The afferent impulse passes directly from the hand to spinal neurons and back to the hand without modulation by the brain. By the time the secondary impulse passes through the thalamus to the somatosensory cortex and the brain registers and localizes pain, the hand has already pulled away from the hot object.

Interruption of the reflex arc at any point (through damage to the nerve as from trauma or from disease, such as peripheral neuritis) abolishes the response.

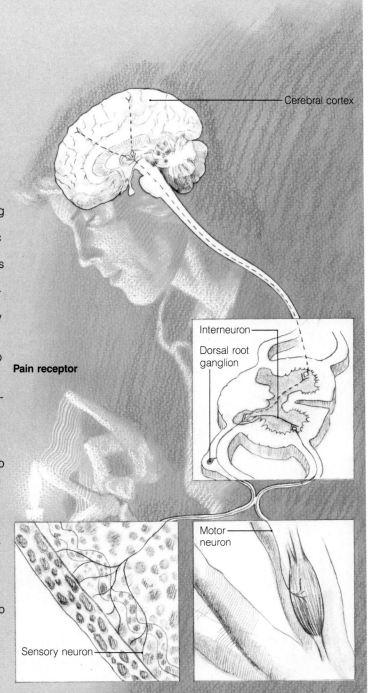

Cerebral cortex

Pain receptor

Interneuron

Dorsal root ganglion

Motor neuron

Sensory neuron

second-order neuron, and the thalamocortical neuron as the third-order neuron. This pathway mediates the corneal reflex (sensory), lacrimal reflex (tearing resulting from conjunctival irritation or drying), sneezing, reflex tongue movements, and the jaw jerk reflex.

Proprioception is mediated through two major pathways. Conscious proprioception involves the dorsal (posterior) columns—fasciculus gracilis and fasciculus cuneatus—that cross the midline to form the contralateral medial lemniscus. Unconscious proprio-

ception involves the spinocerebellar tract.

The reflex arc, a primitive system combining sensory and motor functions, mediates perception of a harmful stimulus and quick removal of the endangered body part without input from the brain (see *The reflex arc*).

MOTOR SYSTEM
This system regulates movement by relaying motor impulses along two major paths from the cerebral cortex through the spinal cord to the muscles. The pyramidal pathway, so

Pyramidal and extrapyramidal motor pathways

Premotor cortex

Motor cortex

Subcortical relay station

Extrapyramidal tract

Medulla oblongata

Decussation of pyramids

Crossed pyramidal tract

Uncrossed pyramidal tract

Lower motor neuron

Anterior white commissure

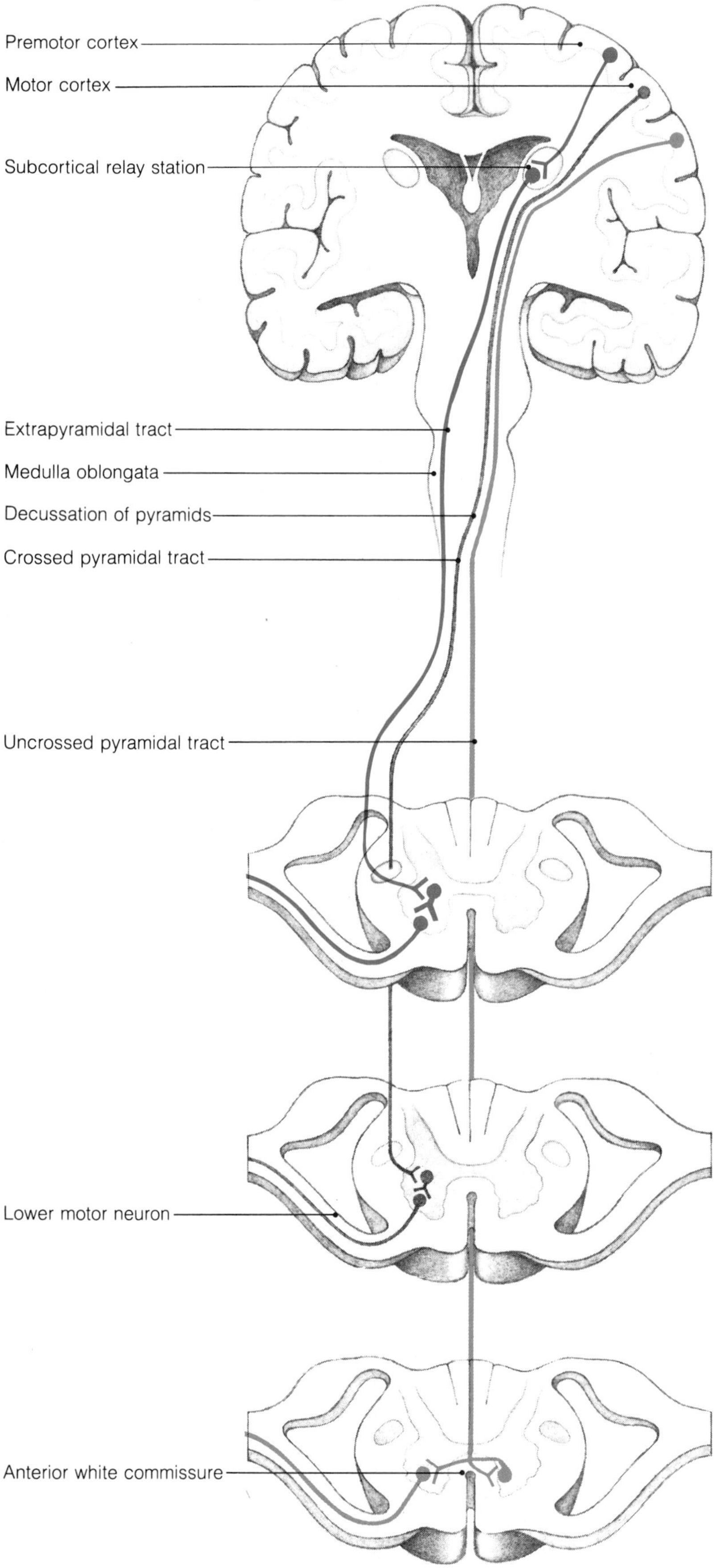

named because it courses through the pyramids of the medulla, controls fine, voluntary movement. The extrapyramidal pathway, consisting of all nonpyramidal structures, controls gross motor movements. (See *Pyramidal and extrapyramidal motor pathways.*)

Pyramidal pathway
This pathway consists of upper and lower motor neurons between cortex and muscle. The upper neuron's cell body lies in the precentral gyrus, while the axon descends to a lower neuron. This lower neuron lies in either a cranial nerve motor nucleus of the brain stem or in the ventral horn of the spinal cord and is the final common pathway for pyramidal, extrapyramidal, and reflex impulses.

The pyramidal pathway contains large myelinated fibers that originate in the cerebral motor cortex. Ninety percent cross contralaterally at the decussation of the pyramids and become the lateral corticospinal tract; the remaining 10% continue ipsilaterally as the anterior corticospinal tract, finally decussating through the anterior white commissure.

Extrapyramidal pathway
This multisynaptic pathway features chains of neurons interposed above the motor neuron that finally contacts the muscle. It includes the basal ganglia and cerebellum—semi-independent pathways that do not themselves project to the spinal cord, ventral horn, or cranial nerve motor nuclei, but which modulate movement by projecting to structures that ultimately affect lower motor neurons. Both the basal ganglia and the cerebellum maintain muscle tone and temper motor responses. Impulses from the basal ganglia reach the cerebral cortex through projections from the thalamus and influence activity in the corticospinal tract. Cerebellar impulses reach the red nucleus of the midbrain and influence activity along the rubrospinal tract, particularly proprioception and balance.

AUTONOMIC NERVOUS SYSTEM
The ANS directs involuntary muscle and gland activity. It's composed of two antagonistic systems: the sympathetic and parasympathetic systems. (See *Distribution paths of the autonomic nervous system,* page 22.)

Sympathetic system
Originating in the thoracic spinal and upper lumbar segments, the sympathetic system prepares the body to expend energy, espe-

cially in stressful situations, by releasing the adrenergic catecholamine norepinephrine. Its preganglionic and postganglionic neurons are scattered throughout the system, with numerous associated ganglia and plexuses.

Sympathetic stimulation produces widespread effects for two reasons. First, each preganglionic neuron synapses with 30 or more postganglionic neurons, which in turn synapse with numerous effector cells. Secondly, the norepinephrine secreted by the postganglionic terminals deactivates slowly, as does the epinephrine and norepinephrine secreted by the adrenal medulla during sympathetic stimulation.

Parasympathetic system

This cholinergic system helps conserve energy by releasing acetylcholine to mediate the pre- and postganglionic synapse and the postganglionic synapse with effector cells. It consists of preganglionic neurons with long axons, located in the brain stem and the sacral spine, and postganglionic neurons with short axons, located in peripheral ganglia or plexuses near or within the innervated structures.

The parasympathetic system affects localized, discrete areas, rather than the whole body, for two reasons. First, it contains only small numbers of pre- and postganglionic neurons and effector cells. Second, the enzyme cholinesterase quickly inactivates acetylcholine, limiting the duration of parasympathetic stimulation.

Hypothalamic control

Although the brain stem, spinal cord, and limbic system stimulate or influence the ANS, the hypothalamus is the major controlling and integrating center for all autonomic function. It's located at the crossroads of ascending and descending tracts. Hypothalamic control of autonomic function is mediated through efferent pathways to the autonomic nuclei in the brain stem and spinal cord. It's also mediated neurochemically through the hypothalamic-pituitary axis in which secretory cells in the hypothalamus produce releasing factors that control anterior pituitary secretions.

By balancing physiologic responses to environmental changes, the hypothalamus maintains homeostatic control within the narrow range necessary for optimal function. For example, certain hypothalamic cells act as thermostats to regulate body temperature, monitoring the temperature of capillary blood and initiating responses necessary for temperature adjustment. These responses include sweating or cutaneous vasodilation to promote heat loss and shivering or cutaneous vasoconstriction to conserve heat. The hypothalamus also regulates hunger and satiety. Cells in the lateral hypothalamus detect lowered blood glucose levels and stimulate appetite. In contrast, cells in the medial hypothalamus detect elevated blood glucose levels and inhibit food intake.

Perhaps the most dramatic example of hypothalamic control is the fight-or-flight response. Here, the balance between sympathetic (preparative) and parasympathetic (restorative) responses tilts toward whichever side will best protect homeostasis. Sympathetic responses, associated with stimulation of the posterior and lateral nuclei, include elevated heart rate and blood pressure, cessation of peristalsis, bronchial dilation, hyperglycemia, pupillary dilation, and peripheral cutaneous vasoconstriction. Parasympathetic responses, associated with anterior hypothalamic stimulation, include lowered heart rate and blood pressure, increased peristalsis, salivation, diaphoresis, and peripheral cutaneous vasodilation. Sympathetic responses usually occur within seconds to minutes; parasympathetic responses take minutes to hours, depending on the cause of the original sympathetic stimulation.

Sensory stimulation

Evidence of homeostatic alterations reaches the hypothalamus through changes in adjacent cells (as with hunger or temperature) or peripherally through sensor cells that access the brain stem from cranial nerves or the spinal cord. Sensor cells include chemoreceptors, which detect chemical changes; mechanoreceptors, which detect changes in tension and stretch; and baroreceptors, which detect changes in pressure. The integrated workings of sensor cells is most apparent in respiratory regulation, which is controlled in the brain stem.

Three major stimuli influence autonomic control of respiration: the presence of carbon dioxide in the brain's respiratory center, the effect of lung distention on mechanoreceptors, and detection of low blood oxygen levels by chemoreceptors in the carotid and aortic bodies. Inspiration begins when serum carbon dioxide levels stimulate neurons in the respiratory center, located in the medial aspect of the medullary reticular formation. Impulses

Distribution paths of the autonomic nervous system

The autonomic nervous system (ANS) functions below the conscious level to direct the involuntary actions of smooth muscles, cardiac muscles, and glands. Beyond the major viscera, the ANS controls muscles of the iris and ciliary body in the eye; smooth muscles in the orbit; lacrimal, salivary, and sweat glands; erector pili muscles; and blood vessels.

Highly integrated with the rest of the nervous system, the ANS maintains homeostasis through the opposing forces of its two subsystems: the sympathetic and parasympathetic divisions. These divisions hold dual sway over all ANS efferents in delicate balance. For example, they modulate exocrine and endocrine secretions, which inhibit or accelerate muscle activity; any impairment may allow nervous activity to exceed or fall short of the needed response.

Key:

 Sympathetic system

 Parasympathetic system

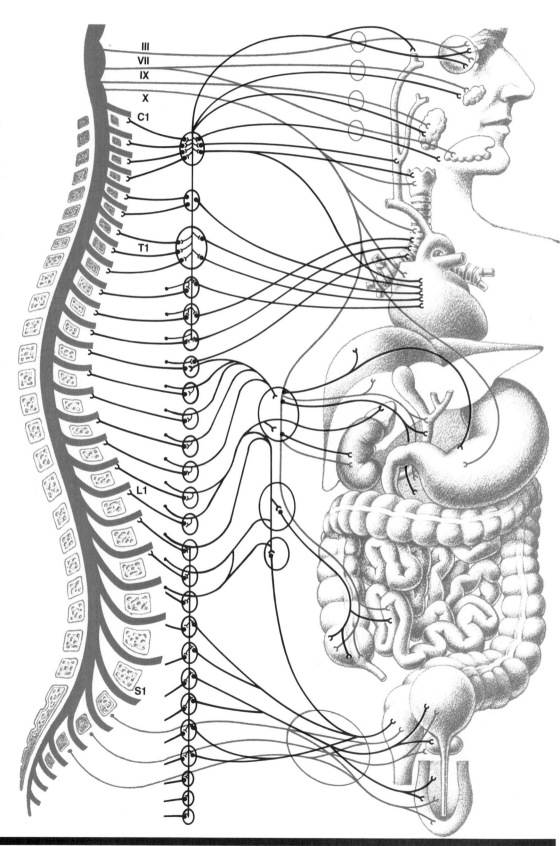

from the respiratory center follow reticulospinal connections to reach lower motor neurons that supply the diaphragm and intercostal muscles, causing these muscles to contract and the lungs to expand. Then, the Hering-Breuer reflex comes into play to limit inspiration: lung excursion stretches local mechanoreceptors and projects impulses along the vagus nerve (CN X) to the medulla, inhibiting neurons of the inspiratory center and those supplying the inspiratory muscles. Expiration, a passive elastic process, follows.

Respiration is also chemically influenced by nerve impulses traveling from the carotid bodies, along the glossopharyngeal nerve (CN IX), and from the aortic bodies, along the vagus nerve, through the brain stem. Nerve terminals in these bodies act as chemoreceptors, sensing blood oxygen levels. At a low PO_2, these terminals send impulses to the brain stem to increase respiratory rate and depth.

RETICULAR ACTIVATING SYSTEM
Guardian of consciousness, the RAS governs arousal from sleep, wakefulness, alertness or direction of attention, perceptual association, and direct introspection. This system consists of neurons whose axons extend from the brain stem and thalamus to the cerebral cortex. Each part controls different functions. The brain stem alerts the entire brain and controls wakefulness. The thalamus alerts only the cerebrum, while parts of the thalamus stimulate given areas of the cortex, perhaps focusing attention on specific mental tasks.

The RAS receives data from almost all sensory systems and has efferent connections, either direct or indirect, with all levels of the CNS. It correlates information from the brain stem, cerebrum, cerebellum, and hypothalamus with impulses from sensory receptors for pain, temperature, touch, and pressure, which are located throughout the body, as well as with those from visceral sensory endings. However, these sensations aren't sharply distinguished: they give only a vague awareness of any particular sensation. When cortical stimulation occurs during sleep, as with stretching of the bladder muscles, changes in brain wave activity are the first sign of an increasing level of consciousness. During wakefulness, stimuli reaching the cortex through the RAS sharpen attentiveness.

Cutaneous stimuli appear to be particularly helpful in maintaining consciousness, while visual, acoustic, and psychic stimulation affect alertness and attention. Impulses from the trigeminal nerve area of the face are particularly strong, as shown when ammonia capsules held to the nose rapidly restore consciousness.

PATHOPHYSIOLOGIC MECHANISMS
Prompt, efficient neurotransmission depends on a structurally intact corticospinal tract, adequate production of neurotransmitter substances at the synapse, and appropriate cellular ion concentration. Any change in these structural or chemical factors can impair or arrest transmission of nerve impulses.

Structural changes
Neurodysfunction can result from structural changes to the myoneural junction, which block transmission or reception of nerve action potentials. Normally, a nerve action potential gravitates along the axon toward the synapse with the motor end plate (surface of the muscle cell). This action potential causes the release of acetylcholine, which diffuses across the synaptic cleft and reacts with acetylcholine receptors on the motor end plate, generating end-plate potentials in the muscle.

Certain neurologic disorders, however, alter these structures. For example, in myasthenia gravis, the number of acetylcholine receptors on the muscle end plate declines, reducing end-plate potentials, and the receptors show marked anatomic changes that interfere with their response to acetylcholine. The muscle surface becomes simplified, and the synaptic cleft widens. Apparently, these changes result from the presence of acetylcholine receptor antibodies that bind to these receptors and accelerate their removal from the membrane.

Nerve death. Irreparable damage to neural cells occurs through primary injury or secondary hypoxia, ischemia, or mechanical displacement of tissue. For instance, hypoxia leads to decreased availability of ATP in the nerve cell. With lowered levels of this important energy source, the cell resorts to anaerobic metabolism, a short-term and inefficient energy source. Prolonged anoxia leads to cellular edema and nerve death.

Damage to an axon usually produces changes in the cell body (axonal reaction) and causes degenerative changes in the nerve fiber distal to the injury (wallerian degeneration). In *axonal reaction*, the nerve fiber between the cell body and the lesion doesn't alter markedly, except for traumatic degenera-

Secondary injury: Expect intracranial hypertension

Typically, secondary neurologic injury results from intracranial hypertension—a complication of head trauma, tumor, central nervous system infection, or other disorder that causes cerebral swelling, elevated cerebrospinal fluid (CSF) volume, or increased cerebral blood volume.

In fact, in head-injured patients who reach the hospital alive, intracranial hypertension is the leading cause of death. Thus, your understanding of intracranial pressure (ICP) and its pathophysiology plays an important part in delivering effective care to the neurologic patient.

Mechanics of intracranial pressure

The skull forms a rigid enclosure containing brain tissue (80%), blood (10%), and CSF (10%). These components are nearly incompressible, nearly constant in volume. Their relation to the semiclosed skull largely determines ICP.

The Monro-Kellie doctrine of relative displacement explains the concept of nearly constant volumes. It says: If the volume added to the cranial vault equals the volume displaced from it, total intracranial volume doesn't change. For example, if 50 ml of blood enters the cranial vault and 50 ml of CSF escapes from it, total volume remains the same. Since loss offsets gain, no change in intracranial dynamics occurs.

Normal ICP ranges from 0 to 15 mm Hg. Transient fluctuations occur normally during coughing, straining, or position changes. However, continued elevation above 20 mm Hg denotes intracranial hypertension.

Compensatory mechanisms

According to the Monro-Kellie doctrine, the brain initially compensates for elevated ICP. Its compensatory mechanisms include shrinkage of brain tissue through loss of intracellular fluid; reduction of CSF volume by narrowing of the ventricular system and subarachnoid spaces or by increased venous absorption of CSF; and reduction in cerebral blood volume. Its compensatory capacity depends on various anatomic and physiologic factors, which may themselves be altered by primary brain injury. However, when the brain's compensatory capacity is exceeded, ICP rises quickly and dangerously. If not corrected, persistent intracranial hypertension can cause fatal brain herniation.

A volume-pressure curve illustrates the Monro-Kellie principle. Up to a point, a rise in intracranial volume—as may occur with hemorrhage, CSF abnormalities, or other space-occupying lesions—causes only a minimal rise in ICP. However, beyond this point, compensatory mechanisms are insufficient, and ICP curves sharply and dangerously upward.

tion immediately adjacent to the lesion. However, the cell body itself swells to a concentric contour within 24 to 48 hours after axon injury, and the nucleus becomes eccentric. The reaction peaks 10 to 20 days after the injury and is most severe when the injury occurs close to the cell body.

Wallerian degeneration refers to the nerve response distal to injury. Separation from the cell body deprives the axon of the cytoplasmic proteins necessary for axon maintenance. That part of the axon distal to the lesion becomes swollen and irregular in the first day after axon injury and fragmentizes by the fourth day. Its myelin sheath first converts to short ellipsoidal segments and then degenerates from the axon, leaving only the outermost (neurilemmal) sheath.

In addition, heat production associated with impulse conduction may also inhibit transmission, especially under anaerobic conditions.

Changes in neurotransmitter substances

Numerous pathologic processes cause neurodysfunction by reducing the production of neurotransmitter chemicals. For example, parkinsonism is associated with low levels of dopamine in the basal ganglia. Both hypoxia and ischemia may reduce the levels of a variety of neurotransmitters. The many ways that neurotransmitter effectiveness can be blocked include interference with neurotransmitter synthesis, transport, storage, release, and receptor interactions.

Ionic changes

Abnormalities in ion concentrations may cause neurodysfunction by altering resting membrane potential and interfering with propagation of action potentials. High extracellular potassium levels and low extracellular calcium levels change the resting potentials of peripheral nerves and increase nerve excitability. Excessive magnesium levels have a general depressant effect on neurologic function. Disruption of the sodium-potassium pump diminishes or prevents the ionic activity crucial to neurotransmission. Impairment of the sodium-potassium pump can result from accelerated neural activities, such as increased muscle activity or increased sympathetic response, which may alter ion concentrations.

Causes of neurodysfunction

Communication between neurons is impaired by a variety of types of tissue damage. Trauma, vascular lesions, infection, tumors, or toxic substances may cause the damage. Typically, primary injury leaves neural cells more susceptible to secondary damage. (See *Secondary injury: Expect intracranial hypertension,* page 24.)

Trauma. CNS tissue trauma is a chief cause of neurodysfunction. Traumatic damage may be localized (as with cerebral contusion) or diffuse, or it may cause frank disruption of tissue (as with spinal cord injury). Spinal injuries can cause permanent paralysis even if they haven't damaged surrounding vertebrae. This happens with central cord syndrome, which is marked by cord contusion, self-destructive cord edema, and eventual bleeding into the central gray area of the spinal cord. Hemorrhagic damage to the medial part of the lateral corticospinal tract and to the ventral (anterior) horn cells results in paralysis of upper limbs while leaving lower limbs relatively unaffected. Similarly, cerebral hemorrhage, as with epidural hematoma, can produce localized ischemia with concomitant impairment of specific functions.

Vascular lesions. Such lesions impair cerebral blood flow by causing localized tissue ischemia or widespread diversion of blood, as with intracranial aneurysm, arteriovenous malformation, or arteriosclerosis. Aneurysms usually produce symptoms by rupture and hemorrhage into the subarachnoid space or by slow expansion, causing compression of adjacent neural structures. Arteriovenous malformation shunts blood from normal cerebrovascular circulation, causing reduced cerebral blood flow in nearby areas.

Arteriosclerotic patches constrict extracranial anterior circulation, especially in the internal carotids, and often result in transient cerebral ischemia with temporary anaerobic conditions at the cellular level. Permanent cerebral ischemia may result if the affected vessels become occluded.

Infectious disease. CNS infections can impair nerve impulse transmission directly by destroying neural tissue or indirectly by increasing CNS metabolic requirements through an inflammatory response. Common CNS pathogens include bacteria, such as meningococcal, pneumococcal, streptococcal, staphylococcal, gonococcal, and tuberculosis organisms, as well as the organisms associated with neurosyphilis, toxoplasmosis, and viruses.

Tumors. Indigenous CNS tumors appear as intracranial masses and as spinal cord tumors. Also, the CNS offers fertile ground for the growth of metastatic carcinomas and sarcomas disseminated from extraneural foci because of the system's intense vascularity and high levels of glucose and oxygen. Regardless of origin, an expanding mass impairs neurotransmission by causing ischemia or by obstructing CSF circulation. For example, a tumor affecting one side of the spinal cord may cause Brown-Séquard syndrome, marked by ipsilateral lower motor neuron paralysis at the level of the tumor, ipsilateral upper motor neuron weakness and loss of proprioceptive vibration sensation and two-point discrimination below the tumor level, and contralateral loss of pain and temperature sensation below the tumor level. The tumor primarily influences the dorsal sensory root, with the effects of compression manifest in most all spinal cord functions.

Toxic agents. Effects of drugs and toxins on neurotransmission vary widely. Many drugs, including ethyl alcohol, methyl alcohol, morphine, and the related alkaloids, directly influence the brain stem and cerebrum, delaying conduction of nerve impulses. Others, such as physostigmine, act at the myoneural junction and delay neurotransmission by inhibiting cholinesterase, thus prolonging parasympathetic activity. Stimulants, such as caffeine and strychnine, greatly increase reflex excitability, especially of the spinal cord, and boost CNS activity.

In addition, toxins released by certain bacteria show an affinity for the nervous system. These bacteria include *Clostridium botulinum, Clostridium tetani,* and *Corynebacterium diphtheriae.* Their toxins produce various cranial nerve dysfunctions, such as paralysis of extraocular and laryngopharyngeal muscles, by local action at the myoneural junction and along nerve tracts.

Effective nursing care

Nursing care in neurologic disorders demands complex and specialized assessment, monitoring, teaching, and special skills. Reviewing your understanding of neurologic anatomy and physiology and of the pathologic effects of trauma, infection, and toxins will help you plan more effective management.

Points to remember

- The neuron, the nervous system's basic structural and functional unit, receives sensory stimuli, transmits motor responses, and coordinates communication between body parts.
- All operations of mind and body rely on nerve impulse transmission from neuron to neuron.
- The nervous system consists of two anatomic divisions—the central and the peripheral nervous systems—and four physiologic divisions—the sensory (afferent) system; the motor (efferent) system, including the pyramidal and extrapyramidal divisions; the autonomic nervous system, including the sympathetic and parasympathetic divisions; and the reticular activating system.
- Efficient transmission of nerve impulses requires structural integrity of the cerebrospinal tract; sufficient blood, oxygen, and other nutrients; production of neurotransmitter substances at the synapse; and appropriate cellular ion concentrations.
- Impairment of impulse transmission accompanies physical changes at the myoneural junction, alteration in production of transmitter substances, nerve death, and change in neural ion concentrations.

2 ASSESSING NEUROLOGIC STATUS

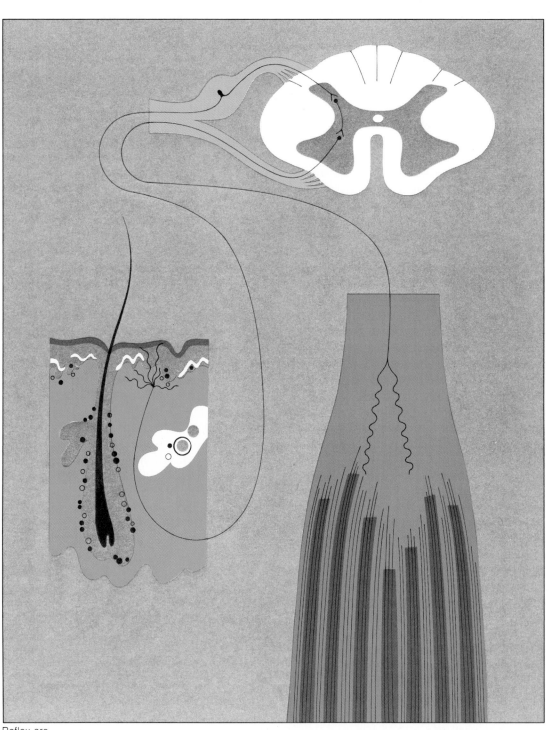

Reflex arc

specially if you don't have occasion to do it very often, you may find neurologic assessment a formidable challenge for several reasons. Doing it thoroughly takes longer than most examinations and requires certain complex skills. Neurologic changes are often elusive: some are quite subtle, while others are typically latent, requiring systematic testing to elicit them. What's most confusing, because the neurologic system is related directly or indirectly to every other body system, neurologic changes can cause or result from disorders of any other system. Consider the patient with food poisoning from *Clostridium botulinum.* Such a patient comes to the emergency department with severe diarrhea, muscle weakness, and lethargy. His muscle weakness and lethargy result from the neurotoxins produced by this pathogen, but identical symptoms could have resulted from severe diarrhea alone, as a result of overwhelming electrolyte losses.

How can you sort out symptoms and causes as confusing as these? Only by following an assessment routine that's detailed enough to uncover both subtle and latent symptoms. You'll need to listen for important clues in the history, develop keen observation skills, and master techniques for evaluating mental status, cranial nerves, reflexes, and sensory and motor functions—just what this chapter explains. With perseverance and patience, you can master these techniques and approach neurologic assessment with confidence.

Prepare the patient

After gathering equipment for the neurologic examination (see *Equipment checklist,* page 28), introduce yourself to the patient. Explain that the examination will evaluate how well his nervous system is functioning. Then let the patient express his feelings about the examination. Do all you can to make him comfortable and relaxed, because tension may interfere with the examination.

As you talk with the patient, try to understand his feelings about his illness and its impact on his life-style. Begin to devise ways of helping him cope with it effectively. Also note areas for patient teaching.

Next, ask the patient to remove his street clothes or pajamas and put on a hospital gown. (This allows you to inspect his body for symmetry and permits him to move freely.) If he appears chilled or tense, cover him with a sheet or blanket.

Plan your approach

Establish an orderly system for performing the examination. Keep in mind that you can assess several areas simultaneously. For example, you can combine assessment of mental status and speech with history-taking and your general survey, and assessment of cranial nerves with examination of the head and neck. You can also combine inspection of the patient's arms and legs with evaluation of the peripheral vascular and musculoskeletal systems.

HISTORY AND OBSERVATION

After planning your approach, begin the patient history. Form an overall impression of the patient's appearance as you interview him. Look especially for clues to neurologic dysfunction.

Observe the patient's body build and note any asymmetry or abnormal posture. Evaluate his nutritional status and determine whether he looks his stated age. When the patient talks, listen carefully for the quality of his voice and the organization and clarity of his thoughts. Note whether he responds promptly or slowly (see *Locating common communication disorders,* page 29). Also watch for any unusual mannerisms or gestures.

Determine the chief complaint

First have the patient describe his chief complaint. Typically, he might report headache, motor disturbances (including weakness, paresis, and paralysis), seizures, sensory deviations, or altered states of consciousness.

Gather as many details as possible about the complaint, including its onset and duration, precipitating factors, and impact on the patient's life-style. If the patient has difficulty communicating, ask his family to supply this information.

Review past history

Ask about these significant health factors when you take the patient's past history:
• *Head injury.* Head injury can lead to persistent headache, seizures, or coma from a fracture or increased intracranial pressure.
• *Birth trauma.* This is a common cause of seizures in children.
• *Recent infections.* Ear and sinus infections can cause headache. Septicemia and pneumonia can cause confusion. Other infections can result in acute idiopathic polyneuritis.
• *Cardiovascular disorders.* In some patients, confusion may result from treatment with

Equipment checklist

Before beginning the neurologic examination, gather this equipment:

Transparent millimeter ruler, to measure pupil size and skin lesions

Snellen's chart, to test visual acuity

Ophthalmoscope, to assess eyegrounds

Penlight or flashlight, to test pupillary reflexes

Tuning fork, to test hearing and vibratory sensation

Otoscope, to examine ears

Tongue depressors, to test gag reflex

Stethoscope, to auscultate for bruits

Toothpaste, tobacco, soap, cloves, or other familiar substances, to assess sense of smell

Sugar, salt, and vinegar or lemon juice, to assess sense of taste

Cotton wisp, to assess light-touch perception

Coins or keys, to test for tactile agnosia

Reflex hammer, to test deep tendon reflexes

Safety pin, to test pain and pressure perception

Test tubes of hot and cold water, to test temperature perception.

antihypertensives. Systemic hypotension reduces cerebral arterial perfusion, causing sensory and motor impairment.

• *Respiratory disorders.* Any severe respiratory disorder can cause hypoxia, leading to confusion and coma.

• *Thyroid disorders.* Abnormal levels of thyroid hormone strongly influence neurologic status. For example, hyperthyroidism commonly causes tremors and extreme hyperactivity— sometimes to the point of mania. Hypothyroidism can cause sluggishness, weakness, and coma. Thyroidectomy can result in myxedematoid symptoms, including lethargy and apathy.

• *Metabolic disorders.* Hypoglycemia can cause confusion, seizures, and unconsciousness; hyperglycemia can cause lethargy and coma.

• *Urinary disorders.* Chronic renal failure can lead to uremia, characterized by confusion, convulsions, and eventually coma.

• *Psychological disorders.* Depression can cause apathy, mental sluggishness, and confusion, which should be clearly distinguished from similar symptoms resulting from organic changes.

• *Drugs.* Ask the patient about use of over-the-counter or prescription drugs for headache, insomnia, and mental disturbances. Note drug names and dosage schedules. Determine if he knows the purpose for each drug.

Drug abuse and chronic alcoholism can cause convulsions, especially during withdrawal, and can produce severe neurologic changes, including neuropathy, delirium tremens, and confusion.

Also ask about drug allergies and his immunization history. Certain innoculations can cause acute idiopathic polyneuritis.

• *Past neurologic testing.* The results of the patient's previous computerized tomography scan, skull X-ray, or other diagnostic tests can usually provide information that will help you evaluate his present symptoms.

Review family history

Ask the patient about a family history of genetic diseases, such as Huntington's chorea, dystrophies, and Duchenne's disease. Keep in mind that the incidence of seizures is higher among patients whose family history shows idiopathic epilepsy, and about 65% of persons suffering from migraine headaches show a family history of the disorder.

Explore the patient's life-style

Have the patient describe his home and work environments and the activities of a typical day. Ask about any recent stress or emotional disturbances. Also ask about exposure to toxic substances, such as carbon monoxide, nitrates, or heavy metal fumes. Toxins can cause neurologic symptoms or exacerbate an existing neurologic disorder.

PHYSICAL EXAMINATION

Begin the physical examination with a general survey of the patient. Check his blood pressure and major arterial pulses bilaterally. Remember that hypertension and bradycardia may signal increased intracranial pressure. Throughout the examination, record your findings on a neurologic examination form.

Observe the size and shape of the patient's head and jaw. Inspect his nostrils and ear canals for patency (necessary to accurately assess cranial nerves I and VIII). Check his skin for any rash, lesions, discoloration, or scars.

Palpate the patient's cranium for bony abnormalities, lumps, tenderness, and soft areas. Then palpate his carotid and temporal arteries for pulsations. Next, percuss his cranium firmly with your index and middle fingers, and then percuss his sinuses and mastoid processes for tenderness.

Moving to the patient's neck, auscultate bilaterally for bruits over the carotid artery: the presence of bruits indicates distortion of a blood vessel that could interfere with blood flow to the brain. Assess the patient's neck for suppleness by asking him to place his chin on his chest and then to turn his head. He should be able to move his head easily.

Finally, inspect the patient's spine for deformities, abnormal posture, and unusual hair growth. Palpate the vertebrae for structural abnormalities and for pain and tenderness.

Evaluate mental status

This part of the neurologic examination assesses level of consciousness, orientation, memory, general knowledge, arithmetic skill, comprehension of abstract relations, and judgment. Take into account the patient's age and education, because inappropriate responses may stem from these factors rather than from neurologic impairment.

Level of consciousness and orientation. Evaluate the patient's awareness of himself and his immediate environment. Does he appear alert or confused? Determine if the patient knows his name, where he is, and the date and time of day.

Locating common communication disorders

Disorder	Clinical findings	Location of lesion	
Broca's aphasia (motor expressive nonfluent)	Patient knows what he wants to say, but has motor impairment, and can't articulate spontaneously. Also, patient understands written or verbal requests but can't repeat words or phrases.	Frontal (posterior)	
Wernicke's aphasia (sensory receptive/expressive fluent)	Patient articulates spontaneously and well, but uses words inappropriately and/or uses neologisms. Also, patient has difficulty understanding written or verbal requests and can't repeat words or phrases.	Temporoparietal (anterior)	
Global aphasia	Patient has profound expressive and receptive deficits and can barely communicate.	Temporoparietal	
Anomia	When given an object, patient can describe its characteristics (color, size, purpose) but cannot name it.	Parietal, subcortical, and/or temporal	
Apraxia	When asked to speak, patient can't coordinate movement of lips and tongue. When left alone, he may be able to do so.	Frontal	
Dysarthria	Patient knows what he wants to say, but has motor impairment, and fails to speak clearly. Also, patient has difficulty swallowing and chewing.	Cerebellar and/or frontal (posterior)	
Perseveration	Patient continually repeats one idea or response.	Throughout cerebrum (primarily anterior)	

Memory. Note the patient's attention span and his recall of the immediate, recent, and remote past.

Immediate past. Give the patient a simple series of numbers to remember; for example, 5, 7, 6, 4, 1, 2. Wait 5 minutes; then ask him to repeat them. Normally, the patient can recall six numbers without much difficulty.

Recent past. Have the patient describe the details of his admission to the hospital.

Remote past. Ask the patient to name the town where he grew up. Then have him relate important dates of his life chronologically.

General knowledge. Question the patient about a well-known current event or ask him to name several presidents.

Arithmetic skill. Tell the patient to subtract 7 from 100 (in his head, not on paper). Then, after each response, tell him to continue subtracting 7 from the remainder.

Comprehension of abstract relations and judgment. Quote a common proverb or saying, such as "people who live in glass houses shouldn't throw stones." Ask the patient to tell

Guide to cranial nerve assessment

Thorough neurologic examination includes assessment of the 12 cranial nerves, which may have sensory or motor functions, or both. Because the functions of nerves III, IV, and VI and nerves IX and X overlap, assess these groups together.

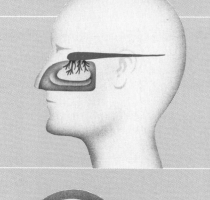

Cranial nerve I
To assess this nerve, which controls sense of smell, have the patient identify familiar odors with his eyes closed.

Cranial nerve II
Before assessing the *optic nerve*, inspect the eyes for cataracts, inflammation, or corneal scarring. Then test visual acuity with a Snellen's chart or newspaper. Also test visual fields.

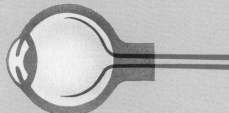

Cranial nerves III, IV, and VI
Cranial nerve III, the *oculomotor nerve,* controls pupillary constriction, upper eyelid elevation, and most eye movements.
   Cranial nerve IV, the *trochlear nerve,* controls downward and inward eye movements.
   Cranial nerve VI, the *abducens nerve,* controls lateral eye movements. To assess this group of nerves, first inspect the eyelids for ptosis. Then assess ocular movements and note any eye deviation. Test accommodation and direct and consensual light reflexes.

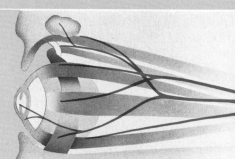

Cranial nerve V
This nerve imparts sensation to the corneas, nasal and oral mucosa, and facial skin. It also controls the muscles of mastication. To assess its function, first have the patient close his eyes. Touch his jaws, cheeks, and forehead bilaterally with a cotton wisp and then with the point of a pin. Next, lightly touch the cornea with a cotton wisp. Have the patient clench his jaw. Palpate the temporal and masseter muscles bilaterally. Try to separate the patient's clenched jaw to test muscle strength. Finally, observe for asymmetry as the patient clenches and unclenches his jaw.

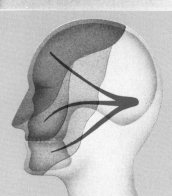

Cranial nerve VII
This nerve controls all facial muscles. It's also responsible for taste perception on the anterior portion of the tongue. To assess its function, have the patient smile, show his teeth, and puff out his cheeks. Then observe for facial symmetry as the patient raises and lowers his eyebrows. Have the patient identify sugar, salt, vinegar, and a bitter substance placed on the anterior portion of the tongue.

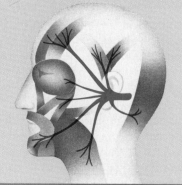

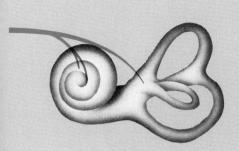

Cranial nerve VIII

The cochlear division of this nerve controls hearing; the vestibular division controls equilibrium, body position, and orientation to space. To screen for hearing loss, occlude one ear and whisper near the other. Ask the patient if he can hear you. To evaluate hearing more precisely, perform the Weber's, Rinne, or Schwabach tests. Have an audiologist perform caloric testing to assess the vestibular division.

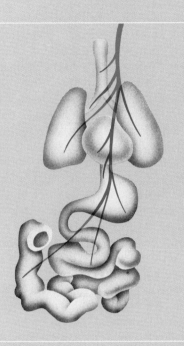

Cranial nerves IX and X

Cranial nerve IX, the *glossopharyngeal nerve*, controls swallowing and supplies sensation to the mucous membranes of the pharynx. It's also responsible for taste perception on the posterior third of the tongue and for salivation.

Cranial nerve X, the *vagus nerve*, controls swallowing, phonation, and movement of the uvula and soft palate. It also supplies sensation to the mucosa of the pharynx, soft palate, tonsils, and viscera of the thorax and abdomen. To assess the function of these nerves, first have the patient identify tastes at the back of the tongue. Then inspect the soft palate. Observe for symmetrical elevation when the patient says "ahh." Touch the mucous membrane of the soft palate with a swab to elicit the palatal reflex. Touch the posterior pharyngeal wall with a tongue depressor to elicit the gag reflex.

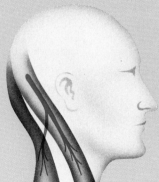

Cranial nerve XI

This nerve controls the sternocleidomastoid muscles and the upper portion of the trapezius muscles. To assess its function, palpate and inspect the sternocleidomastoid muscle as the patient pushes his chin against your hand. Palpate and inspect the trapezius muscle as the patient shrugs his shoulders against your resistance. Also have the patient stretch out his hands toward you.

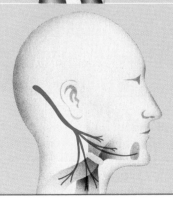

Cranial nerve XII

This nerve controls normal tongue movements involved in swallowing and speech. To assess its function, first observe the tongue for asymmetry, deviation to one side, loss of bulk, and fasciculations. Ask the patient to push his tongue against a tongue depressor. Then have him move his tongue rapidly in and out and from side to side.

Rating scale for muscle strength

To record the patient's muscle strength, use this rating scale:

5/5: Patient moves joint through full range of motion (ROM) against normal resistance and gravity.

4/5: Patient completes full ROM against moderate resistance and gravity.

3/5: Patient completes full ROM against gravity only.

2/5: Patient completes full ROM but not against gravity.

1/5: Patient's attempt at muscle contraction is palpable, but limb doesn't move.

0/5: Patient makes no visible or palpable muscle contraction; muscle is paralyzed.

you what it means. Evaluate his judgment by asking him to analyze and solve a simple problem. For example, ask the patient what he would do if he saw a fire start in a crowded movie theater.

Test cranial nerves

See *Guide to cranial nerve assessment,* pages 30 and 31, for step-by-step instruction on testing these important nerves.

Assess motor function

Begin by observing the patient's gait and posture. Then evaluate the tone and strength of his muscles and his balance and coordination. Proceed from head to toe, examining each muscle group bilaterally for comparison. Find out if the patient is right-handed or left-handed, and remember that the dominant extremity is usually slightly stronger.

Gait and posture. Ask the patient to take 20 steps, walking naturally. Observe the rhythm and regularity of his gait. Also note his posture, balance, arm swing, and any associated motions. Then ask him to walk in a straight line, heel to toe. Again, observe his gait, posture, balance, and arm swing.

Next, perform the Romberg test. Ask the patient to stand with his arms at his sides, his feet together, and his eyes open. Note his posture and balance. Then observe him in the same position with his eyes closed. Stand close to him in case he loses his balance. Slight swaying is normal.

Muscle tone and strength. Before assessing muscle tone or resistance to passive movement, encourage the patient to relax. Then move his joints through passive range of motion (ROM). Palpate the muscles for consistency, passive elasticity, and firmness as you do so. Note any muscle tenderness.

Next, assess muscle strength. Have the patient perform active ROM against your resistance (see *Testing muscle strength,* pages 34 and 35). Record your findings using the five-point scale (see *Rating scale for muscle strength*).

Coordination. These tests evaluate purposeful, fine movements and coordination of the arms and legs.

With the patient seated facing you, begin assessing his coordination by testing his arms. Ask him to touch each finger rapidly with his thumb, rhythmically pat his leg with his hand, and quickly turn his hand over and back. Have the patient perform each maneuver with each hand for about 30 seconds. Then,

ask him to touch your index finger, then his nose, several times. Have him repeat this maneuver with his eyes closed.

To test leg coordination, ask the patient to tap his foot on the floor or on your palm. Then ask him to place the heel of one foot on his other knee and slide the heel down his shin.

As the patient performs all these tests, observe for slowness, tremor, or awkwardness.

Assess sensory function

To assess your patient's sensory function, test these five areas of sensation: pain, touch, vibration, position, and discrimination. Your findings will help you locate the dermatomes where sensations may be absent, decreased, exaggerated, or delayed (see *Mapping sensory function by dermatomes*). Make sure the patient is relaxed before beginning the examination. Have him close his eyes during each of the five tests so he can't see what you're about to do. Because testing every square inch of the patient's body surface is impractical, try to test as many dermatomes as possible by distributing the stimuli over his body. Randomly apply each stimulus so the patient doesn't anticipate it. Give him time to identify the stimulus and its location.

Note whether the patient perceives the stimulus appropriately and symmetrically. When testing pain and touch, compare distal and proximal parts of the patient's arms and legs. Test vibration and position distally. If you locate a dermatome in which sensation is absent or exaggerated, mark it. Then stimulate a nearby area of greater or lesser sensations, moving away from the suspect dermatome until the patient feels a change.

Test pain and touch sense

Use a safety pin to test your patient's pain sensation. Starting at his shoulder, gently stimulate the skin of the arms, trunk, and legs with the sharp end of the pin. Next, apply the blunt end to check the patient's ability to distinguish between sharp and dull sensations. If he responds normally to the pinpricks, you don't need to test his response to temperature, because both of these sensations travel along related pathways.

To test the patient's sense of touch, lightly touch his skin with a piece of cotton. Ask him to tell you where you're touching him each time. Once or twice, pretend you're touching him but don't actually do so—to check if he can tell the difference.

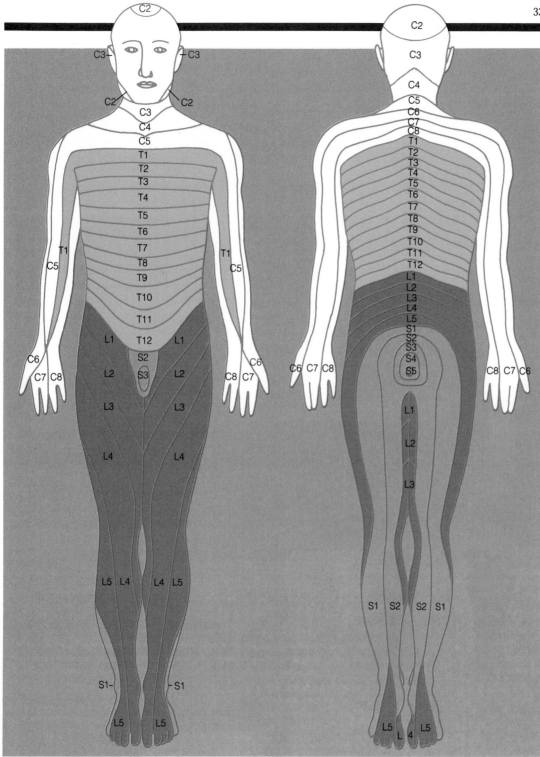

Mapping sensory function by dermatomes

The two figures illustrated at left show the segmental distribution of spinal nerves that transmit pain, temperature, and touch from the skin to the spinal cord.

As you assess the patient's sensory function, use this chart as a reference to document the specific area tested, as well as the test results.

Test vibration and position sense

Use a lightly vibrating tuning fork (128 cycles/second) to test your patient's response to vibration. Place it against a bony prominence on each arm and leg, such as the distal joint of a finger or the middle joint of the great toe. Make sure the patient understands that he's trying to feel a vibration, not just pressure or touch. To evaluate this sense, place the vibrating tuning fork on one of the patient's joints. Then, while the fork is still vibrating,

place your hand on it to stop it and ask the patient if he can feel the difference. If his sense of vibration seems impaired, test more proximal bony prominences.

Next, test the position sense in each arm and leg. Holding one of the patient's fingertips between your thumb and index finger, slowly flex or extend the finger. Ask the patient to tell you when he feels the finger moving and in which direction he thinks it's moving. (Make sure the patient's eyes are closed dur-

Testing muscle strength

Although it's impractical to test all muscles during the neurologic examination, testing the following 10 muscle groups provides an overall assessment of muscle strength. To test the strength of each group, ask the patient to perform active range of motion against your resistance. If the muscle group is weak, decrease or eliminate resistance to permit more accurate assessment. If necessary, position the patient's extremity so he doesn't have to resist gravity, and repeat the test.

Muscles of the arms

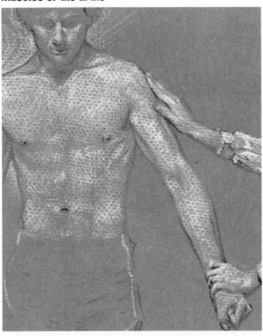

Deltoid muscle
Place one hand over the deltoid muscle and support the patient's straightened arm with your other hand. Have him abduct his arm to a horizontal position against your resistance. Palpate contraction of the deltoid.

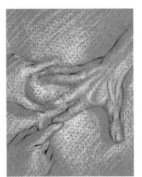

Triceps
Have the patient abduct his arm and hold the forearm midway between flexion and extension. Support his arm at the wrist with your hand. Ask him to extend his arm against your resistance. Observe contraction of the triceps muscle.

Biceps
Place your hand over the patient's hand. Have him flex his forearm against your resistance. Observe contraction of the biceps muscle.

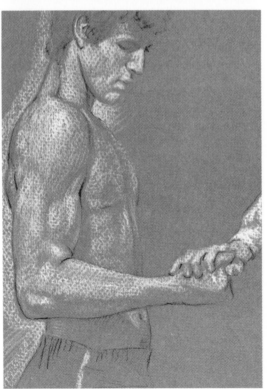

Dorsal interossei
Have the patient extend his fingers and spread them. Tell him to resist your attempt to bring them together.

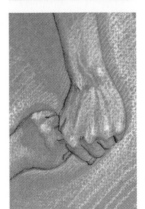

Forearm and hand (grip)
Ask the patient to grasp your index and middle fingers firmly with his hand.

Muscles of the legs

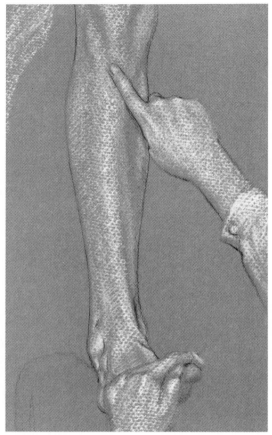

Anterior tibial
Have the patient extend his leg. Then place your hand on his foot and ask him to dorsiflex his ankle against your resistance.

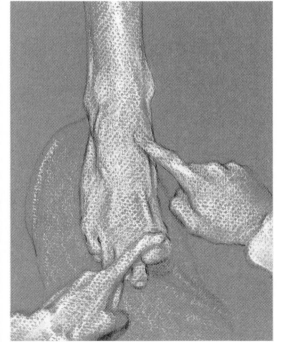

Extensor hallucis longus
Place your forefinger on the patient's great toe and ask him to dorsiflex his toe against your resistance.

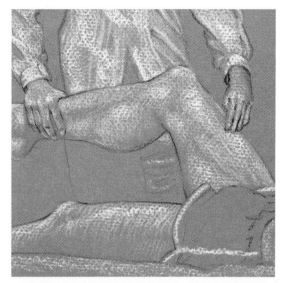

Quadriceps
Have the patient bend his knee slightly while you support his lower leg. Then ask him to extend his knee against your resistance. Palpate contraction of the quadriceps muscle.

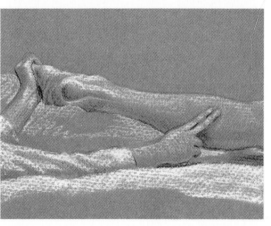

Gastrocnemius
Ask the patient to turn on his side. Then support his foot and have him plantar-flex his ankle against your resistance. Palpate contraction of the gastrocnemius muscle.

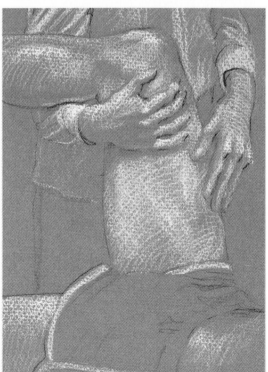

Psoas
Have the patient raise his knee while you support his leg. Ask him to flex his hip against your resistance. Observe contraction of the psoas muscle.

Grading reflexes

When testing your patient's deep tendon and superficial reflexes, use the following grading scales:

Deep tendon reflex grades

0 absent

1+ present but diminished

2+ normal

3+ increased but not necessarily pathologic

4+ hyperactive; clonus may also be present

Superficial reflex grades

0 absent

± equivocal or barely present

+ normally active

Record the patient's reflex scores by drawing a stick figure and entering the scores at the proper location. The figure shown here indicates normal deep tendon reflex activity as well as normal superficial reflex activity over the abdominal area. The arrows at the figure's feet indicate normal plantar reflex activity.

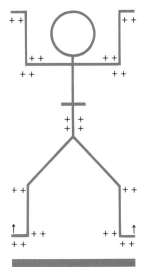

ing this test.) Repeat the maneuver with each great toe.

Test discrimination sense

Discrimination testing assesses the ability of the brain's sensory cortex (in the parietal lobe) to interpret and integrate information. The following tests assess the parietal lobe's ability to interpret these sensations and the posterior column's ability to conduct them.

• *Stereognosis.* Place several small, familiar objects in the patient's hand—keys or coins will do. Ask the patient to identify them, one at a time.

• *Graphesthesia.* With the blunt end of a pen, trace several letters or numbers on each of the patient's palms and ask the patient to identify them.

• *Two-point stimulation.* Gently prick the patient's fingertip or another body area with two safety pins, held several millimeters apart. Ask the patient if he feels one or two pricks. Repeat the procedure several times, occasionally pricking him with only one pin to test the reliability of his responses. Find the minimal distance at which the patient can discriminate one prick from two, and compare it to these normal findings:

    Tongue: 1 mm
    Fingertips: 2.8 mm
    Toes: 3 to 8 mm
    Palms: 8 to 12 mm
    Chest, forearms: 40 mm
    Back: 40 to 70 mm
    Upper arms, thighs: 75 mm.

• *Extinction phenomenon.* Gently prick the patient's skin simultaneously on opposite sides of his body, and ask him if he feels one prick or two. Repeat the procedure several times in different symmetrical areas. Occasionally, apply only one stimulus to test the reliability of the patient's responses.

Assess reflexes

Reflexes are divided into two categories: deep tendon and superficial. You elicit deep tendon (or muscle stretch) reflexes when you apply a stimulus to a tendon, a bone, or a joint. You elicit superficial (or cutaneous) reflexes when you apply a stimulus to a skin surface or mucous membrane. Superficial reflexes respond more slowly to stimuli and fatigue more easily than deep tendon reflexes.

Use a percussion hammer—preferably with a soft rubber end—to elicit deep tendon reflexes. To assess superficial reflexes, touch or scratch the patient's skin surface with an ob-

ject that won't damage the skin, such as a tongue depressor.

Test each reflex bilaterally for comparison before moving down the patient's body. Remember that reflexes should be symmetrically equal. If you note a brisk response on one side of the patient's body, you should find an equally brisk response on the other side.

Record your findings, using a grading scale. In your notes, indicate the particular scale you used (see *Grading reflexes*).

Test deep tendon reflexes

The most commonly assessed deep tendon reflexes are the following:

• *Biceps.* To elicit this reflex, have the patient relax his arm and pronate the forearm slightly, positioned somewhere between flexion and extension. (For best results, ask the patient to rest his elbow in your hand.) Then, percuss the biceps tendon with the reflex hammer. The biceps muscle should contract, followed by flexion of the forearm.

• *Brachioradialis.* Position the patient's forearm in semiflexion and semipronation, resting it either in your hand or on his knee. Tap the styloid process of the radius 1″ to 2″ (2.5 to 5 cm) above the wrist. You should see flexion at the elbow and a simultaneous pronation of the forearm, as well as flexion of the fingers and hand.

• *Triceps.* Position the patient's arm about midway between flexion and extension. If possible, have the patient rest his arm on his thigh or in your hand. Tap the tendon above the insertion on the ulna's olecranon process, 1″ to 2″ (2.5 to 5 cm) above the elbow. The stimulus should elicit muscle contraction of the triceps and elbow extension.

• *Patellar.* Have the patient sit on a table with his legs dangling freely, or have him cross his legs. Place one of your hands over the patient's quadriceps, and use your other hand to tap his tendon just below the patella. A firm tap should draw the patella down and stretch the muscle, causing an extension of the leg at the knee.

• *Achilles.* Have the patient sit on a table with his legs dangling. (If the patient can't sit without support, have him sit or lie in bed.) Flex his leg at the hip and knee, and rotate it externally. If the patient is prone, flex his knee and hip and rotate the leg externally so it rests on the other shin. Then, place your hand under the patient's foot, dorsiflex the ankle, and tap the tendon just above its insertion on the posterior surface of the calcaneus. You

Glasgow coma scale

Test	Reaction	Score
Eyes	Open spontaneously	4
	Open to verbal command	3
	Open to pain	2
	No response	1
Best motor response	Obeys verbal command	6
	Localizes painful stimulus	5
	Flexion-withdrawal	4
	Flexion-abnormal (Decorticate rigidity)	3
	Extension (Decerebrate rigidity)	2
	No response	1
Best verbal response	Oriented and converses	5
	Disoriented and converses	4
	Inappropriate words	3
	Incomprehensible sounds	2
	No response	1
Total		3-15

should see a plantar flexion of the patient's foot at the ankle.

Test superficial reflexes
The most commonly assessed superficial reflexes are the following:
• *Upper abdominal.* To test this reflex, have the patient lie down and relax. Move a tongue depressor downward and outward from the tip of his sternum. You can also stroke the area horizontally, moving medially toward the umbilicus. The abdominal muscles should contract, and the umbilicus should deviate toward the stimulus.
• *Lower abdominal.* With the patient lying down, stroke his skin in an upward and outward movement from the symphysis or horizontally in the lower quadrants. The umbilicus should deviate toward the stimulus, along with abdominal contraction.
• *Cremasteric* (males only). Lightly stroke the inner aspect of the upper thigh with a tongue depressor. The testis on the same side as the stimulus should rise.
• *Gluteal.* Stroke the skin over the patient's buttocks, and observe for tense muscles in this area.
• *Plantar.* Firmly stroke the lateral surface of the dorsum of the patient's foot with the end of a percussion hammer. A normal response is plantar flexion of the foot and toes.

• *Pathologic reflex.* Babinski's sign, or reflex, is the opposite of the normal plantar reflex. When you firmly stroke the lateral aspect of the patient's sole with a blunt object, the great toe extends, or dorsiflexes, as the other toes fan out.

PATIENT MONITORING
After you complete the physical examination, you have a firm baseline for subsequent patient monitoring. Detecting and interpreting changes from the baseline requires practice and skill. Obviously, the alert, cooperative patient can be a help by reporting new or varying symptoms. But if the patient's unconscious, you must rely on your assessment alone to uncover baseline changes. Use of the Glasgow coma scale provides a standard method for recording such changes (see *Glasgow coma scale*). A decreased reaction score in one or more categories warns of impending neurologic crisis.

Besides level of consciousness, monitor pupillary size and light responses and vital signs. Pupillary dilation and poor or absent response to light result from compression of the third cranial nerve and signal uncal herniation.

Altered vital signs may reflect an ominous increase in intracranial pressure. Watch for increased systolic pressure, an early sign of increased intracranial pressure, and then for bradycardia and abnormal respiratory patterns due to brain-stem compression.

NURSING DIAGNOSES
Using the data gathered from baseline assessment and subsequent patient monitoring, you can establish the nursing diagnosis. A nursing diagnosis describes a set of signs and symptoms that indicate an actual or potential health problem requiring nursing intervention. For the patient with neurologic dysfunction, health problems may involve almost any aspect of daily living, from impairment of basic body functions to derangement of complex thought processes. When writing a nursing diagnosis, describe the patient's problem, clearly relating it to its cause. Then outline appropriate goals to solve each problem and construct your care plan around them. With this approach, your nursing care will be well-organized and purposeful. Most important, it will be specific and personal, reflecting your keen assessment and effective management of the individual patient's changing health status.

Points to remember
• Thorough neurologic assessment helps you identify and assess early signs and symptoms of neurologic dysfunction, which can be life-threatening.
• To achieve accurate assessment, make the patient as relaxed and comfortable as possible.
• The most common chief complaints in neurologic disorders are headache, motor disturbances (including weakness, paresis, and paralysis), seizures, sensory deviations, and altered states of consciousness.
• Neurologic assessment involves evaluation of mental status, cranial nerves, sensory and motor functions, and reflexes.
• The Glasgow coma scale, an invaluable aid for assessing unconscious patients, grades consciousness in relation to eye opening and motor and verbal responses.
• Assessment data provide the basis for nursing diagnoses—the building blocks of your care plan. Always aim to help the patient cope effectively with his illness and modify his life-style, as necessary.

3 UPDATING DIAGNOSTIC METHODS

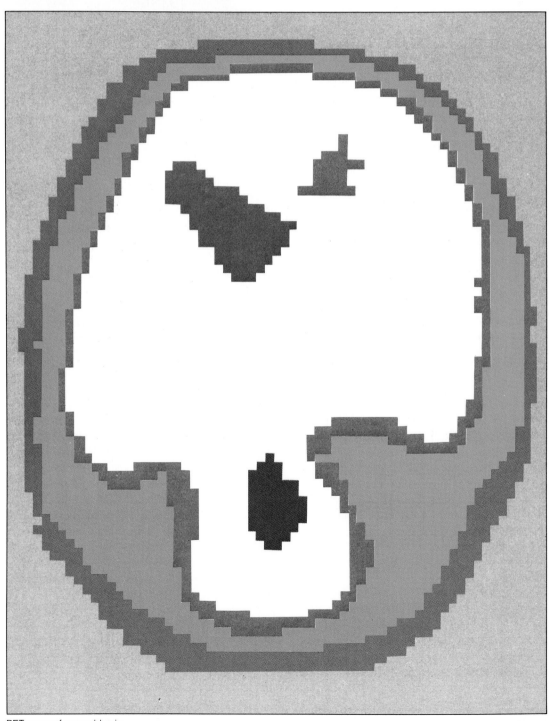

PET scan of normal brain

oday, highly sophisticated computers and X-ray scanners make viewing the brain's interior a remarkably simple procedure, providing reliable information with little risk to the patient. That's clearly been the major goal of the new neurodiagnostic technology, and the resulting improvements have been impressive. The revolutionary computerized tomography (CT) scan of the early 1970s eliminated the overlapping detail seen on plain X-rays, providing clear radiographic images of cross sections of the head. Magnetic resonance imaging (MRI), an equally promising technique of the 1980s, eliminates exposure to radiation, using magnetic and radio waves to study cranial and spinal structures.

Even if you don't routinely perform or assist with neurodiagnostic tests, you should know what they are and understand how they fit into the patient's care plan. It's often your responsibility to adequately prepare the patient for such tests and to care for him after they're complete. To prepare the patient, you must be able to explain the purpose of the test and describe the procedure in detail so the patient knows what to expect. This chapter will help you to understand the available diagnostic tests and prepare you to anticipate and participate in their effective use.

RADIOLOGIC TESTS
Radiologic tests are the most common neurodiagnostic tests and have an important place in virtually every neurodiagnostic workup. These tests, from plain X-rays to the more complicated and invasive tests, localize and reveal the structural dimensions of many neurologic disorders. Invasive vascular tests highlight the cerebral vessels; invasive non-vascular tests highlight the ventricles and subarachnoid space.

Plain X-rays of skull and spine
The oldest noninvasive neurologic test, plain X-rays are frequently the second step, after routine neurologic examination, in a complete neurologic workup. In patients with head injuries, X-ray films of the skull offer limited information about skull fractures. Nevertheless, they are extremely valuable for detecting increased intracranial pressure (ICP), abnormalities of the base of the skull and the cranial vault, congenital and perinatal anomalies, and many systemic diseases that produce bone defects of the skull. X-ray films of the spine are useful for identifying vertebral fracture or displacement, which may impinge on the spinal cord or nerve roots. Typically, a complete examination requires several radiographic views of the skull or spine.

Cerebral angiography
Cerebral angiography allows radiographic examination of the cerebral vasculature after injection of a contrast medium. The femoral and brachial arteries are the most common puncture sites; however, the carotid and vertebral arteries may also be used but with greater risk. The usual clinical indication for this test is a suspected abnormality of the cerebral vasculature, often as suggested by a CT or radionuclide scan of the brain. Angiography commonly confirms the presence of aneurysm, arteriovenous malformation, thrombosis, stenosis, or occlusion. It may also identify vascular changes caused by cranial tumor, hematoma, cyst, edema, herniation, arterial spasm, or hydrocephalus.

Myelography
Myelography combines fluoroscopy and radiography to evaluate the spinal subarachnoid space after injection of a contrast medium via lumbar puncture. Because the contrast medium is heavier than cerebrospinal fluid (CSF), it will flow through the subarachnoid space to the dependent area when the patient, lying prone on a fluoroscopic table, is tilted up or down. The fluoroscope allows visualization of the flow of the contrast medium, the outline of the subarachnoid space, and any abnormalities that may be present. Simultaneously, radiographs are taken for a permanent record. This test can demonstrate lesions, such as tumors and herniated intervertebral disks, that partially or totally block the flow of CSF in the subarachnoid space. It also aids detection of arachnoiditis, spinal nerve root compression or injury, or tumors in the posterior fossa of the skull.

Pneumoencephalography
Pneumoencephalography allows radiographic examination of the cerebral ventricles and cisterns after injection of air (or oxygen) into the subarachnoid space, usually by lumbar puncture. The injected air acts as a contrast agent, filling the cavities in the brain as the patient is rotated in a motorized chair. Pneumoencephalography is a painful and dangerous procedure—now it's virtually obsolete, having been replaced by the CT scan. However, pneumoencephalography may be used

Viewing the brain's interior

A dvances in research and technology continue to refine and develop safer, more rewarding methods for studying the nervous system. Computerized tomography (CT), positron emission tomography (PET), and, more recently, magnetic resonance imaging (MRI) and digital subtraction angiography (DSA) are major strides in neurodiagnostic testing.

Computerized tomography
CT is a noninvasive test that provides clear, cross-sectional images of the head and spine, based on computer reconstruction of radiation levels absorbed by various tissues. The reconstructed image displays tissue density within a black-to-white spectrum. Black areas on the CT scan correspond to air density; white areas, to bone and blood density. Shades of grey correspond to cerebrospinal fluid and soft-tissue density. Valuable for diagnosing intracranial and spinal lesions, the CT scan also helps identify hydrocephalus, cerebral atrophy, and cerebral edema. Using an I.V.-injected radiopaque contrast agent with the CT scan helps define abnormalities.

Positron emission tomography
Like CT scanning, PET provides cross-sectional images of the head but involves a different technique. This experimental test maps the brain's metabolic activity by recording gamma rays produced by the union of an injected biochemical—typically glucose—tagged with a radioisotope and negatively charged electrons in the brain. Abnormal isotope concentration identifies brain areas damaged by stroke or contusion or areas involved in seizure activity. Current research aims to understand the interaction of neurotransmitters in the brain. Locating dopamine and its receptor sites, for example, may provide an effective treatment or cure for Parkinson's disease.

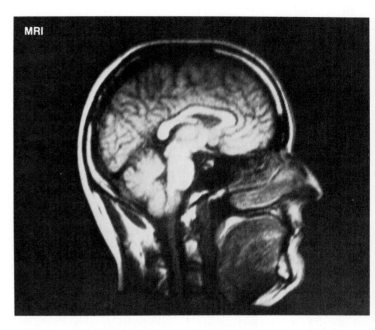

MRI

Magnetic resonance imaging
MRI, also known as nuclear magnetic resonance, is a noninvasive test that detects structural and biochemical abnormalities by directing magnetic and radio waves at body tissues to determine the response of a test element. MRI relies on the natural magnetic properties of atoms in the body. Certain particles that form any atom possess an electrical charge, either positive (protons) or negative (electrons). Hence, the particles act as tiny magnets. Some MRI studies, called proton MRI, focus on hydrogen protons because of their abundance in the body. These hydrogen protons align themselves within the external magnetic field created by the MRI magnet. Then, the protons are briefly bombarded with radio-frequency signals that deflect them from their induced alignment. When the radio signals stop, the energized protons emit a return signal. The MRI computer analyzes this signal, which varies with the tissue concentrations of the test element and the time it takes the protons to return to their original alignment. These "relaxation" times differ for each type of body tissue but may be prolonged for malignant tissue. Use of MRI in neurologic testing is still evolving, but it may aid diagnosis of stroke, other cerebrovascular disorders, and multiple sclerosis. Soon MRI may be able to provide information *in vivo* about cellular processes.

Digital subtraction angiography
DSA is a type of intravenous arteriography. It combines X-ray detection methods and a computerized subtraction technique with fluoroscopy for real-time visualization without interference from adjacent structures, such as bone or soft tissue.

A radiologist injects contrast medium through a catheter threaded into the superior vena cava. As the contrast medium circulates through the arteries, serial X-rays are taken. A computer then "subtracts" structures that block a clear view of the arteries and projects the enhanced image onto a screen. Using direct arterial injection for DSA also provides angiographic information, but it requires much less contrast medium.

DSA is currently used in neurologic testing to visualize cerebral blood flow and to detect vascular abnormalities.

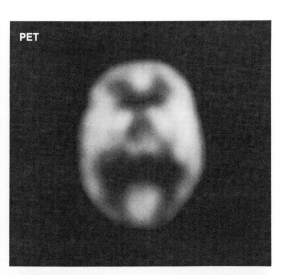

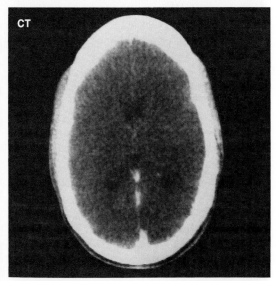

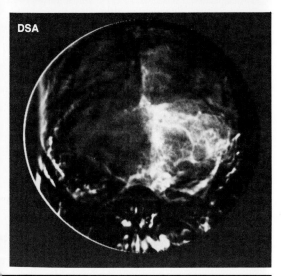

in selected patients with suspected aqueductal stenosis or tumors of the cerebral ventricles and cisterns and of the pituitary gland.

Ventriculography

Ventriculography, a variation of pneumoencephalography, involves the direct replacement of CSF in the ventricles with air or another contrast medium, followed by serial X-rays. Although this test may be done when increased ICP contraindicates pneumoencephalography, it's been largely replaced by CT scanning.

CEREBROSPINAL FLUID ANALYSIS

CSF is a unique distillate of blood that originates in the choroid plexuses of the brain and circulates in the subarachnoid space. It protects the brain and spinal cord from injury and transports products of neurosecretion, cellular biosynthesis, and cellular metabolism through the central nervous system (CNS). For laboratory analysis, CSF is obtained most commonly by lumbar puncture (usually between the third and fourth lumbar vertebrae) and, occasionally, by cisternal or ventricular puncture. A sample of CSF is frequently obtained during other neurologic tests, including myelography and pneumoencephalography. CSF analysis helps identify various CNS disorders, such as tumors, subarachnoid or intracranial hemorrhage, demyelinating diseases, viral or bacterial meningitis, neurosyphilis, and chronic CNS infections (see *Characteristics of cerebrospinal fluid,* page 42). Measuring CSF pressure just before removal of a sample helps detect CSF obstruction.

Infection at the puncture site contraindicates removal of CSF. In a patient with increased ICP, CSF should be removed with extreme caution because the rapid reduction in pressure that follows withdrawal of fluid can cause cerebellar tonsillar herniation and medullary compression.

INTRACRANIAL PRESSURE MONITORING

ICP monitoring measures the pressure exerted by brain tissue, blood, and CSF against the skull. Indications for this procedure include head trauma with bleeding or edema, overproduction or insufficient absorption of CSF, cerebral hemorrhage, and space-occupying brain lesions. Such monitoring can detect elevated ICP early, before clinical danger signs develop. Prompt intervention can then help avert or diminish neurologic damage caused by cerebral hypoxia and shifts of brain mass.

Characteristics of cerebrospinal fluid

Test	Normal	Abnormal	Implications
Pressure	50 to 180 mm H$_2$O	Increase	Increased intracranial pressure due to hemorrhage, tumor, thrombosis, meningitis, or edema caused by trauma
		Decrease	Spinal subarachnoid obstruction above puncture site
Appearance	Clear, colorless	Cloudy	Infection (elevated white blood cell [WBC] count or many microorganisms) or elevated protein level
		Pink, red, or bloody	Subarachnoid, intracerebral, or intraventricular hemorrhage; subarachnoid obstruction; traumatic tap (usually noted only in initial specimen)
		Brown, orange, or yellow (xanthochromic)	Elevated protein, red blood cell (RBC) breakdown (blood present for at least 3 days)
Protein	15 to 45 mg/100 ml	Marked increase	Tumors, trauma, hemorrhage, diabetes mellitus, bacterial or fungal meningitis, polyneuritis, blood in cerebrospinal fluid (CSF), demyelinating disease (such as multiple sclerosis)
		Marked decrease	Rapid CSF production
Gamma globulin	3% to 12% of total protein	Increase	Demyelinating disease (such as multiple sclerosis), neurosyphilis, Guillain-Barré syndrome
Glucose	40 to 80 mg/100 ml (60% to 80% of blood glucose)	Increase	Systemic hyperglycemia
		Decrease	Systemic hypoglycemia, bacterial fungal infection, meningitis, mumps, postsubarachnoid hemorrhage
Cell count	0 to 5 WBCs	Increase	Active disease: meningitis, acute infection, onset of chronic illness, tumor, abscess, infarction, demyelinating disease (such as multiple sclerosis)
	No RBCs	RBCs	Hemorrhage or traumatic tap
VDRL and other serologic tests	Nonreactive	Positive	Neurosyphilis
Chloride	118 to 130 mEq/liter	Decrease	Infected meninges (as in tuberculosis or meningitis)
Gram stain	No organisms	Gram-positive or gram-negative organisms	Bacterial meningitis

The three basic ICP monitoring systems use a ventricular catheter, subarachnoid screw, or epidural sensor.

Ventricular catheter monitoring, which monitors ICP directly, involves insertion of a small polyethylene or silicone rubber catheter into the lateral ventricle through a burr hole. This method measures ICP most accurately and is the only ICP monitoring method that allows for evaluation of brain compliance and drainage of significant amounts of CSF. However, it has two disadvantages: it carries the greatest risk of infection, and placing the catheter may be difficult, especially if the ventricle is collapsed or displaced.

Subarachnoid screw monitoring involves the insertion of an ICP screw into the subarachnoid space through a burr hole in the skull behind the hairline. Placing an ICP screw is easier than placing a ventricular catheter, especially if a CT scan has revealed shifting of the cerebrum or collapsed ventricles. This type of ICP monitoring also carries less risk of infection and parenchymal damage because the screw doesn't penetrate the cerebrum.

In ventricular catheter and subarachnoid screw monitoring, a fluid-filled line connects the catheter or screw to a pressure dome transducer. Elevated ICP exerts pressure on the fluid in the line, depressing the dome's diaphragm. The transducer then transmits pressure readings to a monitor for display. If desired, the readings can also be transmitted to a recorder for permanent readout strips.

Epidural sensor monitoring, the least invasive method with the lowest incidence of infection, uses a fiber-optic sensor inserted into the epidural space through a burr hole. A cable connects the sensor to a monitor and, if desired, to a recorder. Unlike a ventricular catheter or subarachnoid screw, the sensor can't become occluded with blood or brain tissue. However, epidural monitoring provides less reliable information because it doesn't measure ICP directly from a cranial space filled with CSF.

The three basic waveforms used to describe abnormal ICP are A, B, and C waves. See *Interpreting intracranial pressure waveforms,* to learn how to recognize such waves.

ELECTROPHYSIOLOGIC TESTS

Several neurodiagnostic tests identify neurologic disorders by measuring electrical activity in the brain, spinal cord, or peripheral nerves.

Electroencephalography

In electroencephalography (EEG), electrodes attached to standard areas of the patient's scalp record a portion of the brain's electrical activity. These electrical impulses are transmitted to an EEG machine, which magnifies them 1 million times and records them as brain waves on moving strips of paper. Some waves are irregular, while others demonstrate frequent patterns (see *EEGs: Recording the brain's electrical activity,* page 44).

Especially valuable in assessing patients with seizure disorders, EEG is also used to evaluate patients with symptoms of brain tumors, abscesses, and cerebral damage due to other causes.

In patients with epilepsy, EEG patterns may identify the specific disorder. In patients with *petit mal epilepsy,* the EEG tracing shows spikes and waves at a frequency of 3 cycles/second. In *grand mal epilepsy,* it typically shows multiple, high-voltage, spiked waves in both hemispheres. In *temporal lobe epilepsy,* the EEG tracing usually shows spiked waves in the affected temporal region; in focal seizures, it usually shows localized, spiked discharges.

In patients with intracranial lesions, such as tumors or abscesses, the EEG tracing may show slow waves (usually delta waves, but possibly unilateral beta waves). Vascular lesions, such as cerebral infarcts and intracranial hemorrhages, typically produce focal abnormalities in the injured area. In patients who are depressed or apathetic or who show

Interpreting intracranial pressure waveforms

Normal ICP waveform

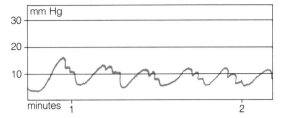

A waves (plateau waves)

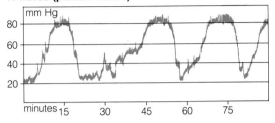

B waves

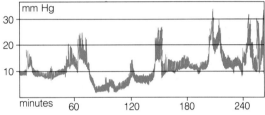

C waves

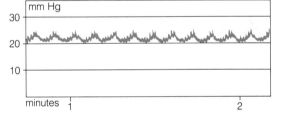

other signs of mental dysfunction, a normal EEG tracing may verify mental retardation or a psychiatric disorder, such as schizophrenia.

Generally, any condition that causes a depressed level of consciousness changes the EEG pattern, which will show reduced electrical activity in proportion to the degree of consciousness lost. For example, in a patient with a severe inflammation (as in meningitis or encephalitis) or rising ICP, the EEG recording shows brain waves that are generalized, diffuse, and slow. The most pathologic finding of all is the absence of electrical activity, the so-called EEG flat tracing, which may indicate brain death.

Electromyography

Electromyography is the recording of the electrical activity of selected musculoskeletal

When your patient's receiving intracranial pressure (ICP) monitoring, you'll be expected to accurately identify and interpret the waveforms shown here. A *normal ICP waveform* has a steep upward systolic slope followed by a downward diastolic slope with dicrotic notch. This waveform typically occurs continuously, indicating an ICP measurement between 4 and 15 mm Hg. *A waves* are the most clinically significant ICP waveforms. These waves plateau for more than 5 minutes before dropping sharply and may reach elevations of 50 to 100 mm Hg. Recurring A waves indicate a rapid, dangerous rise in ICP and a reduced ability to compensate. Sustained A waves may be associated with irreversible brain damage. *B waves* appear sharp and rhythmic, with a sawtooth pattern. They occur every 1½ to 2 minutes and may reach elevations of 50 mm Hg. The clinical significance of B waves isn't clear, but they seem to occur more frequently with decreasing compensation. These waves sometimes accompany erratic or abnormal respirations caused by fluctuations in intrathoracic pressure or PCO_2 that influence intracranial pressure. *C waves* are rapid and rhythmic and appear less sharp than B waves. They may fluctuate with respiration or systemic blood pressure and aren't considered clinically significant. Transient spikes in ICP waveforms may result from temporary rises in thoracic pressure. These spikes rarely last longer than 1 to 2 minutes but may reach elevations above 50 mm Hg.

EEGs: Recording the brain's electrical activity

In electroencephalography (EEG), electrodes attached to the patient's scalp, as shown, detect electrical impulses generated by the brain's nerve cells. Lead wires then transmit these impulses to an EEG machine, which translates them into waveforms. Among the basic waveforms are the alpha, beta, theta, and delta rhythms. Alpha waves occur at frequencies of 8 to 12 cycles/second in a regular rhythm and are most prominent in the occipital region of the brain. They're present only in the waking state when the patient's eyes are closed but he's mentally alert; usually, they disappear with visual activity or mental concentration. Beta waves (13 to 30 cycles/second)—generally associated with anxiety, depression, or sedative drugs—are seen most readily in the frontal and central regions of the brain. Theta waves (4 to 7 cycles/second) are most common in children and young adults and appear in the frontal and temporal regions. Delta waves (0.5 to 3.5 cycles/second) normally occur only in young children and during sleep.

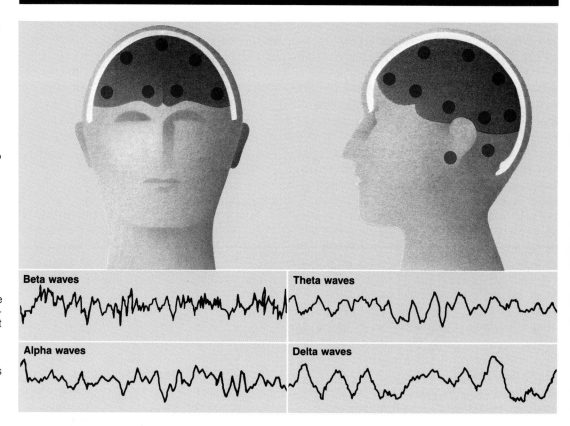

Beta waves

Theta waves

Alpha waves

Delta waves

groups at rest and during voluntary contraction. In this test, a needle electrode is inserted percutaneously into a muscle. The electrical discharge (or motor unit potential) of the muscle is displayed and measured on an oscilloscope screen. The amplitude and duration of the motor unit potential are directly proportional to the force of muscle contractions.

Electromyography is a useful diagnostic technique for differentiating primary muscle disease from lower motor neuron disease. In primary muscle disease, such as the muscular dystrophies, motor unit potentials are short (of low amplitude), with frequent, irregular discharges. In disorders such as amyotrophic lateral sclerosis (as well as in peripheral nerve disorders), motor unit potentials are isolated and irregular but show increased amplitude and duration. In myasthenia gravis, motor unit potentials initially may be normal during short-term effort by the patient but progressively diminish in amplitude with continuing contractions. The interpreter must distinguish between waveforms that indicate a muscle disorder and those that indicate denervation by correlating electromyographic findings with the patient's history and clinical status and the results of other neurodiagnostic tests.

Electronystagmography

Electronystagmography is the technique for monitoring nystagmus, the involuntary oscillating eye movement caused by the vestibulo-ocular reflex. The battery of tests used to elicit the nystagmus includes calibration, gaze, pendulum tracking, optokinetics, positional methods, and caloric tests. Electronystagmography relies on the corneoretinal potential—the difference of 1 millivolt between the positive charge of the cornea and the negative charge of the retina—to record nystagmus through electrodes placed near the eyes. As the eyes move horizontally or vertically, the electrodes pick up the corneoretinal potential and feed it to a recorder, which amplifies the signal and charts it. Abnormal nystagmus can result from lesions of either the vestibular or ocular system; however, it's the primary sign of vestibular disturbances, along with the symptom of vertigo.

Evoked potentials

Stimulation of the sense organs or peripheral nerves produces a discrete electrical response, or evoked potential, along a neurologic pathway to the brain. Measuring such potentials, also known as short latency evoked potentials (SLEP), evaluates the integrity of visual, auditory, and somatosensory pathways. It's especially valuable for assessing neurologic status of infants, comatose patients, and those under anesthesia or with latent neurologic symptoms. Evoked potentials are recorded via surface electrodes attached to standard sites and then maximized by computer for accurate measurement. Visual-evoked responses, produced by applying a flashing-light stimulus or a rapid series of visually identifiable shapes to the eye, help evaluate demyelinating disease, posttraumatic injury, and puzzling visual complaints. Brain stem auditory-evoked responses, produced by delivering clicks to the ear, help locate auditory lesions and evaluate brain stem integrity. Somatosensory-evoked responses, produced by electrically stimulating a peripheral sensory nerve, help diagnose peripheral nerve disease and locate lesions of the brain and spinal cord.

NUCLEAR MEDICINE TESTS
These tests, including the brain scan and the newer positron emission tomography scan (see *Viewing the brain's interior,* page 40), involve the injection of a radionuclide followed by externally tracing its dispersal through the brain. Areas of abnormal distribution reflect parenchymal or vascular disorders.

Brain scan
This test uses a gamma scintillation camera or rectilinear scanner to provide images of the brain after an I.V. injection of a radionuclide. The scintillation camera or scanner detects rays emitted by the radionuclide and converts them into images, which are then displayed on an oscilloscope screen. Normally, the radionuclide can't permeate the blood-brain barrier. However, if pathologic changes have destroyed the barrier, the radionuclide may concentrate in or around the abnormal area. Immediately after injection of the radionuclide, rapid-sequence images may be taken to evaluate cerebral blood flow. However, the images displayed on the oscilloscope screen are inferior by arteriographic standards.

Especially valuable when combined with CT findings, the scan is typically used to detect an intracranial mass or vascular lesion or to locate areas of ischemia, cerebral infarction, and intracerebral hemorrhage. It's also useful for evaluating the course of certain lesions postoperatively and during chemotherapy. A scan with negative results must be correlated with the patient's clinical picture to confirm or eliminate the need for further testing.

NURSING RESPONSIBILITIES
Even though doctors or technologists perform most neurodiagnostic tests, you're responsible for adequately preparing the patient beforehand and for performing post-test care. Preparation involves explaining the purpose and procedure of the test in words that the patient can readily understand. Tell him who will perform the test and where and how long it will take. Let the patient know what he should expect to see, hear, smell, taste, and feel during the test. For example, describe the formidable equipment in the angiographic suite and, if possible, show the patient a picture of it. If the test involves contrast enhancement, check the patient's history for hypersensitivity to shellfish, iodine, or other contrast media. Also maintain adequate hydration. Warn the patient that he may feel flushed and warm and may experience a transient headache, a salty taste, or nausea and vomiting after injection of the dye. Make sure the patient or responsible family member has signed a consent form, if necessary. Just before the test, obtain baseline neurologic status and vital signs for post-test patient monitoring.

After the test, watch for residual side effects from the contrast medium, and encourage fluids. Administer analgesics or antinauseants, as ordered. Watch for signs of complications, such as fever, excessive drainage, or altered level of consciousness, which may indicate meningitis or brain herniation following lumbar puncture. Also observe post-test instructions, especially proper positioning of the patient. For example, if iophendylate is used for myelography, keep the patient lying flat for 24 hours. (This contrast medium isn't water-soluble and must be aspirated after the procedure.) However, if metrizamide is used instead, keep the patient's head elevated 30° or more for at least 8 hours. (This contrast medium is water-soluble and, after it's absorbed into the bloodstream, is excreted by the kidneys. In the meantime, the head-elevated position prevents this contrast medium from irritating the cerebral cortex, causing focal or generalized seizures.)

Test results: Good news—or bad?
Whether the patient undergoes one test or many in his neurodiagnostic workup, you can expect abnormal test results to trigger intense emotion. A definitive diagnosis of a brain tumor or Huntington's chorea, for example, can be devastating. Your ability to provide emotional support and reassurance after the test can be a pivotal contribution and significantly influence the patient's response to his newly diagnosed disorder.

Points to remember

- Neurodiagnostics is a relatively young, fast-changing field that aims to perfect safe, effective methods for studying the nervous system.
- Neurodiagnostic testing is not a substitute for a careful, detailed history and physical examination.
- Even though doctors or specially trained technicians perform most neurodiagnostic tests, you're responsible for adequately preparing the patient beforehand and performing post-test care.

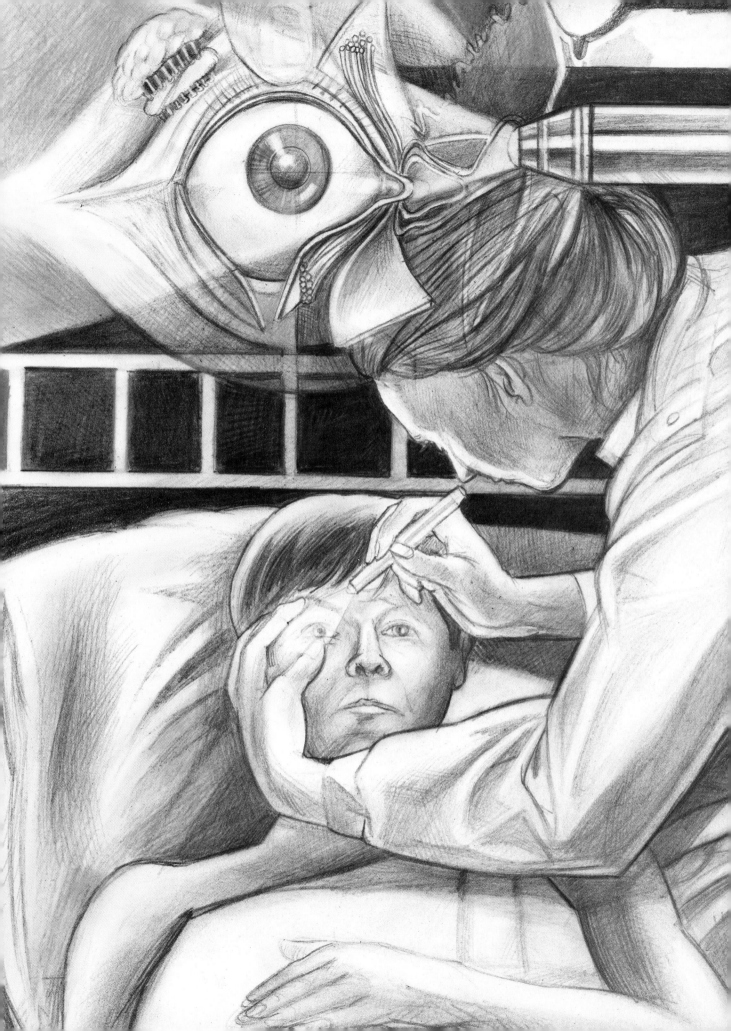

DISORDERS OF CONSCIOUSNESS

4 IMPROVING PROGNOSIS IN HEAD INJURY

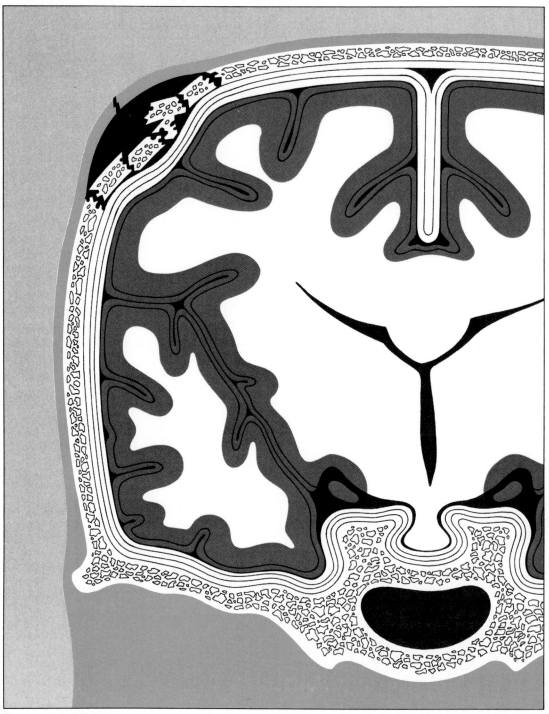

Depressed skull fracture

Considering the statistics, it's no surprise that head injury is the neurologic disorder you see most often. More than 7 million head injuries occur in the United States alone each year, ranging from minor concussions to life-threatening parenchymal damage. Severe head injuries account for the majority of trauma deaths; in fact, roughly 70% of patients with fatal head injury die within the first 48 hours.

What can you do about such disheartening statistics? Unfortunately, not much about primary brain injury. But you can do a great deal to upgrade first aid and acute care, which can minimize secondary brain injury. The most common cause of secondary brain injury is intracranial hypertension. It develops in about 50% of hospitalized patients with head injury and is perhaps the greatest obstacle to recovery. Your skill in recognizing and monitoring rising intracranial pressure can often make a life-saving difference and prevent devastating neurologic deficits. This chapter will help you master the nursing skills you need to manage head-injured patients with confidence.

Classifying head injury

Before discussing the pathophysiology of head injury, it's important to review its classification. Head injury can be broadly classified as open or closed. Open injury—a break in the scalp, skull, and dura—exposes the brain to environmental contaminants. Although closed head injury involves no such break in this protective barrier, it's typically more serious because of the risk of associated intracranial hypertension. Head injury may be further classified by the severity of damage.

Skull fractures are classified as linear, comminuted, or depressed. A linear fracture, a single clean break, accounts for approximately 70% of all skull fractures. A comminuted fracture splinters or crushes the skull into many bony fragments. A depressed skull fracture pushes these bony fragments toward the brain.

Skull fractures are also classified by location within the cranial vault. As its name implies, basilar fracture occurs at the base of the skull and usually involves the anterior and middle fossae. (See *Locating basilar fractures,* page 50.) It's typically more serious than fractures located elsewhere in the cranial vault since it carries significant risk of meningitis or associated parenchymal injury.

Parenchymal injury damages the brain tissue itself and includes concussion, contusion, and laceration. A concussion results from a blow to the head that jostles the brain, causing it to strike the skull. Although concussion results in temporary neural dysfunction, it causes no structural damage. A contusion results from a more severe blow, which bruises the brain and disrupts neural function. A laceration is the traumatic tearing of the cerebral cortex. It usually affects the brain's central areas adjacent to the floor of the anterior and middle fossae.

PATHOPHYSIOLOGY

One of the body's most fragile tissues, the brain depends on a constant supply of oxygen and glucose to function properly. Head injury can interfere with brain function by causing neuronal death—either by direct destruction of brain tissue (primary brain injury) or by interruption of oxygen and glucose delivery (secondary brain injury).

Primary brain injury includes any immediate neuronal death or temporary dysfunction caused by head injury. Because the central nervous system (CNS) has limited regenerative capacity, neuronal death is typically irreversible; so there's little, if anything, that can be done to correct primary brain injury.

Fortunately, this grim prognosis doesn't apply to secondary brain injury, which includes any neurologic damage that increases morbidity or mortality after the initial injury. Such damage usually results from intracranial hypertension, hypoxemia, hypercapnia, or hypotension.

Causes of primary brain injury

Primary brain injury results from physical stress within the brain tissue caused by penetrating or blunt trauma. Its signs and symptoms depend on the site of injury and the extent of neuronal dysfunction.

Penetrating trauma. Knife and gunshot wounds are the most common penetrating injuries. A knife wound creates a clean laceration surrounded by some hemorrhage and edema. A gunshot wound typically causes more extensive damage—resulting from shock waves that precede the bullet's path through the brain. Shock waves cause tissue damage directly or by compressing the brain against the skull, which may result in contusion. The most intense shock waves and the greatest tissue damage result from high-velocity gunshot wounds.

A characteristic profile

To identify potential victims of head injury and to promptly institute preventive measures, you'll have to become familiar with the typical head-injured patient—a profile described by Rimel. He's male, single, and under age 30. He's likely to be driving or riding in a motor vehicle that's exceeding the speed limit and, in about 80% of cases, he isn't wearing a seat belt. What's worse, he probably has positive blood alcohol levels and, in approximately 55% of cases, he's legally drunk. In many instances, he has a history of alcohol abuse and central nervous system trauma. With this grim demographic data in mind, don't hesitate to refer alcohol-abusing patients to a rehabilitation program and, if appropriate, to a safe-driving program. Also provide comprehensive discharge teaching to help prevent repeated hospitalizations for head injuries.

Locating basilar fractures

Basilar fractures usually occur in the anterior or middle fossa. Fractures in the middle fossa are most common and typically involve the petrous portion of the temporal bone, as shown. These fractures may be linear, comminuted, or depressed.

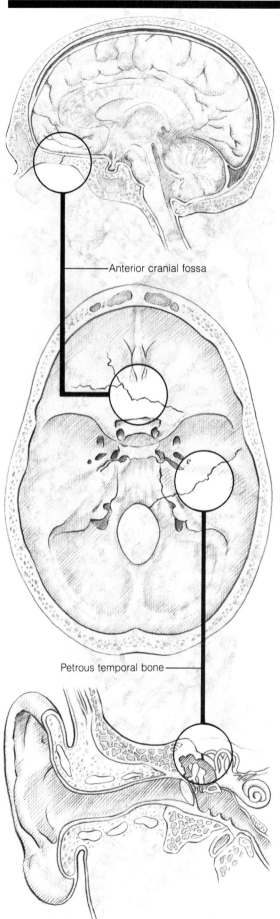

Anterior cranial fossa

Petrous temporal bone

Blunt trauma. Any severe blow to the head can produce injury on contact or by deceleration. Direct contact may result in local (or coup) injury at the impact site. Shock waves radiating from this site cause additional damage. Deceleration, the gross movement of the brain after impact, produces shearing and rotational forces that disrupt neuronal function. Deceleration may result in contrecoup injury, which affects areas of the brain on the side opposite the impact site.

Intracranial injuries resulting from blunt trauma include laceration, contusion, and diffuse axonal damage.

Causes of secondary brain injury

Secondary brain injury complicates a clinical picture that's often already grim. As you'll recall, it can result from intracranial hypertension, hypoxemia, hypercapnia, or systemic hypotension. Intracranial hypertension, however, is the leading cause of death in head-injured patients who reach the hospital alive.

Intracranial hypertension results from an increase in the volume of one or more intracranial components (brain tissue, blood, cerebrospinal fluid [CSF]) that exceeds the brain's compensatory capacity. Its severity depends on the size and rate of the volume increase, the total volume of the intracranial vault, and the relative volumes of other intracranial components available for displacement. Causes of intracranial hypertension include hemorrhage, edema, hyperemia, impaired autoregulation, and hydrocephalus. Understanding each of these causes helps promote early detection and guides treatment.

Hemorrhage. Caused by vascular damage from head injury, intracranial hemorrhage ranges from small intracerebral collections to large intra- or extracerebral clots. Its major types include epidural, subdural, and intracerebral hematomas (see *Effects of intracranial hematoma,* pages 52 and 53). These hematomas act like other space-occupying lesions, compressing surrounding cerebral structures and, at times, markedly raising intracranial pressure. Typically, edema surrounds the hematoma, contributing further to rising intracranial pressure.

A closer look at the major types of hematomas reveals their distinguishing characteristics. Epidural hematoma involves accumulation of blood between the dura mater and the inner table of the skull. It commonly results from laceration of the middle meningeal artery during skull fracture but occasionally results from venous laceration. Occurring in about 2% of head injuries, it affects children and adolescents more often than adults because the dura isn't yet firmly attached to the bony table.

Subdural hematoma, the accumulation of blood between the dura mater and the arachnoid, occurs in 10% to 15% of head injuries. It's classified as acute, subacute, and chronic. In acute hematoma, symptoms appear within 3 days of injury. In subacute hematoma, they appear 3 days to 3 weeks after injury. In chronic hematoma, they appear more than 3 weeks after injury and, in up to 50% of patients, there's no reported history of trauma.

Intracerebral hematoma, the accumulation of blood within the cerebrum itself, occurs in 2% to 3% of head injuries. This hematoma may be a single pocket of blood, resulting from contusion or laceration, or multiple pockets of blood, resulting from blunt trauma.

Edema. Like hemorrhage, cerebral edema increases brain tissue volume. It's classified as vasogenic or cytotoxic (see *Understanding cerebral edema,* page 54).

Vasogenic edema, the most common type, results when vascular damage disrupts the tight junctions between the capillary endothelial cells, increasing the permeability of the blood-brain barrier. Consequently, protein-rich plasma filtrate leaks into the extracellular space, triggering an influx of water into brain tissue. Typically, vasogenic edema surrounds contusions and hematomas.

Cytotoxic edema is the accumulation of fluid within the brain cells (neurons and glia) and the capillary endothelium. Frequently, it follows cellular ischemia, which alters cellular metabolism as well as cell membrane permeability.

Impaired autoregulation. Unlike edema and hemorrhage, which increase brain tissue volume, impaired autoregulation raises blood volume. Normally, autoregulation maintains constant cerebral blood flow, despite variations in systemic blood pressure, by dilatation or constriction of the cerebral arteries. Loss of autoregulation may follow local or diffuse vascular damage. Cerebral blood flow then fluctuates with systemic blood pressure. As a result, systemic hypertension can increase cerebral blood flow and thus increase intracranial pressure.

Hyperemia. One of the more common causes of intracranial hypertension in children with head injury, hyperemia also increases cerebral blood flow. For reasons still unclear,

it develops less frequently in adults.

Hydrocephalus. This abnormal increase in CSF volume may also cause intracranial hypertension. It results from obstruction or impaired reabsorption of CSF.

Other factors in secondary injury

Like intracranial hypertension, hypoxemia, hypercapnia, and systemic hypotension may also contribute to secondary brain injury. These factors may occur alone or in conjunction with intracranial hypertension.

Hypoxemia. A common finding in head injury, hypoxemia may result from primary brain injury or from associated multiple trauma. However, the patient may maintain a normal breathing pattern and show minimal signs of respiratory distress.

Severe hypoxemia—a PO_2 less than 50 mm Hg—triggers cerebral vasodilatation, which increases cerebral blood flow. Moderate hypoxemia may worsen the effect of existing brain tissue ischemia and increase neuronal death. Ischemia slows or interrupts oxygen and glucose delivery to the brain cells, altering cellular metabolism and cell membrane permeability. As a result, sodium and water accumulate within the brain cells, causing cytotoxic edema.

Hypercapnia. Like hypoxemia, hypercapnia causes marked cerebral vasodilatation. It may result from impaired cerebral metabolism due to poor perfusion or from impaired respiration due to brain stem injury or associated multiple trauma.

Systemic hypotension. Hypotension often accompanies trauma due to hemorrhage or shock. But when head injury impairs autoregulation, hypotension is especially significant, because systemic blood pressure directly influences cerebral perfusion. Normally, cerebral perfusion pressure (CPP) is 80 to 90 mm Hg, determined by the equation: mean systemic arterial pressure (MSAP) − intracranial pressure (ICP) = CPP. When it falls below 50 mm Hg, brain tissue becomes ischemic. As you'll recall, ischemia may trigger or enhance cytotoxic edema, which contributes to intracranial hypertension.

An inside look at intracranial hypertension

Briefly consider what happens within the skull as intracranial hypertension develops. An excessive or unrelenting increase in intracranial volume soon exhausts the brain's compensatory reserve, and intracranial pressure

Effects of intracranial hematoma

Intracranial hematoma, a potentially life-threatening complication of head injury, is the accumulation of blood within the epidural or subdural space or the cerebrum itself. By compressing adjacent brain tissue, such hematomas increase intracranial pressure and cause shift of midline structures.

Epidural hematoma

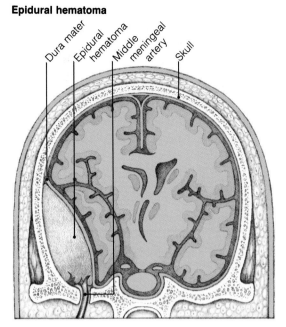

Subdural hematoma

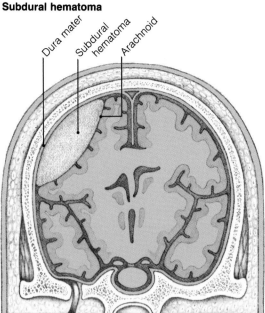

rises. Increased intracranial pressure impairs cerebral blood flow, which causes critical tissue hypoxia and upsets cell metabolism. As a result, lactate accumulates in the tissues and CSF. Decreased cerebral blood flow and increased intracranial pressure activate the CNS ischemic response, which raises systemic blood pressure in an effort to bolster cerebral blood flow. However, blood can flow through the brain only if arterial pressure exceeds intracranial pressure. Increased cerebral blood flow further increases intracranial pressure, triggering a vasomotor response, and the cycle repeats itself. Without emergency cerebral decompression, steadily increasing intracranial pressure may force the swollen brain through the tentorial notch. This often life-threatening herniation of brain tissue compresses the brain stem, affecting the vital centers and cranial nerves located there. Uncal herniation—displacement of the medial aspect of the temporal lobe (the uncus)—is most commonly seen in head injury. (See *Herniation: Shifting of brain tissue under pressure,* page 55.) But the effect of a relentless increase in intracranial pressure on cerebral blood flow is more devastating. Eventually, arterial pressure no longer exceeds intracranial pressure, and cerebral blood flow ceases.

MEDICAL MANAGEMENT
After head injury, medical management involves emergency treatment to stabilize the patient's vital signs, neurologic examination and diagnostic tests to determine the type and severity of head injury, and treatment to

promote optimal neurologic recovery. Typically, emergency care and neurologic examination occur simultaneously, but the ABCs of emergency care take top priority.

A for airway
Ensuring airway patency is the immediate priority after head injury; however, remember that about 20% of all head-injured patients also have cervical spine injury, so avoid hyperextension of the neck until X-rays rule out this possibility. Use the jaw thrust to open the patient's airway and intubation to maintain airway patency. Insert the endotracheal tube through the mouth, not the nose, if you suspect basilar skull fracture.

B for breathing
After establishing airway patency, evaluate respiratory rate, depth, and rhythm. If spontaneous respiration is inadequate, as is often the case in severe head injury, begin mechanical ventilation immediately to avoid hypoxemia and hypercapnia, which may trigger cerebral vasodilatation and increased intracranial pressure. Carefully regulate the fraction of inspired oxygen (FIO_2) to maintain the PaO_2 between 80 and 100 mm Hg. Later, positive end-expiratory pressure (PEEP) may be instituted if an FIO_2 of 60% or less fails to maintain adequate PaO_2. Recognize that PEEP raises central venous pressure, which, in turn, may raise intracranial pressure; so elevate the head of the bed to enhance jugular venous drainage when using PEEP. Hyperventilate the patient to achieve a $PaCO_2$ of 25 to 30 mm

Intracerebral hematoma

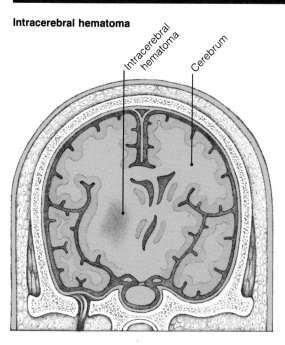

Intracerebral hematoma

Cerebrum

Hg, which will trigger vasoconstriction. This most valuable, fast-acting treatment for intracranial hypertension reduces intracranial pressure by reducing cerebral blood flow. However, since damaged vessels don't consistently constrict in response to decreasing $PaCO_2$, blood flow to these damaged areas may actually improve. Failure of hyperventilation to affect intracranial pressure implies widespread vascular damage and carries a poor prognosis.

C for circulation—and for cervical spine
Hemodynamic stability ensures delivery of oxygen and nutrients to the brain and other tissues. In the head-injured patient, hemodynamic stability refers to a constant blood pressure sustaining a cerebral perfusion pressure of more than 50 mm Hg. Measures taken to achieve this stability include the use of volume infusion, medical antishock trousers (a MAST suit), and vasopressors.

Although strict fluid restriction was once advocated to prevent fluid overload and a subsequent rise in intracranial pressure, current therapy involves only mild dehydration—achieving serum osmolality of 310 mOsm or lower. Mild dehydration maintains adequate vascular volume, an indispensable factor for maintaining adequate cerebral perfusion pressure. However, fluid replacement is crucial when hemorrhage from other injuries complicates head injury. Without such replacement, hypotension compromises cerebral perfusion, causing further brain tissue damage due to ischemia. Treatment involves blood transfusion and administration of colloid and crystalloid solutions. However, avoid using dextrose 5% in water because it lacks electrolytes and promotes fluid accumulation in the brain, causing edema. Check the patient's urine output hourly to evaluate renal perfusion, which is a good indicator of the adequacy of volume replacement.

In the ABCs of emergency assessment, "C" also stands for cervical spine—a critical consideration since approximately 20% of all head-injured patients also have cervical spine injury. Until X-rays rule out such injury, maintain neutral alignment and spinal stability to prevent further neurologic damage.

Evaluating head injury
Rapid neurologic examination of the patient on admission provides the first clues to the type and severity of head injury. It identifies focal neurologic deficits and establishes a baseline for subsequent neurologic checks.

The Glasgow coma scale (GCS), which grades level of consciousness in relation to eye opening and motor and verbal responses, is a useful tool for evaluating the severity of head injury and predicting its outcome. A GCS score of 14 to 15 indicates minor head injury; a score of 9 to 13, moderate head injury; and a score of less than 8, severe head injury. Mortality typically increases with lower GCS scores, reaching 30% to 50% with scores of less than 8. The International Data Bank for Head Injury uses both the GCS score and the Glasgow outcome category (see *Glasgow outcome categories*) to characterize the neurologic deficits caused by head injury. Typically, gross deficits accompany severe head injury, while subtle, sometimes puzzling deficits accompany minor head injury. Even slight structural injury can cause distressing residual lapses in concentration, memory, and judgment.

Diagnostic tests, particularly computerized tomography (CT) scan and intracranial pressure monitoring, also furnish valuable information. The CT scan has largely replaced skull X-rays and arteriography for evaluating head injury. This sensitive, noninvasive test can quickly identify skull fractures, focal lesions like epidural or subdural hematomas, foreign bodies, and even cerebral edema.

During the CT scan, the size and location of the ventricles often guide interpretation of results. For example, shifting of the ventricles from midline indicates a unilateral focal lesion or unilateral edema. Decreased ventric-

Glasgow outcome categories
Use the following categories to help describe the outcome of head injury:

Good outcome
Patient regains independence with minimal, if any, cognitive deficit and returns to full-time employment at his previous or a comparable job.

Moderate disability
Patient regains independence but fails to return to full-time employment at his previous or a comparable job.

Severe disability
Patient depends on others for some aspects of daily living.

Vegetative state
Patient exhibits no obvious cortical function.

Death

Understanding cerebral edema

Cerebral edema—the accumulation of fluid within the brain after head injury—takes one of two forms: vasogenic or cytotoxic. Vasogenic edema results from leakage of plasma filtrate into extracellular spaces. Cytotoxic edema involves swelling of brain cells with extracellular fluid.

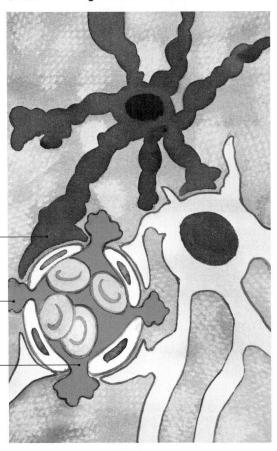

Astrocyte foot

Leakage of plasma filtrate

Opened tight junctions between capillary endothelial cells

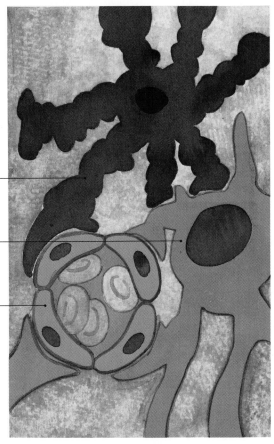

Edematous astrocyte

Edematous neuron

Edematous capillary endothelial cell

ular size—the result of CSF shunting from the ventricles to the spinal subarachnoid space during compensation—points to generalized edema.

Intracranial pressure monitoring helps detect intracranial hypertension. In fact, it allows early detection of critically high pressures before the onset of telltale clinical signs. Consequently, it helps ensure prompt intervention and may significantly reduce mortality.

Two electrodiagnostic tests—EEG and brain stem auditory evoked response (BAER)—occasionally prove useful in head injury. The EEG may help confirm brain death or document posttraumatic epilepsy. Although diagnosis of brain death varies from state to state, an isoelectric EEG tracing is a widely used criterion (see *Defining brain death,* page 56). In posttraumatic epilepsy, a common sequela of head injury, the EEG can identify the epileptogenic foci triggering seizure activity.

The BAER—the recording of electrical potentials triggered by an auditory click delivered to the ear—can detect and evaluate primary or secondary brain stem injury. In secondary brain stem injury, which results from increased supratentorial pressure, BAER typically returns to normal before clinical signs improve. Consequently, serial BAER may help determine prognosis.

Restoring neurologic function

Although treatment varies with the type of head injury, the goal remains the same: to promote optimal neurologic recovery. Considering the complexity of the nervous system and its intimate ties with other body systems, this is no easy goal. Treatment must address the head injury itself as well as aim to control intracranial pressure and prevent complications. First, let's see how specific head injuries are commonly treated.

Scalp lacerations. Treatment involves careful cleansing and debridement of the laceration, followed by suturing, if necessary.

Concussion and contusion. Although there's no specific treatment for concussion, close observation is necessary for 24 hours to detect altered neurologic status. Contusion, however, requires comprehensive supportive care and frequent assessment for changes in neurologic status.

Skull fractures. Linear fracture typically heals without specific treatment, although mild analgesics help relieve headache. If linear fracture extends into the sinuses or middle ear, as often occurs in basilar skull fractures, antibiotic therapy may be given to prevent CNS infection. Note that CSF leaks associated with basilar skull fractures usually seal spontaneously. However, persistent drainage or recurrent meningitis may indicate the need for surgical repair.

Although treatment of comminuted fracture varies with its severity, depressed fracture typically requires surgical removal or elevation of splintered bone and repair of dural and venous sinus tears. Cranioplasty to repair the resulting cranial defect may be delayed for about 6 months to allow postoperative swelling to subside.

Hematomas. Acute epidural hematoma requires prompt aspiration through a craniotomy to prevent fatal complications. Acute subdural hematoma usually requires the same surgical approach. However, surgical removal of subacute or chronic subdural hematoma and of intracerebral hematoma depends on the patient's neurologic status. If his status is stable or improving, surgery may be delayed. But if it's deteriorating and the hematoma is amenable to surgery, immediate removal is indicated.

Controlling intracranial hypertension
Intracranial hypertension occurs in roughly 50% of all hospitalized patients with severe head injury. You need to know how to treat it or—better yet—prevent it. (See *Managing intracranial hypertension*, page 57, for the most common interventions.)

Besides intracranial hypertension, the head-injured patient is susceptible to many other complications. Potentially, neurologic trauma can affect all body systems—from the most basic body functions to highly complex thought processes. Consequently, supportive care of the patient is often extensive, its success hinging on the combined efforts of the entire health-care team.

NURSING MANAGEMENT
Nursing management begins with a skillfully taken patient history and a thorough physical examination to establish how head injury occurred and to determine its severity.

Reconstruct the scene of injury
Begin the patient history by collecting details about the head injury. If the patient is groggy or unconscious when you first see him, question the paramedics or those who witnessed the injury. Obtain the following information:
• Determine the type of accident. Was the

Herniation: Shifting of brain tissue under pressure

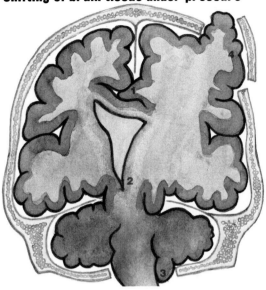

Brain herniation—the life-threatening displacement of brain tissue—may result from an unrelenting increase in intracranial pressure. In cingulate, or falx, herniation (1), the cingulate gyrus and hemisphere force beneath the falx to the opposite side. In uncal, or transtentorial, herniation (2), the medial aspect of the temporal lobe (the uncus) squeezes through the tentorium, causing midbrain compression. In cerebellar, or tonsillar, herniation (3), the cerebellar tonsils squeeze through the foramen magnum, causing cervicomedullar compression. In postoperative, or traumatic, herniation (4), brain tissue escapes through a craniotomy site or traumatic break in the skull.

patient in a motor vehicle accident? Was he wearing a seat belt? If not, was he thrown from the car or through the windshield?
• Establish the elapsed time between the accident and institution of life-support measures, either at the scene or in the hospital.
• Determine the patient's neurologic status at the accident scene. Did he briefly lose consciousness and then experience a lucid period? Were any focal neurologic findings present? Also determine the patient's general physical condition after the accident. Did he ever stop breathing? Was he hypotensive? Hypotension may cause inadequate CPP, depleting the brain's supply of oxygen and nutrients.
• On admission, ask the alert patient if he can remember the accident. Also determine if he's under the influence of alcohol or other drugs that could cloud neurologic findings. Draw blood for an alcohol screen or obtain a urine specimen for a drug screen, if indicated.

Complete the patient history
After the patient receives emergency treatment, complete the history:

Defining brain death

Doctors, lawyers, and legislators have yet to agree on a national definition of brain death. As a result, many states have adopted statutory law definitions of brain death while others have left such definitions to local authorities or individual hospitals. Despite the absence of a uniform definition of brain death, the following criteria are generally accepted as evidence of brain death.

• *Presence of irreversible coma of established cause.* Coma resulting from drug overdose or profound hypothermia must be ruled out.

• *Absence of cerebral function.* Assessment reveals lack of spontaneous movement and no verbal or motor response to any stimulus. Occasionally, spinal reflexes remain intact. A flat (isoelectric) EEG or cessation of cerebral blood flow also provides confirming evidence.

• *Absence of brain stem function.* Assessment reveals no pupillary reaction to light; no corneal, oculocephalic, oculovestibular, oropharyngeal, or tracheal reflexes; no decerebrate or decorticate response to noxious stimuli; and no spontaneous respirations.

These criteria must be met during two or more examinations performed 24 hours apart.

Compassion for the living
Besides aiding in the diagnosis of brain death, your nursing role includes much more. Of course, you'll need to provide emotional support for the patient's family. Brain death may be difficult for them to grasp when they see the patient breathing with ventilator assistance and his heartbeat displayed on a monitor. Your human touch and kind explanations can provide much-needed comfort.

Also, if the patient is a potential organ donor, strictly adhere to your institution's donor protocol to help assure successful transplantation.

• Explore the patient's medical history. Look for factors that may have lead to the possible cause of the accident, such as transient ischemic attack or myocardial infarction. And, although unrelated to the head injury, current health problems can significantly influence recovery. For example, the patient with a respiratory infection stands a greater chance of developing pulmonary compromise because of prolonged immobility after head injury. Modify your care plan to take such health problems into account.

• Ask the patient if he's taking any prescription or over-the-counter drugs. Note drug names and dosages.

• Find out if the patient is allergic to any drugs or foods, pets, dust, or pollen. Has he ever been treated for an allergy?

• Ask the patient if he smokes. If he does, obtain a history in pack-years. Also ask about the patient's drinking habits.

• Determine the patient's dominant hand. Later, when you're evaluating his neurologic status, expect grip strength to be slightly stronger in the dominant hand.

• Explore the patient's current life-style. Where does he live and with whom? Does he have any pets? What are his hobbies or favorite pastimes? What are his plans and aspirations for the future?

• Evaluate the patient's emotional response to the injury. Find out how he's coped with stress in the past.

• Assess the patient's family. How many members are there? What are their roles? How does the patient relate to individual family members? Find out how well the family understands the patient's injury. Are they familiar with the hospital setting? Determine the impact of the patient's injury on their lives. For example, is a family member missing work to care for small children? How has the family coped with stress in the past? Explore existing social supports, such as friends, relatives, and religious counselors. While gathering the history, maintain a warm, personal approach. Remember, the goal is to get to know the person who happens to have a head injury, not to plan care for an anonymous head-injured patient whose name happens to be John.

Perform the physical examination next
Begin this part of the nursing assessment with a comprehensive neurologic examination. Use this data later as a baseline for neurologic checks at bedside. The frequency of neurologic checks will vary with the patient's condition. Generally, they should be performed at least every 4 hours, and perhaps hourly, for the first 72 hours.

Neurologic findings vary with the type of injury, its location and severity, and the degree of associated intracranial hypertension. Although a characteristic clinical description exists for concussion, contusion, and other common head injuries, the patient will probably demonstrate some, but not all, of the symptoms (see *Signs and symptoms of common head injuries,* pages 58 and 59). Because the brain regulates the function of many other body systems, you should also perform periodic head-to-toe examinations to supplement neurologic checks. Such examinations may uncover evidence of hypoxemia and hypotension, physiologic changes that adversely affect brain function.

Watch for intracranial hypertension
Because intracranial hypertension can be disastrous for the head-injured patient, be constantly alert for its signs and symptoms during the physical examination.

 Check for decreased level of consciousness, the most sensitive sign of increased intracranial pressure. Always notify the doctor of any change in the patient's level of consciousness. Clearly document other possible causes for such a change—for example, sedation, hypoxemia, hypoglycemia, or hyponatremia.

 Expect changes in motor function when increased intracranial pressure causes compression of the cerebral peduncles. Typically, motor changes are contralateral to the lesion. The patient initially responds by purposeful withdrawal, then decorticate posturing, and ultimately, decerebrate posturing.

 Evaluate pupillary size, equality, and response to light. Also check for deviation from the midline. Pupillary changes are an ominous, but late, sign of intracranial hypertension, indicating uncal herniation through the tentorium. The resulting pressure on the third cranial nerve initially causes the ipsilateral pupil to enlarge and react poorly to light, then, eventually, to become fixed and dilated.

 Monitor vital signs. Increasing pulse pressure, a reliable but late sign of intracranial hypertension, occurs when intracranial pressure equals diastolic blood pressure. The resulting cerebral ischemia triggers increased systolic pressure, which, in turn, increases pulse pressure. Although bradycardia typically accompanies intracranial hypertension, alternating tachycardia and bradycardia is also possible.

 Watch for abnormal respiratory patterns. Brain stem compression may also influence respiratory patterns (see *Abnormal respiratory patterns,* page 61). Recognize that the patient is often intubated before these patterns develop fully. Monitor respiratory rate, depth, and rhythm during each neurologic check,

Managing intracranial hypertension

Treatment	Purpose
Mechanical ventilation	• To maintain PaO_2 between 80 and 100 mm Hg and to avoid cerebral vasodilatation • To maintain $PaCO_2$ between 25 and 30 mm Hg and to promote cerebral vasoconstriction
Patient positioning	• To improve venous drainage from the brain
Fluid management	• To achieve mild dehydration while maintaining adequate vascular volume and cardiac output
Antihyperthermia measures (cooling blankets or rectal acetaminophen)	• To reduce fever and prevent increased cerebral blood flow due to higher metabolic demands
Vasopressors	• To regulate systemic arterial pressure and to maintain cerebral perfusion pressure at 50 mm Hg or greater
Paralytics and narcotics	• To prevent spontaneous decorticate and decerebrate posturing, which increases systemic arterial pressure • To avoid agitation or stress, which increases systemic arterial pressure
Anticonvulsants	• To prevent seizures, which increase cerebral metabolism and blood flow
Hyperosmotics	• To reduce cerebral edema by drawing water out of brain tissue • To improve cerebral blood flow by decreasing intracranial pressure (restricted in children for 24 hours after head injury since about 50% have diffuse edema from hyperemia)
Corticosteroids	• To possibly reduce intracranial pressure by decreasing capillary permeability or inhibiting CSF production (role is unclear) • To possibly minimize cellular death by stabilizing lysosomal membranes
Barbiturates	• To reduce intracranial pressure of more than 20 mm Hg when conventional measures fail • To decrease cerebral metabolism and blood flow
Loop diuretics	• To decrease cerebral edema • To possibly inhibit CSF production
Antibiotics	• To prevent infection in patients with open fractures or CSF leaks or in those undergoing surgery

Signs and symptoms of common head injuries

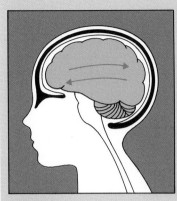

Concussion
Headache
Retrograde amnesia
Transient loss of consciousness
Nausea
Dizziness
Irritability
Lethargy

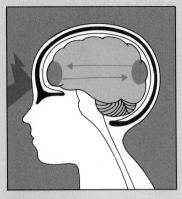

Contusion
Loss of consciousness
Speech disturbance, such as
  temporary aphasia
Sensory or motor disturbance, such
  as slight hemiparesis or unilateral
  numbness

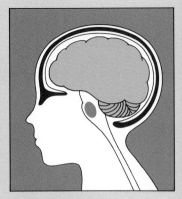

Brain stem contusion
Coma
Cranial nerve dysfunction
Impaired oculocephalic/
  oculovestibular reflexes
Respiratory and cardiovascular
  instability

and note the muscles used for respiration. Other signs and symptoms of intracranial hypertension include hyperthermia, papilledema, headache, and vomiting. Hyperthermia, a relatively late sign of intracranial hypertension, results from increased pressure on the hypothalamus. However, because hyperthermia also accompanies infection, it's a nonspecific sign. Although papilledema is a reliable sign, it typically occurs several days after the onset of intracranial hypertension. Headache is a variable symptom and, although frequently linked with intracranial hypertension, vomiting isn't a reliable sign.

Shape data into nursing diagnoses
Once you've completed the physical examination, you're ready to shape the collected data into nursing diagnoses—the building blocks of your care plan. The following nursing diagnoses are commonly seen in the head-injured patient.

Potential for intracranial hypertension. Factors associated with intracranial hypertension are many and varied, making prevention of this complication a formidable task. For example, routine care procedures like suctioning, positioning, and clustering care procedures can increase intracranial pressure; so can emotional upset. Suctioning can increase in-

tracranial pressure by causing hypoxemia or hypercapnia, or by inducing coughing. Positioning can increase intracranial pressure by impairing jugular venous outflow, which increases the total volume within the cranial vault. Fortunately, modifying patient care can do much toward preventing increased intracranial pressure. To prevent hypoxemia and hypercapnia during suctioning, hyperventilate the patient's lungs for a full minute with an Ambu bag before and after suctioning. Also limit suctioning to 10 seconds. Lightly sedate the patient before suctioning, if ordered, to prevent undue coughing.

To enhance venous outflow during positioning, elevate the head of the patient's bed 15° to 30°. Also maintain head and neck alignment to prevent occlusion of the jugular vein. To maintain alignment, avoid placing large, fluffy pillows under the patient's head. When he's supine, place towel rolls on either side of the patient's head or make a support using a 2-ft² piece of foam mattress. Cut a space in the mattress to frame the back of the patient's head, then place the cut mattress on the bed around his head. The mattress will be firm enough to maintain alignment, yet soft enough to avoid skin irritation. When repositioning the patient, use a turning sheet and logroll him.

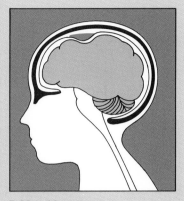

Epidural hematoma
Brief loss of consciousness followed
    by lucid interval (30% to 40% of
    patients)
Increasingly severe headache
Rapidly deteriorating level of
    consciousness
Vomiting
Possible seizures
Ipsilateral pupillary dilation
Contralateral hemiparesis

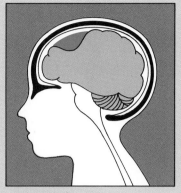

Subdural hematoma
Altered level of consciousness
Headache
Focal neurologic deficits
Personality changes
Ipsilateral pupillary dilation
    progressing to fixation

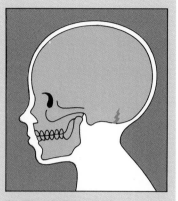

Basilar skull fracture
Cerebrospinal rhinorrhea and
    otorrhea associated with dural
    laceration
Periorbital ecchymosis (Raccoon's
    eyes)
Mastoidal ecchymosis (Battle's
    sign)

To prevent emotional distress, remember that the comatose patient may react to external stimuli, such as conversations or touch, even though he appears unresponsive. So follow this rule of thumb: Never say anything in the presence of the comatose patient that you wouldn't say if he were alert and well-oriented. Continue to explain care procedures to the patient, talking *to him* instead of *over him*. Also use touch to convey warmth and concern.

Avoid clustering care procedures, which can increase intracranial pressure by producing a cumulative stimulant effect.

When head injury causes loss of autoregulation, measures to prevent systemic hypertension can also keep the patient's intracranial pressure within normal limits. Recognize factors that increase systemic blood pressure, including sudden loud noise, isometric muscular contraction, and Valsalva's maneuver.

Unfortunately, intracranial hypertension may develop despite your best efforts to prevent it. If it does, your responsibilities will likely include administering drugs, assisting in diagnostic procedures, or, perhaps, preparing the patient for surgery. When administering mannitol, an osmotic diuretic that's frequently used in such patients, monitor serum osmolality closely; an increase to more than 310

mOsm may disrupt the blood-brain barrier. Also monitor fluid and electrolyte balance, and watch especially for hypokalemia and hypo- or hypernatremia. Use an in-line filter when giving mannitol by I.V. drip, and store this drug in a warm place to prevent crystallization. If the doctor orders high-dose barbiturates, anticipate the need for artificial ventilation and cardiac and hemodynamic monitoring. Consider your nursing goal met if the patient shows no signs or symptoms of intracranial hypertension. If the patient's intracranial pressure is being monitored, watch for an intracranial pressure of less than 15 mm Hg at rest that doesn't exceed 20 mm Hg for more than 15 minutes during care procedures.

Potential for impaired gas exchange. The head-injured patient is at risk for impaired gas exchange for several reasons. The primary reason is ineffective secretion clearance due to decreased level of consciousness or immobility. Mild dehydration may also impair ventilation by making secretions thick and more viscous. Ineffective breathing patterns due to primary or secondary brain stem injury can also impair gas exchange.

Your nursing goal is to maintain optimal oxygenation and ventilation because impaired gas exchange can cause cerebral ischemia and increase intracranial pressure. If the patient has difficulty clearing secretions, determine why. Is his cough ineffective? Are his secretions thick and viscous? Monitor intake and output closely for signs of dehydration. If necessary, instill sterile saline solution to help liquefy secretions. To stimulate coughing in the alert, cooperative patient, encourage deep breathing or the use of incentive spirometry. In the patient with decreased level of consciousness, tracheal suctioning may be necessary to remove secretions.

Perform chest physiotherapy to help prevent or treat pulmonary congestion. You'll have to modify this procedure slightly for the head-injured patient. As a general rule, avoid placing the patient in Trendelenburg's position, which impairs venous outflow and can trigger intracranial hypertension. In fact, even a flat position may impair venous outflow. Consider each patient's sensitivity to position changes before beginning chest physiotherapy. Sedate the patient, if ordered, to avoid undue stress. Remember to observe proper suctioning technique to prevent hypoxemia and hypercapnia.

Consider your nursing interventions effective if the patient:
• has normal breath sounds with a clear chest X-ray
• shows no sign of pulmonary infection
• maintains a PaO_2 between 80 and 100 mm Hg and a $PaCO_2$ between 25 and 30 mm Hg.

Potential for injury related to seizures or severe agitation. When planning nursing interventions to prevent such injury, recognize that all head-injured patients are considered at risk for seizures. Seizures can produce injury by triggering uncontrolled, violent muscular activity or by increasing cerebral metabolism. Increased cerebral metabolism increases cerebral blood flow, expanding the volume of an already critically full cranial vault.

To protect the patient from injury related to seizures, institute seizure precautions and administer drugs, as ordered. Phenytoin, the antiepileptic most commonly used after head injury, is less likely to mask neurologic findings than depressant drugs, such as phenobarbital, which may alter the sensorium.

Eliminate or minimize environmental or physiologic stimuli that may provoke seizures. Such stimuli may include loud noises, hypoxemia, hypoglycemia, CNS infection, and uncontrolled withdrawal from alcohol or drugs.

Severe agitation also increases the potential for injury. As the head-injured patient awak-ens from coma, he's typically confused and goes through a period of severe agitation. Agitation raises blood pressure, which can raise intracranial pressure.

To protect the patient from injury related to agitation, keep the bed in a low position with padded side rails up. Because restraints may increase agitation, avoid using them if possible. Orient the patient by explaining where he is and how you're trying to help him. Attempt to minimize noxious environmental stimuli. Provide carefully selected stimuli, guided by the patient's interests or personality. A tennis match on TV may satisfy one patient, while a Bach cantata on the radio may satisfy another. Always approach the patient in a calm, quiet manner; avoid unexpected or rapid movement toward him. Speak to the patient in a gentle, soothing tone and keep your directions short and simple. Help the patient's family cope with his agitation by suggesting that they also maintain a calm, soothing attitude. Assure them that the patient's irrational behavior stems from neurologic injury and isn't purposeful.

Consider your nursing interventions effective if the patient:
• avoids physical injury
• experiences no seizure activity.

Potential for alteration in nutrition. The head-injured patient is at risk for impaired nutrition due to decreased level of consciousness, dysphagia, or prolonged tracheostomy with mechanical ventilation. Maintaining adequate nutrition first requires consultation with the hospital dietitian to determine the patient's needed daily caloric intake. Then, unless the patient has abdominal injuries, use the enteral route—by tube or by mouth—for feeding. Tube feeding is best for patients at risk for aspiration, such as those with decreased level of consciousness or prolonged intubation. To decrease the risk of aspiration during tube feeding:
• check residuals every 2 to 4 hours. Discontinue tube feeding if it's not being absorbed properly.
• elevate the head of the bed 45° during, and for 30 minutes after, feeding.
• avoid scheduling chest physiotherapy within an hour of feeding.

Feeding the dysphagic patient by mouth is a challenge requiring patience and skill. For best results, conduct the feeding in an unhurried manner. Offer the patient pureed or soft foods, like custard or gelatin, which are easier to swallow than liquids.

Abnormal respiratory patterns

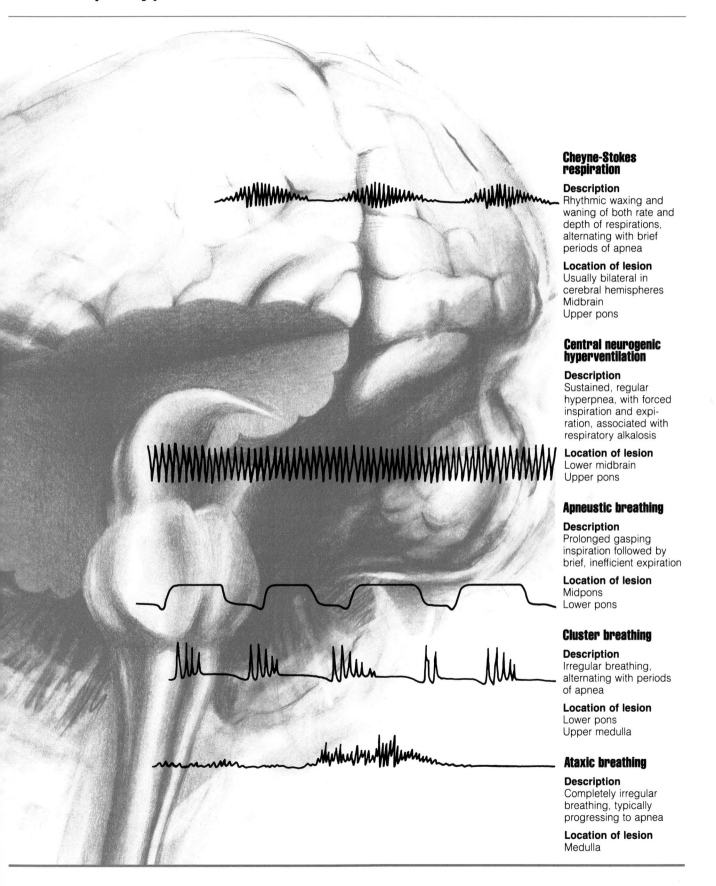

Cheyne-Stokes respiration

Description
Rhythmic waxing and waning of both rate and depth of respirations, alternating with brief periods of apnea

Location of lesion
Usually bilateral in cerebral hemispheres
Midbrain
Upper pons

Central neurogenic hyperventilation

Description
Sustained, regular hyperpnea, with forced inspiration and expiration, associated with respiratory alkalosis

Location of lesion
Lower midbrain
Upper pons

Apneustic breathing

Description
Prolonged gasping inspiration followed by brief, inefficient expiration

Location of lesion
Midpons
Lower pons

Cluster breathing

Description
Irregular breathing, alternating with periods of apnea

Location of lesion
Lower pons
Upper medulla

Ataxic breathing

Description
Completely irregular breathing, typically progressing to apnea

Location of lesion
Medulla

Preventing CNS infection

Because central nervous system (CNS) infection can increase morbidity and mortality, its prevention ranks high among your nursing goals for the head-injured patient. Prevention begins with recognizing major routes of CNS infection.

Open head injury breaks the barrier of the scalp, skull, and dura, exposing the brain to environmental contaminants. And if this injury is also penetrating, as in a stab or bullet wound, nonsterile debris—skin, hair, bony fragments—enter the brain itself. A cerebrospinal fluid (CSF) leak resulting from a dural tear provides a less noticeable route for bacterial invasion through the nasopharynx or middle ear. Monitoring or drainage devices and surgery also violate the brain's protective layers and may introduce infection.

Preventive measures
To help prevent CNS infection, maintain sterile technique when changing dressings or caring for monitoring or drainage systems. If the patient has a CSF leak, place him in the semi-Fowler position. Avoid obstructing the flow of drainage and packing the nostrils or ear canal to absorb fluid. Instruct the patient to wipe his nose, not to blow it. And refrain from inserting tubes or suction catheters through the nose. Administer antibiotics, as ordered, and observe good handwashing technique at all times.

Signs of success
Consider your nursing interventions successful if the patient:
• maintains normal temperature
• has clear, odorless CSF
• demonstrates a normal white blood cell count/differential
• shows no evidence of nuchal rigidity
• heals properly at incisions and drainage sites.

Recognize that enteral feeding requires proper bowel function. Monitor bowel function closely and administer a stool softener or daily suppository, as necessary.

Consider your nursing interventions effective if the patient:
• maintains body weight within 10% of admission weight
• has normal serum albumin levels, indicating adequate protein intake
• meets required daily caloric intake.

Potential for impaired skin integrity. Immobility, persistent spontaneous posturing, spasticity, and inadequate nutrition are among the factors that contribute to skin breakdown in the head-injured patient. To maintain skin integrity, perform skin assessment at each shift change and with each position change. Place a foam mattress or alternating pressure pad on the patient's bed to reduce pressure on the skin. Use special devices, such as a Roto Rest bed or Clinitron therapy unit, if appropriate. Because these beds allow only limited elevation of the head, they may be unsuitable in early injury when the risk of intracranial hypertension is greatest. Turn the patient every 2 hours and massage bony prominences to promote circulation. Place the patient in the prone position only after the risk of intracranial hypertension subsides. Pad adjacent bony parts and apply heel and elbow protectors. When spasticity or spontaneous posturing is a problem, place sheepskin or a gel pad under the heels instead; otherwise, contact between the heel protectors and the sole of the foot may stimulate posturing or spasticity. Administer antispasmodics or sedatives, as ordered, to control abnormal movement. Also monitor the patient's nutritional status.

Consider your nursing interventions effective if the patient shows no signs of skin breakdown.

Potential for ineffective family coping. Head injury is typically a crisis situation, abruptly confronting the patient's family with unexpected, often devastating life-style changes. Just as you strive to restore optimal function in the head-injured patient, so you must support his family through their crisis. When planning interventions to achieve this goal, carefully assess the family. How do the members relate to one another? What are their individual roles and responsibilities? If possible, work consistently with them, either by yourself or with the same group of nurses, to develop a trusting relationship. Recognize the most common needs of a family in their predicament. First, they need to know what's going on. Offer kind and clear explanations. Next, they need to know what to expect. Dealing with the uncertainty of their loved one's survival and the quality of life he may have should he survive is extremely difficult. Be willing to discuss realistic expectations. Of course, offer emotional support at all times.

Encourage gradually increased participation in the patient's care. Urge the family to talk to and touch the patient even if he appears unresponsive. Also give the family certain tasks to help them feel useful at a time when they're likely to feel powerless. Such tasks may include bringing pictures from home, making a tape of family members' voices for the patient's room, or calling the insurance company.

Because recuperation from head injury can be a long and arduous process, encourage the family not to neglect themselves. Suggest that they rotate the vigil at the patient's bedside so each can obtain much-needed rest. Help them draw on social supports, such as friends, relatives, or religious counselors, and encourage them to talk to each other. Communication tends to dwindle in an effort to avoid sharing painful feelings. Assure the family that the anger they may feel toward the patient for disrupting their lives is a common reaction, and they need not feel guilty about it. Identify positive coping mechanisms and reinforce them.

Consider your nursing interventions effective if the patient's family:
• demonstrates effective coping mechanisms
• participates in decision making and patient care
• shows regard for their own needs and care.

Potential for disturbance in self-concept. As the head-injured patient realizes what has happened to him and what his new deficits are, his self-concept may be shattered or, at least, significantly affected. Your nursing goals are to encourage a positive self-concept and to help the patient achieve the highest possible quality of life.

When planning nursing interventions to meet these goals, recognize that everyone needs to feel that he's a productive member of society. Permanent neurologic deficits may interfere with the patient's ability to fulfill this need. To make matters worse, health-care personnel and family members tend to focus on what the patient has lost instead of on what he can do. Before intervening to encourage a positive self-concept, carefully consider the patient's personality and special needs. First, assure the patient that he's still a valued human being, and encourage his family to do the same. Identify the patient's strengths and explore ways to build on them. Also help him develop his unexplored potential instead of planning his life solely around his limitations. Acknowledge, yet avoid judging, the patient's emotional response to head injury. For example, he may feel anger against his

family yet be afraid to express it because of his new dependence on them. Offer support and a listening ear. Above all, avoid encouraging regression or passivity. Involve the patient's family in decision making and care to help reintegrate the patient into society. Don't hesitate to suggest family counseling. Also advise the patient to contact local self-help groups. These groups offer information and support to help the patient cope with major life-style changes.

Consider your nursing interventions effective if the patient realistically acknowledges his neurologic deficits yet displays a positive self-concept and shows responsible independence.

Potential for inability to function independently. As discharge draws near, the patient's degree of independence assumes paramount significance. The inability to function independently can result from various deficits that may follow head injury: incontinence, impaired coordination, poor memory, and inability to think abstractly are but a few.

Your nursing goal is to discharge the patient safely at his optimal level of independence. Begin by carefully reviewing the patient's physical, cognitive, or emotional deficits that impede independence. For accurate evaluation, consult with all involved health-care personnel as well as the patient's family. Develop a list of activities that the patient should avoid for his own safety or should strive to participate in for optimal independence. Review this list of do's and don'ts with the patient and his family.

Prepare the patient and his family well before discharge for the anticipated level of dependence. Try to arrange a day or weekend pass for a trial run at home. Afterward, arrange a meeting to evaluate its success and to discuss unforeseen problems. Determine a schedule for follow-up visits, and designate a nurse that the family can contact to discuss problems that arise after discharge.

Consider your nursing interventions effective if the patient functions at his optimal level of independence without jeopardizing safety.

An unmatched reward
Head injury typically strikes healthy, active persons—and its outcome can be devastating. No amount of nursing expertise can erase the effects of primary brain injury. However, skillful nursing care can prevent or minimize secondary brain injury and thereby save the patient's life and limit permanent neurologic deficits.

Points to remember

• Head injury causes the majority of trauma deaths.
• Major causes of head injury include motor vehicle accidents, violent crimes, falls, birth trauma, and industrial and sporting accidents.
• Head injury is broadly classified as open or closed, depending on whether the protective barrier of the scalp, skull, and dura is violated.
• Primary brain injury includes immediate neuronal death or temporary dysfunction caused by penetrating or blunt trauma.
• Secondary brain injury includes any damage occurring after head injury that increases morbidity or mortality. Major causes of such damage include intracranial hypertension, hypoxemia, hypercapnia, and systemic hypotension.
• Intracranial hypertension is the most common cause of death in head-injured patients who reach the hospital alive. Its causes include hemorrhage, edema, hyperemia, impaired autoregulation, and hydrocephalus.
• Medical and nursing interventions aim to promote neurologic recovery by treating the head injury itself, controlling intracranial pressure, and preventing complications.
• Nursing care must address many complex physical, psychological, and social problems associated with the neurologic deficits of head injury.

5 PROVIDING SUPPORTIVE CARE IN BRAIN TUMORS

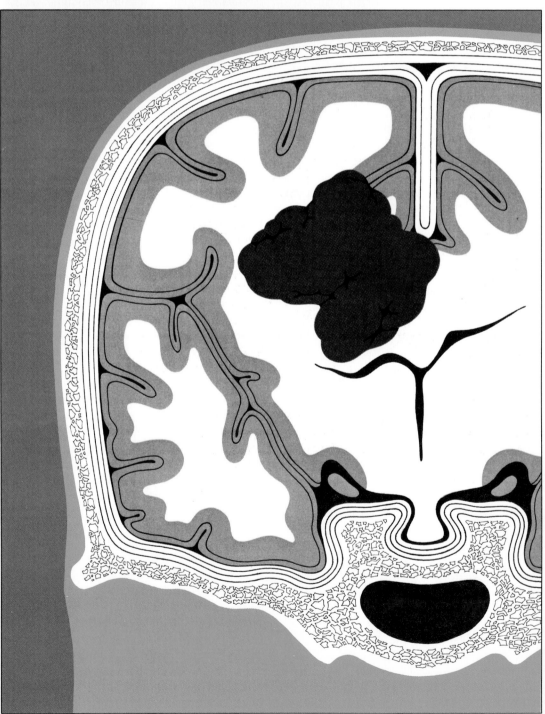

Brain tumor

either predictable, preventable, nor readily treatable, brain tumor surely ranks among the most dreaded diagnoses. And it's not reliably linked to specific risk factors or high-risk groups. Unlike many other tumors, it eludes early diagnoses during routine examination; moreover, early detection of a malignant tumor rarely helps prognosis. Even when a tumor is benign, surgical removal is typically both risky and difficult. When malignant, brain tumor is relentlessly progressive and can be fatal within 18 months of detection.

Despite this grim prognosis, there's much you can do to help the patient with a brain tumor. By understanding the types and characteristic effects of brain tumors, you can help pinpoint the tumor's location. By reviewing current tests and treatments, you can provide the patient with clear explanations of anticipated procedures, their risks, and their expected outcomes. But, most important, by sympathetically listening to the patient's and his family's problems, you may be able to help him accept and cope with his condition.

Contributing factors
Although brain tumor may occur at any age, it typically strikes patients between the ages of 5 and 10 or 35 and 50. It affects slightly more men than women and slightly more whites than blacks. Its cause is unknown, but genetic factors, infection, radiation, trauma, and immunosuppression may contribute to its formation. Genetic factors, for example, may be related to astrocytoma and characteristic defects of neurofibromatosis. Severe viral infection of the central nervous system (CNS) may increase the risk of brain tumor. Exposure to ionizing radiation damages DNA, inducing the development of genetically linked abnormalities. Both immunosuppressive therapy and acquired immune disorders can also contribute to brain tumor.

PATHOPHYSIOLOGY
No matter what causes brain tumor, abnormal intracranial cells begin to proliferate. These cells may arise from supportive brain structures, the meninges, and occasionally from neurons. As the tumor grows, it directly destroys adjacent tissue. Also, the tumor may cause extensive damage by increasing intracranial pressure (ICP) and eventually compressing the brain, leading to fatal herniation. Sometimes, tumors obstruct cerebrospinal fluid (CSF) and cerebral blood flow, contributing to increased intracranial pressure.

Cerebrospinal fluid obstruction
A tumor within the interior ventricular system or one encroaching on the exterior ventricular system, such as a third ventricular or posterior fossa tumor, may obstruct CSF pathways. When this occurs, CSF accumulates inside the intracranial compartment, increasing pressure, obstructing blood flow, and increasing central venous pressure.

Increased intracranial pressure
Because there's no room for tissue growth within the cranial vault, an expanding tumor increases ICP. Initially, the brain compensates by shunting CSF to the spinal cord, by autoregulating blood, and, after an extended period, by reducing CSF production. Eventually, these compensatory mechanisms fail, and ICP continues to increase, compressing cerebral vessels and decreasing blood flow. This produces hypoxia to brain tissue and ischemia, which initially causes local swelling and, later, diffuse edema. Edema further increases ICP, setting in motion another ominous cycle that can lead to brain herniation.

Brain herniation
Most deaths from brain tumor stem from uncal (transtentorial) or central herniation. Cingulate (falx) herniation is another form of brain herniation.

Cingulate (falx) herniation forces the cingulate gyrus underneath the falx cerebri, displacing brain tissue across the midline under the falx. Such herniation may compress brain tissue, compromise local blood flow, produce edema and ischemia, and further increase ICP.

Uncal herniation causes the uncus of the temporal lobe to herniate through the tentorium, thereby compressing the posterior cerebral artery and causing occipital lobe ischemia or infarction and edema.

Central herniation displaces intracranial components downward, compressing the medulla into the foramen magnum and stopping blood flow to the brain stem.

Brain herniation, particularly central herniation, places increased pressure on the respiratory centers in the medulla oblongata, causing abnormal respirations, such as ataxic or Kussmaul's respirations. It also causes bradycardia, hypotension, and, eventually, cardiac and respiratory arrest.
(continued on page 68)

Three major therapies

The major therapies used to treat brain tumors are surgery, radiation, and chemotherapy. The type of therapy depends on the tumor's histologic type, its radiosensitivity, and its anatomic location.

Surgery: Preferred therapy

Surgery may remove a resectable tumor or reduce a nonresectable tumor. Two surgical approaches are commonly used—craniotomy for a supratentorial tumor; craniectomy for an infratentorial tumor or a supratentorial tumor when intracranial expansion is suspected.

In a craniotomy, the surgeon makes a large incision in the cranium, forming a bone flap that can remain attached or be detached during surgery. He may freeze the detached bone so he can later replace it. Next, he incises the dura and opens it in the opposite direction (see illustration at right below). Then he removes the tumor and sutures the dura, skull, and skin flap back in place.

In a craniectomy, the surgeon removes part of the skull, anywhere from a small burr hole to a larger area. When needed, he enlarges the opening with a bone forceps (see illustration at left below). Then he removes the tumor.

Radiation

Typically used along with surgery or chemotherapy, radiation aims to alter the membranes of rapidly dividing cancer cells and to destroy them, while minimizing damage to normal cells. It's delivered by a cobalt machine or by a linear accelerator—an electrical device that creates ionizing radiation by making electrons move at incredibly high speeds. When electrons hit a target within the accelerator, they stop abruptly and their energy is converted to photons (X-rays). The higher the speed of the electrons, the greater the penetration of the X-rays, allowing radiation to reach tumors located deep within the brain behind the skull bones.

To minimize damage to normal tissue, radiation must be aimed accurately, especially if critical structures, such as the eye, are to be spared. However, avoiding damage to normal tissue is difficult since radiation, to be effective, must bombard the entire tumor, which is imprecisely defined. One solution to this problem is the cross-fire technique: rotation of the linear accelerator to create multiple fields of radiation, ensuring that normal tissue receives a smaller dose of radiation than the tumor. Another solution is to give radiotherapy in multiple doses (called fractions) over an extended period rather than in one large dose. Because cells deep within a tumor may be hypoxic and radiation is more damaging to oxygen-rich cells, giving radiotherapy in fractions enables hypoxic cells to obtain oxygen and improves the effectiveness of subsequent radiation treatments.

Adverse reactions to radiation vary. Acute reactions are related to cell renewal failure in irradiated areas and include nausea and vomiting, drowsiness, itching, and scalp and ear discomfort. Delayed reactions include anorexia, lethargy, and fatigue. Rarely, a fatal reaction results from brain tissue necrosis or cerebral vasculature damage.

Surgery

Craniectomy

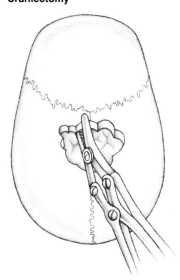

Craniotomy

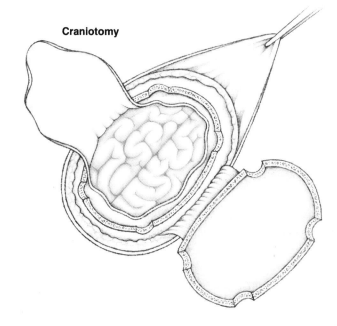

Radiation

Cross-fire technique

Irradiated area

Chemotherapy

Cell cycle disruption

G$_0$ cell

Cell division

Postmitosis

Mitosis

G$_1$ phase

G$_2$ phase

S phase

Premitosis

Methotrexate

Cell death

Chemotherapy

This form of drug therapy attacks stem cells during their reproductive cycle. In malignant brain tumor, only 10% to 40% of stem cells actively reproduce, or proliferate. The remaining cells, called G$_0$ cells, remain in a resting state—the result of undernutrition, hypoxia, or decreased temperature. However, when temperature rises or other conditions change, these cells become active and reproduce. Because all stem cells eventually reproduce, chemotherapy affects normal stem cells as well as malignant ones.

Types of chemotherapy include cell-cycle-specific drugs, such as the antimetabolite methotrexate, and cell-cycle-nonspecific drugs, such as the nitrosoureas lomustine (CCNU) and carmustine (BCNU). Cell-cycle-specific drugs try to interrupt a specific phase of mitosis, while nonspecific drugs produce their effects independently of mitotic phases.

With both types, the safe chemotherapeutic dose depends on the extent of drug damage to normal cells. Usually the higher the dose, the greater the number of both normal and malignant cells destroyed. With most chemotherapeutic drugs, intermittent, divided high doses are more effective than prolonged administration of low doses. Each dose seems to destroy a fixed percentage rather than a fixed number of cells.

Along with damage to normal cells, other factors must be considered in prescribing chemotherapy. For example, most malignant cells are in a resting state and all have a long generation time. As a result, these cells are difficult to treat with cell-cycle-specific drugs. Also, most malignant brain tumors contain many cell types, so more than one drug may be needed to attack all types.

To increase the effectiveness of chemotherapy, a combination of drugs that differ in action and toxicity should be given.

Key

Phases of the cell cycle

G$_1$ Preparation for DNA synthesis
S   DNA synthesis
G$_2$ Preparation for cell division

Tumor types and their locations

Type of tumor	Common locations
Acoustic neuroma	8th cranial nerve Cerebellopontine angle Cranial nerves adjacent to the 8th (compress 5th, 7th, 9th, and 10th)
Astrocytoma, grades I and II	Cerebral hemispheres (frontal, parietal, and temporal lobes) Cerebellum in children
Astrocytoma, grades III and IV (glioblastoma multiforme)	Frontal lobe Corpus callosum
Craniopharyngioma	Sella turcica
Ependymoma	Ventricular system (especially the 4th ventricle)
Hemangioblastoma	Cerebellum Cerebral hemispheres Medulla
Medulloblastoma	Cerebellum 4th ventricle Spinal cord
Meningioma	Near the venous sinuses on the convexity of the brain Anterior, posterior fossae floors
Neurofibromatosis (von Recklinghausen's disease)	Throughout the central and peripheral nervous systems
Oligodendroglioma	Cerebral hemispheres (frontal and temporal lobes)
Pituitary adenoma	Sella turcica
Spongioblastoma	Optic nerves

MEDICAL MANAGEMENT

For the patient with suspected brain tumor, a thorough medical history and physical examination should precede diagnostic tests. Then, both invasive and noninvasive tests will help detect the location of the lesion and the progression of the disease and direct the course of treatment.

Locating the lesion

Diagnostic tests reliably pinpoint the location of a lesion, but precise diagnosis requires direct histologic study.

Skull X-rays identify the shape and size of skull bones and can detect tumors containing calcium, such as a meningioma or an oligo-

dendroglioma. In a pituitary tumor, skull X-rays may show bony erosion of the sella turcica. In a tumor of the cerebral hemisphere, X-rays may show calcification and displacement of the pineal gland.

The *computerized tomography (CT) scan,* perhaps the most frequently used test for brain tumor, often eliminates the need for hazardous invasive tests, such as pneumoencephalography and cerebral angiography. It's especially valuable in evaluating patients with focal neurologic abnormalities or other clinical features that suggest an intracranial lesion. The CT scan identifies the specific location of the lesion as well as the shape. Serial CT scans show the progression of a tumor as well as the effects of therapy.

The *nuclear medicine brain scan* can help clarify questionable CT scan findings. However, it may fail to demonstrate certain benign and low-grade malignant tumors because of poor uptake of the injected radioisotope.

Cerebral angiography occasionally follows inconclusive CT or brain scans when a vascular abnormality is suspected. This test reveals vessel displacement, reflecting the presence, location, and size of a tumor, and may also reveal tumor blush—circulation within a tumor.

Pneumoencephalography, now virtually replaced by the CT scan, may be helpful in evaluating a tumor in the posterior fossa or ventricular system.

Lumbar puncture shows increased protein levels, increased pressure, and, occasionally, tumor cells in the CSF. This test is contraindicated if the patient has known or suspected increased intracranial pressure because of the potentially serious complication of brain stem herniation.

Electroencephalography, commonly used in evaluating epilepsy, can also reveal evidence of intracranial lesions by demonstrating areas of abnormal electrical brain activity.

Two promising tests

Magnetic resonance imaging, a noninvasive test with little known risk, discriminates between normal and diseased tissue with greater sensitivity than a CT scan. For example, it can detect small lesions that have biochemical properties similar to those of surrounding normal tissue. A CT scan, in contrast, would fail to detect such a lesion unless the lesion had changed the size and shape of surrounding structures.

Xenon cerebral blood flow studies, another

promising test, can show abnormal perfusion patterns that correlate with the location of a lesion which may or may not be shown by a CT scan.

Traditional treatments

Treatment of brain tumor typically includes surgery, radiation, and drug therapy. Surgery, usually the primary treatment, can alleviate symptoms, provide definitive diagnosis through biopsy of the lesion, and, occasionally, effect a cure. Radiation and chemotherapy are used generally as adjunctive treatment unless the brain tumor is inoperable. (See *Three major therapies,* pages 66 and 67.)

Palliative drug therapy. Drugs help alleviate brain tumor symptoms. Analgesics relieve the headache commonly associated with brain tumor; anticonvulsants control or prevent seizures; and corticosteroids, such as dexamethasone, seem to control cerebral edema by stabilizing cellular membranes. Dexamethasone causes less sodium retention and fewer adverse effects than other corticosteroids and may even stimulate antitumor activity. However, all corticosteroids may induce cushingoid symptoms and GI ulceration. Concomitant use of medications that decrease gastric acidity, such as antacids or cimetidine, can minimize the risk of GI bleeding. When corticosteroids are discontinued, slow tapering is necessary to avoid adrenal insufficiency.

New treatments

New techniques for surgical, drug, and radiation therapy offer new hope for patients with a brain tumor. *Laser neurosurgery,* for example, allows precise tumor resection and access to formerly inoperable areas, reduces brain manipulation, and decreases postoperative cerebral edema.

New drugs, such as nitromidazoles, are now being given before radiation therapy to sensitize normally hypoxic tumor cells. (Hyperbaric oxygenation provides another method for sensitizing hypoxic cells.) According to a new dosage schedule, traditional drugs such as mannitol may be given before chemotherapy to alter the blood-brain barrier, allowing for easier passage of chemotherapeutic agents into brain tissue, and so reduce the effective dose of chemotherapeutic drugs. Also, use of an implantable cerebrospinal reservoir allows injection of chemotherapeutic drugs directly into the ventricular system.

Radiation therapy itself is changing. Some centers are using fast-neutron radiation, a much more precise and powerful form of delivering radiation. Unfortunately, fast-neutron radiation may cause extensive damage to both normal and malignant cells, so calculating the optimal dose is difficult. Other centers are using brachytherapy or bradytherapy, in which radioactive seeds are implanted into the tumor for a limited time delivering a precise radiation dosage to a very localized area, thereby minimizing destruction of surrounding tissue.

NURSING MANAGEMENT

Effectively managing a patient with a brain tumor obviously requires that you understand the complex pathophysiology involved and that you master special techniques for appropriate physical care. But, perhaps more important, you must recognize the emotional strain that prognosis for the brain tumor places on the patient and his family. Your ability to offer understanding and emotional support as they struggle with the diverse problems that stem from this devastating disorder can help them cope more effectively.

Patient history: Involve the family

Because the patient with a brain tumor can't always remember or communicate his history, be sure to involve his family in your history taking. Of course, document both the patient's and the family's answers.

First, ask about the patient's chief complaint. How long has it troubled him? Does it occur in any special pattern? Does it vary with time of day or activity level?

Always ask about headaches. This symptom affects about 70% of patients with a brain tumor and is the chief complaint in about 20%. Headaches are usually moderately intense and generalized, rather than severe and localized. Typically, they worsen in the morning because the compensatory mechanism controlling blood flow and CSF flow out of the brain functions poorly in the recumbent position assumed during sleep.

Ask about symptoms of increased ICP, such as projectile vomiting and visual disturbances. In about 75% of patients, increased ICP causes papilledema manifested by decreased visual acuity, double vision, and visual field deficits.

Ask about hallucinations. Visual hallucinations are most common, but auditory and olfactory hallucinations may also occur. Recognize that the patient may be reluctant to report hallucinations.

Classifying brain tumors

Brain tumors can be classified as malignant or benign, as primary or secondary, by cellular origin, by cellular differentiation, or by location.

Malignant or benign
Distinguishing *malignant* from *benign* brain tumors is difficult. Brain tumors can be benign in their tissue type but malignant because of their location in a vital area.

Primary or secondary
Almost 90% of brain tumors are *primary*, arising from central nervous system (CNS) tissue. Primary tumors rarely metastasize outside the CNS, but they often infiltrate another area of the CNS. The remaining 10% of brain tumors are *secondary*, metastasizing from the lungs, GI tract, breasts, ovaries, or kidneys.

Cellular origin
Brain tumors arise from *neuroectodermal* or *mesodermal* cells. They can be further divided by *specific cell type.* For example, tumors that arise from astrocyte cells are called astrocytomas.

Cellular differentiation
Grading—a measure of cellular differentiation—takes into account the resemblance of tumor tissue to normal cells. *Grade I* shows well-differentiated cells; *grade II,* moderately differentiated; *grade III,* poorly differentiated; and *grade IV,* very poorly differentiated. Typically, grade III and IV tumors are malignant.

Location
Although this classification doesn't provide information on tumor type or prognosis, it does prove helpful for detecting localizing signs. Supratentorial tumors usually develop in the cerebral hemispheres and occasionally in the corpus callosum. Infratentorial tumors develop in the posterior fossa, cerebellum, cerebellopontine angle, and brain stem.

Ask about seizures. How often do they occur? What are they like? What medication does the patient take for them? Does it work? About 30% of patients with a brain tumor experience seizures, and about 15% report them as their chief complaint. Suspect brain tumor when an apparently healthy, middle-aged adult has a first seizure, particularly a localized (simple partial) one.

Ask about a personal and family history of neurologic symptoms. Such symptoms may stem from cardiovascular, respiratory, or other systemic disorders. Also ask about a family history of neurofibromatosis, astrocytoma, or other neurologic disorders.

Gather pertinent psychosocial information. Ask about previous hospitalizations for depression or other psychological disorders since such disorders may actually be symptomatic of brain tumor. Also ask about behavior or personality changes and whether they're mild or severe. For example, a previously mild-mannered patient may become aggressive, or an energetic patient may become apathetic. Determine if the patient has experienced unusual stress at home or at work. Finally, find out if the patient's condition interferes with the activities of daily living.

Physical examination: Determine tumor location

First, assess the patient's level of consciousness by checking his orientation to person, place, and time. Confusion may be an early indicator of a decreased level of consciousness. Also evaluate the patient's memory of recent and remote events as well as his concentration, judgment, and problem-solving ability. Note if the patient seems to be experiencing hallucinations or seizures.

Next, assess the patient's motor function. (See *Brain tumors: Sites and symptoms.*) Identifying specific motor deficits can help pinpoint tumor location. Hemiparesis, for example, occurs with cerebral hemisphere involvement, especially of the frontal and parietal lobes. It always affects the extremities on the side opposite the tumor. Its onset may be slow or sudden, progressing rapidly to paralysis and indicating severe decompensation. Impaired coordination and control of movement occur with cerebellar tumors and, occasionally, midbrain tumors. Severe impairment may produce ataxia in which the patient's broad-based, unsteady gait makes him appear intoxicated.

To further pinpoint the tumor's location,

assess sensory function. Sensory disturbances include hyperesthesia (increased tactile sensitivity), hypalgesia (decreased sensation), paresthesia (abnormal sensation), loss of discrimination (point, texture, right-left), and astereognosis (inability to recognize an object by touch). These disturbances usually result from tumors of the sensory cortex of the parietal lobe.

Evaluate the patient's speech for content, clarity, and coherence and, if indicated, arrange for a speech pathologist to perform a comprehensive speech evaluation. Speech disturbances, which are usually associated with involvement of the left frontal, parietal, or temporal lobes, include difficulty in speaking and writing (expressive aphasia), inability to understand written or oral expression (receptive aphasia) and slurred or garbled speech (dysarthria). Expressive aphasia may occur with frontal tumors; receptive aphasia may occur with posterior fossa tumors affecting the cranial nerves.

Check for symptoms of cranial nerve involvement. Supratentorial tumors may compress the 3rd, 4th, and 6th cranial nerves, causing problems with eye movement, pupillary size, and reaction and eyelid elevation. Infratentorial tumors may surround the 9th, 10th, and 12th cranial nerves, causing problems with speech, swallowing, and cough and gag reflexes. Also, assess the patient's appearance to detect endocrine imbalance from pituitary tumor. For example, a growth hormone–secreting tumor may produce acromegaly.

Formulate nursing diagnoses

Use information obtained from the patient history and physical examination to formulate appropriate nursing diagnoses. These diagnoses should take into account any residual neurologic deficit as well as the prognosis.

Headache related to increased ICP. Your goals are to keep the patient comfortable and to relieve pain. To achieve these goals, administer analgesics as ordered. Watch for the pattern of headache so you can anticipate his recurring pain and administer the scheduled analgesic for it. Encourage the patient to report headaches. If he's unable to communicate, watch for telltale signs, such as restlessness or crying.

To promote cerebral venous outflow, elevate the head of the bed 15° to 30°. Also ask the patient to tell you (or watch his behavior carefully to identify) the comfort measures,

Brain tumors: Sites and symptoms

Brain tumors—whether they are benign or malignant—produce specific signs and symptoms, depending on their location. Knowing these typical effects of major neuro- logic deficits helps identify the site of brain lesions and helps in planning preoperative or post- operative care including recog- nizing life-threatening compli- cations and preparations for discharge. The following list in- cludes the characteristic effects of increased intracranial pres- sure and potential symptoms associated with a lesion in a specific location. Patients with brain lesions may exhibit all, some, or none of these effects.

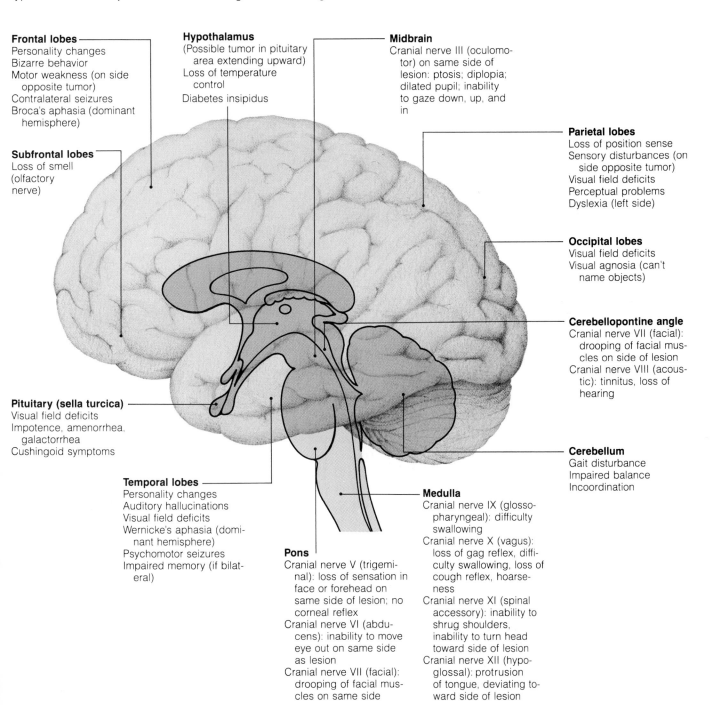

Frontal lobes
Personality changes
Bizarre behavior
Motor weakness (on side opposite tumor)
Contralateral seizures
Broca's aphasia (dominant hemisphere)

Subfrontal lobes
Loss of smell (olfactory nerve)

Hypothalamus
(Possible tumor in pituitary area extending upward)
Loss of temperature control
Diabetes insipidus

Midbrain
Cranial nerve III (oculomo- tor) on same side of lesion: ptosis; diplopia; dilated pupil; inability to gaze down, up, and in

Parietal lobes
Loss of position sense
Sensory disturbances (on side opposite tumor)
Visual field deficits
Perceptual problems
Dyslexia (left side)

Occipital lobes
Visual field deficits
Visual agnosia (can't name objects)

Cerebellopontine angle
Cranial nerve VII (facial): drooping of facial mus- cles on side of lesion
Cranial nerve VIII (acous- tic): tinnitus, loss of hearing

Pituitary (sella turcica)
Visual field deficits
Impotence, amenorrhea, galactorrhea
Cushingoid symptoms

Temporal lobes
Personality changes
Auditory hallucinations
Visual field deficits
Wernicke's aphasia (domi- nant hemisphere)
Psychomotor seizures
Impaired memory (if bilat- eral)

Pons
Cranial nerve V (trigemi- nal): loss of sensation in face or forehead on same side of lesion; no corneal reflex
Cranial nerve VI (abdu- cens): inability to move eye out on same side as lesion
Cranial nerve VII (facial): drooping of facial mus- cles on same side

Medulla
Cranial nerve IX (glosso- pharyngeal): difficulty swallowing
Cranial nerve X (vagus): loss of gag reflex, diffi- culty swallowing, loss of cough reflex, hoarse- ness
Cranial nerve XI (spinal accessory): inability to shrug shoulders, inability to turn head toward side of lesion
Cranial nerve XII (hypo- glossal): protrusion of tongue, deviating to- ward side of lesion

Cerebellum
Gait disturbance
Impaired balance
Incoordination

Caring for the neurosurgical patient

Intracranial surgery requires special preoperative and postoperative care. Preoperative care centers on psychological support and establishing an accurate baseline assessment; postoperative care centers on careful monitoring for life-threatening complications.

Preoperative care

Reinforce the doctor's explanation of the surgery, and answer the patient's questions. Arrange for the patient to visit the intensive care unit, and explain postoperative care measures.

Tell the patient that his head will be shaved before surgery and that he'll awaken with a large bandage on his head, temporary swelling and discoloration around his eye on the affected side, and possibly a headache. Inform him that he'll receive pain medication.

Postoperative care

Position the patient on the unaffected side to avoid placing pressure on the brain. To prevent increased intracranial pressure (ICP), keep his head higher than the rest of his body.

If the patient has had a supratentorial incision, elevate the head of the bed 30°, and turn him every 2 hours to facilitate breathing and venous return. If he has had an infratentorial incision, keep him off his back for at least 48 hours and elevate the head of the bed 30°, as ordered. With the help of another nurse, use a turning sheet to reposition him every 2 hours, making sure to support the head and maintain body alignment.

Observe the patient's respirations closely, and immediately report any signs of respiratory distress. Make sure arterial blood gases are measured regularly.

• Monitor fluid and electrolyte status. To reduce the risk of increased ICP, restrict fluids to 1,500 ml every 24 hours and avoid overly rapid I.V. infusions. Withhold oral fluids since they may provoke vomiting, which could, in turn, raise ICP.

Watch for signs of diabetes insipidus (severe thirst, frequent urination, dehydration) or inappropriate antidiuretic hormone secretion (decreased urination, hunger and thirst, irritability, decreased level of consciousness, muscle weakness). Report these signs immediately and adjust fluid balance, as ordered.

• Monitor the patient's neurologic status (level of consciousness, pupil checks) every half hour or as ordered until the patient's condition stabilizes. Later, monitor his status every 2 hours. Watch for and report seizures, deteriorated level of consciousness, increased ICP (characterized by headache, vomiting, altered level of consciousness, visual disturbances, or fixed dilated pupils.

• Check the patient's dressing at least hourly and report any abnormalities. If the patient has a surgical drain, note the amount, color, and odor of drainage. Notify the doctor if bleeding is excessive, if drainage is clear or yellow (possible cerebrospinal fluid leakage), or if signs of infection appear.

• Give drugs, as ordered. The doctor will probably order steroids to prevent cerebral edema, anticonvulsants to prevent seizures, stool softeners to prevent increased ICP from straining during defecation, and mild analgesics to control pain.

• Provide hair and scalp care. To help prevent infection, apply antiseptic to the incision site. If ordered, apply antibacterial ointment to keep skin along the suture line supple. After suture removal, usually about a week after surgery, thoroughly wash the patient's scalp and hair.

• Apply ice to swollen eyelids. Also, lubricate the lids and the area around the eyes.

such as massage or soft music, that help him the most. Observe and record the patient's responses to analgesics and comfort measures. Consider your interventions successful if the patient appears comfortable.

Impaired level of consciousness resulting from increased ICP. Your goal is to prevent complications from increased ICP. To achieve this goal, use the Glasgow coma scale to assess and record the level of consciousness. Pace your monitoring according to the patient's condition. Identify and report changes in level of consciousness and any corresponding changes in vital signs. Avoid procedures that raise ICP, such as suctioning, turning, isometric exercise, and Valsalva's maneuver. Consider your interventions effective if the patient is alert and oriented and shows no change in level of consciousness.

Potential for injury related to seizures or sensorimotor deficit. To prevent injury, pad side rails and keep them elevated. When appropriate, use a restraint. If the patient is ambulatory, remove unused equipment, tables, or other objects from the patient's room to prevent falls.

Keep suction and intubation equipment readily available. If a seizure occurs, maintain airway patency and summon help. Afterward, record its type, duration, and location.

Before the patient is discharged, explain to the patient and his family necessary seizure precautions, such as driving restrictions and family responsibilities during a seizure. Emphasize the importance of adhering to the prescribed therapy. With effective intervention, the patient can escape injury.

Impaired speech related to damage to the speech center. To promote effective communication, obtain advice from a speech pathologist. Identify the extent of the speech disorder, and set up guidelines to help the patient and family communicate. If the patient is aphasic, suggest and explain the use of a communication board, gestures, letter board, blinking, or nodding. You've intervened successfully if the patient can communicate his needs without frustration.

Sensory or perceptual loss related to the effects of brain tumor. Because brain tumor can cause loss of memory, sensation, and visual fields, your goals are to maintain the patient's orientation to person, place, and time; to provide sensory input; and to prevent injury. To achieve these goals, continually reinforce the patient's orientation to reality, and, when he has a sensory deficit, provide needed stimulation. If the patient has a visual field loss, take care to approach him within his visual field. Inspect areas of sensory loss daily for injury, and teach the patient and his family to do so as well. Also, involve the patient and his family in devising ways to compensate for sensory loss and prevent injury. Consider your interventions successful if the patient maintains his orientation and avoids injury.

Altered body and self-image related to neurologic deficit and hair loss. Your goal is to help the patient cope with and accept this altered image. Since a brain tumor is often associated with residual neurologic deficits, begin rehabilitation early.

Enhance the patient's self-image by gradually promoting independence in daily activities. As needed, provide self-care aids, such as special eating utensils. Encourage the patient to be concerned about his physical appearance. Arrange for family members to bring in his favorite clothes and personal grooming items. After surgery, suggest the use of a head covering such as a turban or scarf or, after the incision is well healed, a toupee or wig. Compliment the patient on his appearance when appropriate.

Continually assess the patient's and the family's coping mechanisms. Help them to identify and cope with any fears, and strengthen their supportive relationships. Coping is successful if the patient and his family acknowledge and accept the patient's diagnosis and his changed appearance.

Knowledge deficit related to brain tumor and its treatment. Your goal is to increase the patient's and family's knowledge, particularly about brain tumor and its effects. Explain relevant diagnostic tests, and help allay the patient's anxieties about testing, treatment, and progression of the disease.

If surgery is scheduled, explain the planned approach as well as preoperative and postoperative care. Be informative and honest. Make sure the patient understands the potential risks and the expected outcome. (See *Caring for the neurosurgical patient.*) Even though you can't guarantee recovery, you can help instill confidence in the surgeon and the recommended approach.

If the patient is receiving drug therapy, explain the purpose, dosage, and schedule of prescribed drugs. Also explain the potential side effects of these drugs, and instruct him to report side effects, such as dyspnea on exertion from congestive heart failure, a side effect of corticosteroids.

If the patient is scheduled for radiation therapy, explain the procedure to him. Instruct him to report any adverse reactions, such as nausea and vomiting. Also advise him to cover his head when he is outdoors because skin exposed to radiation is more susceptible to sunburn.

Teach early signs of recurrence and pertinent self-care procedures. Reinforce your teaching with written materials. Encourage the patient and his family to ask questions, and urge their compliance with therapy. When appropriate, refer them to support groups, such as the American Cancer Society and the Association for Brain Tumor Research. Consider your teaching successful if the patient and his family understand and can explain brain tumor and its treatment and can perform self-care procedures.

Summing it up
Because the location, size, and effects of brain tumor vary so widely, you'll have to tailor your nursing care plan to fit your patient's individual needs. Throughout the patient's hospitalization, you'll need to perform regular neurologic assessments to detect changes in his condition. You'll also need to explain his disorder, its treatment, and its expected outcome. But, most important, you'll need to provide continuous emotional support for both the patient and his family, helping them cope with the devastating effects of brain tumor and its often grim prognosis.

Points to remember

• Brain tumors can be classified as malignant or benign, as primary or secondary, by cellular origin, by cellular differentiation (grade I to grade IV), or by location.
• Brain tumors cause central nervous system changes by invading and destroying tissues and by secondary effect: compression of the brain, cranial nerves, and cerebral vessels; cerebral edema; and elevated intracranial pressure.
• The major therapies used to treat brain tumors are surgery, radiation, and chemotherapy.
• New diagnostic tests, such as magnetic resonance imaging and xenon cerebral blood flow studies, allow earlier detection of brain tumors. New treatments, such as laser neurosurgery, may improve prognosis for certain brain tumors.

6 COMBATING NEUROLOGIC INFECTIONS

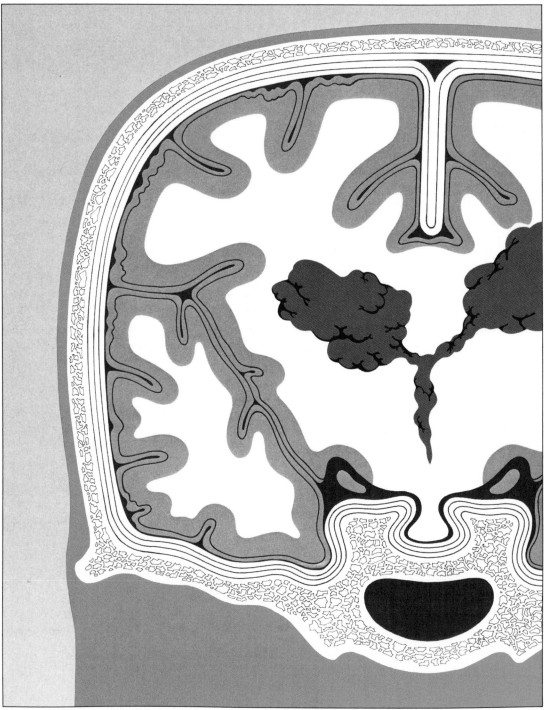

Brain abscess with meningeal involvement

However often you've had to deal with central nervous system (CNS) infections in your practice, you surely find them a formidable challenge every time. And not just because such infections demand intense and special supportive care. In few other conditions does the quality of your care influence the patient's chances for survival so directly and profoundly. For example, your ability to monitor intracranial pressure (ICP) correctly and to recognize early clues to rising ICP can make the difference between death and complete recovery. Your ability to offer the competent care that makes this difference requires a thorough understanding of neuroinfective pathophysiology and a mastery of the special skills required to detect, monitor, and treat these perilous infections.

PATHOPHYSIOLOGY
CNS infections are so perilous because, within this closed system, the edema they cause threatens permanent secondary damage and is potentially fatal. These infections are associated with mortality as high as 95% (for brain abscesses, mass lesions, and some types of meningitis).

Who's at risk?
CNS infections threaten all age-groups but are especially prevalent and dangerous in the very young, the very old, or the nutritionally deficient (such as alcoholics with vitamin deficiency); in persons who are chronically ill, immunodeficient (such as those with acquired immune deficiency syndrome), or leukopenic (for example, associated with reticuloendothelial malignancy, chemotherapy, and radiation therapy); or in those who have preexisting infection. CNS infections are also more prevalent among populations who live in crowded conditions in endemic areas and who are exposed to contact with nonhuman carriers, such as farm animals, ticks, and fleas.

CNS infections may result from bacteria, viruses, parasites, or fungi (see *Major pathogens*; see also *Distinguishing neuroinfective diseases,* page 76). These groups gain entry to a compromised host in different ways.

Bacteria: Primarily inhaled
Bacteria usually enter the body through the nasopharynx or lungs but also commonly enter through skin furuncles, cuts, and the genitourinary tract. Bacteria reach the fetus by crossing the placenta from contaminated amniotic fluid or during fetal passage through a contaminated vagina.

Once in the body, bacteria can multiply and enter the bloodstream. They can then penetrate the blood-brain barrier and gain access to the subarachnoid space. Normally, most blood-borne bacteria are blocked from access to the nervous system by the pulmonary filtering system. However, any condition that impairs pulmonary filtration (such as a damaged lung) or causes a right-to-left circulatory shunt that bypasses the pulmonary filtering system (as in children with cyanotic congenital heart disease) lets bacteria bypass this defense to enter the nervous system. Bacteria from host sources, such as an infected endocardium or a pelvic abscess, can spread to the CNS as septic emboli.

Bacteria also spread to the nervous system by direct extension from an adjacent bony focus of infection. This is the common source of bacterial parameningeal infections, such as brain abscess, subdural empyema, and cerebral or spinal epidural abscess, which usually spread from infections of the ear, teeth, mastoids, sinuses, scalp, face, skull, or vertebrae. Such abscesses spread from the bony focus through the meninges and into the brain or spinal cord parenchyma. Parameningeal infections may be secondary to hematogenous spread of organisms, especially in patients with lung diseases, such as pneumonia with lung abscesses.

Bacteria may enter CNS tissue directly through a penetrating craniocerebral injury; compound depressed skull fracture, including basal skull fractures; craniotomy; intracranial drains and monitoring devices; and intracranial foreign objects.

Viruses: Variable spread
Viruses enter the body in several ways. They may spread from person to person through exposure to airborne droplets or contaminated secretions that are taken in through the nasopharynx, lungs, and gastrointestinal tract. They may spread from infected animals to man through contact with infected saliva or contaminated soil, water, or animal tissue. Viruses may also spread from an infected blood-sucking arthropod to man. Occasionally, latent viruses, such as those causing Guillain-Barré syndrome and postvaccinal encephalomyelitis, may be activated by prophylactic inoculation, as for mumps, measles, or rabies.

Most viruses reach the CNS through the

Major pathogens

Bacteria
Clostridium
Escherichia coli
Hemophilus influenzae
Klebsiella
Mycobacterium tuberculosis
Neisseria meningitidis
Proteus
Pseudomonas
Salmonella
Shigella
Staphylococcus aureus
Streptococcus, Groups A and B
Streptococcus pneumoniae
Treponema pallidum

Fungi
Actinomyces israelii
Aspergillus fumigatus
Blastomyces dermatitidis
Candida albicans
Candida tropicalis
Coccidioides immitis
Cryptococcus neoformans
Histoplasma capsulatum

Parasites
Entamoeba histolytica
Schistosoma haematobium
Schistosoma japonicum
Schistosoma mansoni
Taenia echinococcus
Taenia solium
Toxoplasma gondii
Trichinella spiralis

Viruses
Adenoviruses
  Lymphocytic choriomeningitis virus
  Rabies virus
Enteroviruses
  Coxsackie viruses, Groups A and B
  Echoviruses
  Polioviruses
Herpesviruses
  Cytomegalovirus
  Epstein-Barr virus
  Herpes simplex, Types 1 and 2
  Varicella-zoster
Myxoviruses and paramyxoviruses
  Influenza
  Measles (rubeola)
  Mumps
  Parainfluenza

Distinguishing neuroinfective diseases

Disease	Description	Cause
Bacterial		
Meningitis	Meningeal infection	Neonates: gram-negative bacilli or anaerobic streptococci Children: *Hemophilus influenzae* Adults: *Neisseria meningitidis* or *Streptococcus pneumoniae*
Encephalitis	Brain parenchymal infection	Secondary to bacterial meningitis; injury resulting in invasion by clostridia (anaerobic) or staphylococci (aerobic)
Brain abscess	Free or encapsulated pus in brain parenchyma	Secondary to direct invasion (meningeal, ear, sinus, scalp, or bone infection) or blood-borne (distant infection); anaerobes predominate
Subdural empyema	Pus between dura mater and arachnoid membrane	Secondary to paranasal sinus or middle-ear infection
Cerebral epidural abscess	Pus in epidural space of brain	Secondary to head, face, bone, or paranasal sinus infection
Spinal epidural abscess	Pus in epidural space of spinal cord	Secondary to vertebral body infection; metastatic spread from bacteremia
Neurosyphilis	Meningeal infection; occasional extension into brain parenchyma	*Treponema pallidum*
Viral		
Meningitis	Meningeal infection	Various viruses
Encephalitis	Brain parenchymal infection	Frequent progression of viral meningitis; may be very severe
Herpes zoster (shingles)	Infection of ganglia and innervation area	Varicella virus
Poliomyelitis	Infection involving anterior horn of the gray matter in the spinal cord or medulla	Poliovirus
Rabies	Acute central nervous system (CNS) infection	Rabies virus in saliva of infected host
Reye's syndrome	Acute encephalopathy (brain swelling, fatty infiltration, and liver dysfunction)	Possible complication of viral infections treated with aspirin
Creutzfeldt-Jakob disease	Encephalopathy with dementia and degeneration of pyramidal and extrapyramidal systems; rare, always fatal	Slow virus; can be transmitted by experimental animals or contaminated surgical instruments or corneal grafts
Subacute sclerosing panencephalitis	Subacute encephalitis with white matter deterioration and demyelination	Defective measles virus
Progressive multifocal leukoencephalopathy	CNS demyelination; rare	Opportunistic papovavirus infection in compromised patient
Parasitic		
Amebiasis	Multiple abscesses, usually in frontal lobes and basal ganglia (necrosis and cavitation)	*Entamoeba histolytica*
Toxoplasmosis	Protozoan encephalitis	*Toxoplasma gondii* in compromised patient
Cysticercosis	Parasitic brain infection by way of the intestinal wall (multiple cystic lesions)	*Taenia solium*, present in uncooked, infective pork
Fungal		
Candidiasis	Granulomatous meningitis with multiple abscesses and brain parenchymal lesions	*Candida albicans, Candida tropicalis* in compromised patient
Histoplasmosis	Cerebral lesions spread from other sites (miliary granulomas, meningitis, histoplasmomas)	*Histoplasma capsulatum* in compromised patient

bloodstream (viremia). Some invade by centripetal growth or by movement along the peripheral or cranial nerves, as with herpesvirus and rabies virus. Latent or slow viruses, such as those causing subacute sclerosing panencephalitis and those believed to cause multiple sclerosis, may not produce symptoms until several years after CNS invasion. Such viruses remain dormant until something triggers an acute process.

Parasites: Exposure by ingestion
Parasites usually spread from animal to man through ingestion of contaminated meat, dairy, or other animal products, or contaminated soil or water. Person-to-person spread occurs by the fecal-oral route. Ingested parasites proliferate in the intestines and are hematogenously disseminated to other sites, commonly the liver and lungs. However, the larval forms of some parasites, such as *Taenia solium* (pork tapeworm), may infest CNS tissue.

Fungi: Commonly airborne
Fungi are most often inhaled from the environment and then spread hematogenously from the lungs to the nervous system. Also, some normal flora in the body become pathogenic when carried to sites other than their usual ones. Fungi may be introduced into the bloodstream by extension from a contiguous focus (such as the sinuses), a drug abuser's dirty or contaminated needle and syringe, or iatrogenic spread during oral, facial, maxillary, ENT, or neurosurgical procedures.

Two natural defenses
All microorganisms are potentially dangerous once they invade the body. Some release harmful enzymes that cause cell damage; others give off toxins that disrupt all organ systems and stress the immune system. They're opposed by nonspecific inflammatory and specific immune responses.

Inflammatory response. White blood cells form the first internal defense against an invading pathogen; the inflammatory response varies in intensity proportional to the degree of infection or injury. Cell injury leads to release of inflammation mediators that attract neutrophils and macrophages to the site, and these phagocytes proceed to immobilize and ingest the pathogens. In bacterial infections pus forms, consisting of dead neutrophils and macrophages and necrotic tissue.

At the time of injury, damaged cells release vasoactive substances, such as histamine, serotonin, and bradykinin. These agents promote blood flow to the area and increase capillary permeability. This causes fluid and proteins, including fibrinogen, to leak into surrounding tissues, producing local edema. Extracellular fluid and lymph wall off the infected area.

Specific immune response. Identification and neutralization of specific pathogens and development of resistance to them help to eliminate the infectious agent and to safeguard the body from repeated infection by the same organism. Two specific immune mechanisms originate in the lymphatic system: humoral immunity and cellular immunity.

Humoral immunity. Based on the antibody system, this defense relies primarily on B lymphocytes, which have specialized surface receptors for particular antigens. When an antigen binds to a B cell, the cell divides and forms plasma cells that secrete large quantities of antibodies (immunoglobulins) into the circulation. The combination of antibodies with antigen activates the complement system and sets off a chain of events that lyses the cells, opsonizes bacteria, attracts leukocytes to the area, and releases histamine.

Cellular immunity. The primary opposition to viruses and fungi, this defense is mediated by T cells (lymphocytes derived from the thymus), which become activated on contact with invading pathogens. One group of T cells, known as "killer" cells, enlarge, divide, and release *lymphokines,* which attack cell membranes of the invading pathogens, activating macrophages and stimulating the synthesis of additional T cells. Once activated, the T cells can lyse antigen without the aid of the complement system.

Many cells attacked by viruses form interferon, a natural antiviral protein that helps inactivate the attackers. The infected cells release interferon, which body fluid carries to other sites, thus preventing the transmission of the virus to other cells. Although some viruses, such as those causing influenza, begin to recede when interferon levels peak, the mechanism remains obscure.

CNS involvement
When inflammatory and specific immune responses fail to contain and quell an invasion, pathogens may spread to the CNS.

Bacteria. Penetration of the subarachnoid space affords bacteria free access to the entire space, with subsequent meningeal irritation and swelling. Resulting headache and neck extensor muscle spasm produce nuchal rigidity and, in extreme cases, opisthotonos. The infection spreads into the brain substance by extending along the spaces around the blood vessels (perivascular spaces) that penetrate the pia mater to supply the underlying tissue. Involved blood vessels become engorged and may rupture or thrombose. Exudate accumulates in the ventricles and cisterns and over the convexities, resulting in increased ICP as swelling mounts.

If ICP continues to rise, brain stem decompensation results in widening pulse pressure, bradycardia, and irregular respirations. Cingulate, central, or transtentorial (uncal) brain herniation may also result. Upper brain stem compression may cause decreased level of consciousness, pupillary dilation or constriction, alteration in light reflex, loss of sensory or motor function, headache, and vomiting. The inflammatory reaction may also impair the normal venous absorption of cerebrospinal fluid (CSF), leading to an excess of CSF (hydrocephalus) and further elevation in ICP. As adjacent brain tissue becomes affected, neuronal cell death may occur.

If bacteria (from the bloodstream or from direct spread) lodge in the brain parenchyma and neutrophils accumulate over the cortex, a focal or generalized motor seizure may occur. The area becomes edematous and congested and may eventually contain a central zone of necrosis and liquefaction. A fibroglial capsule then forms. Single or even multiple areas of cavitation and pus (brain abscess) may develop over several weeks. Such infection tends to spread lesions deeply into the brain. In the relatively hypoxic abscess cavity, a mixed infection with several bacteria types usually occurs, with anaerobic organisms predominating. Abscesses may also localize between the dura mater and the arachnoid membrane (subdural empyema) or outside the dura (epidural abscess). (See *Common infections of the brain and spinal cord.*)

Viruses. Viruses produce nonsuppurative inflammation involving the cortex, white matter, and meninges and result in meningeal irritation (as shown by headache and nuchal rigidity). Viruses may also trigger autoimmune reactions to myelin, causing degeneration and cortical neuron destruction with subsequent demyelination. Depending on the specific virus, areas of hemorrhage, necrosis, and cavitation may develop. Perivascular diffuse brain edema occurs with increasing ICP.

Slow viruses may induce CNS damage by invading cells without eliciting an obvious inflammatory or immune response. A cell- and antibody-mediated immune reaction directed against virus-infected cells may cause some further cell destruction. These infections run a course over months or years.

Parasites. In response to parasitic invasion, the host releases enzymes that cause tissue destruction. If parasites have access to systemic circulation, they may cause peripheral thrombi or be embolized to the cerebral vasculature, as in cysticercosis. These emboli can occlude cerebral vessels, obstruct blood flow, and cause infarction and associated infection that resembles an abscess. Moderate-to-severe cerebral edema may occur in adjacent tissue, thus increasing ICP. Meningeal irritation may also occur.

Fungi. Fungi readily form abscesses that are associated with extensive fistula formation. This formation is usually accompanied by an intense fibrotic reaction that blocks spread of the infection but presents a formidable barrier to pharmacologic treatment.

CNS invasion by any of the pathogens commonly leads first to meningeal irritation and then to meningitis. Progressive CNS involvement diminishes the level of responsiveness and leads to seizures or focal symptoms, such as hemiparesis.

MEDICAL MANAGEMENT

Despite the many precise diagnostic procedures that are available today, the neurologic history and physical examination are still the primary sources of reliable diagnostic information about CNS infections. History may reveal important predisposing conditions or past exposure to pathogens. Physical examination establishes signs and symptoms that help pinpoint involved areas.

Diagnosis: Consider intracranial pressure
Increased ICP, which usually accompanies CNS infections, contraindicates certain diagnostic tests. For instance, lumbar puncture in a patient with increased ICP (especially with an abscess or brain tumor) can precipitate brain herniation, so ICP should be evaluated by intracranial monitoring and through assessment of clinical signs and symptoms before other tests begin.

Tests used to diagnose neuroinfective disease may include CT scan, angiography, X-ray, lumbar puncture, and brain biopsy. (See *Diagnostic tests,* page 80, and *Managing fungal and parasitic infections,* page 81.)

Common infections of the brain and spinal cord

Meningitis

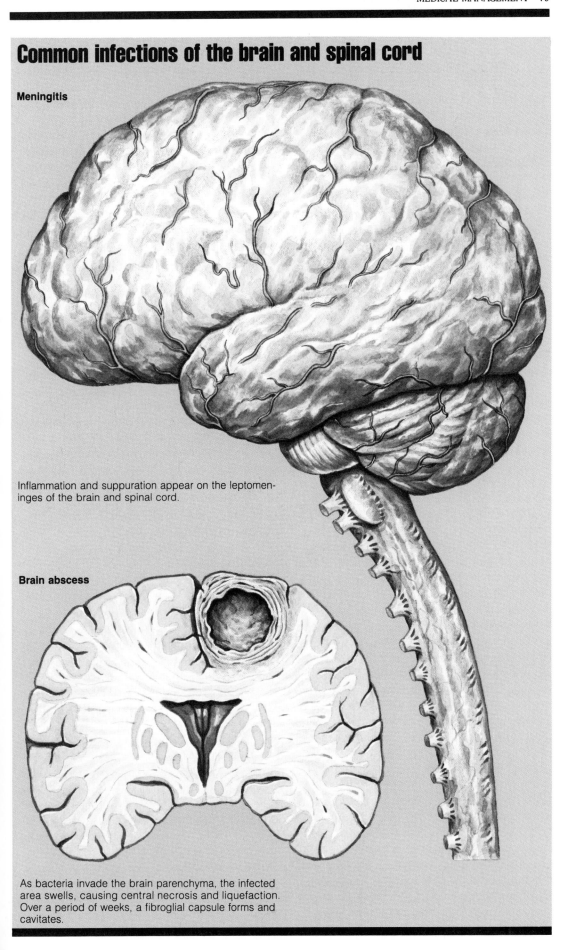

Inflammation and suppuration appear on the leptomeninges of the brain and spinal cord.

Brain abscess

As bacteria invade the brain parenchyma, the infected area swells, causing central necrosis and liquefaction. Over a period of weeks, a fibroglial capsule forms and cavitates.

Diagnostic tests

These tests help diagnose neuroinfective diseases.

Computerized tomography (CT) scan

• May show altered tissue density and increased or displaced vascularity to help identify abscess, calcification, cerebral edema, hydrocephalus, infarction, tumor, middle ear/sinus pus collections
• May use contrast medium for sharper image

Cerebral angiography

• Serves as definitive diagnostic tool for vascular conditions
• Detects and defines space-occupying (even avascular) lesions
• Evaluates vessel lumen for patency, thrombosis, occlusion
• Detects vessel displacement, indicating mass effect from abscess, brain herniation, cerebral edema

X-ray study

• Identifies disease foci
• May show sinus/mastoid disease, pineal shift, signs of chronic elevated intracranial pressure (ICP), gas in abscess cavity

Lumbar puncture

• Helps diagnose CNS infections, especially meningitis
• Gives direct ICP information from CSF pressure readings
• Can identify causative organism through stains and cultures
• Measures protein, glucose, and red and white blood cells through laboratory analysis
• Helps identify causative organism and susceptibility to specific antibiotics through culture and sensitivity tests
• May be contraindicated in meningitis with increased ICP (danger of herniation). Preliminary CT scan advised in suspected abscess

Brain biopsy

• Identifies cause of fungal/parasitic infections
• May be only way of diagnosing some viral infections, such as herpes simplex encephalitis

Bactericidal treatment

Antimicrobial therapy should be bactericidal, not merely bacteriostatic. Antibiotic selection must take into account penetration rates of blood-brain and blood-CSF barriers. Because meningeal inflammation impairs the blood-CSF barrier, antibiotic penetration increases unpredictably and variably.

Penicillins. Penicillinase-susceptible penicillins (penicillin G, ampicillin, and carbenicillin) can achieve high blood levels and effectively penetrate the blood-CSF barrier. They are effective against *Clostridium, Enterobacter, Neisseria, Proteus, Pseudomonas,* staphylococci, streptococci, and *Treponema pallidum.* In high doses, however, penicillins can cause seizures.

Penicillinase-resistant penicillins (methicillin, oxacillin, and nafcillin) are used against group A beta-hemolytic streptococci, pneumococci, and penicillin G–sensitive and penicillin G–resistant staphylococci.

Cephalosporins. Like penicillins, cephalosporins are bactericidal and effective against group A and viridans streptococci, *Streptococcus pneumoniae,* penicillin G–sensitive and penicillin G–resistant staphylococci, *Neisseria,* and gram-negative bacteria, such as *Escherichia coli, Proteus mirabilis, Klebsiella, Bacterioides fragiles, Shigella,* and *Hemophilus influenzae.*

Aminoglycosides. The aminoglycosides (neomycin, kanamycin, gentamicin) cross the blood-CSF and blood-brain barriers so poorly that they're effective only when intravenous and intrathecal therapy are combined. Aminoglycosides are usually effective against *Proteus, Pseudomonas, Klebsiella, Escherichia coli,* and *Enterobacter* infections.

Chloramphenicol. An antibiotic that significantly penetrates the blood-brain barrier, chloramphenicol also crosses the blood-CSF barrier exceedingly well. It's generally effective in treating *Hemophilus influenzae* and *Bacterioides* infections. *Bacterioides* infections frequently resist penicillin, but nearly all strains succumb to chloramphenicol.

At present, antiviral agents have proved ineffective against all CNS viral infections except herpes simplex encephalitis. Corticosteroids, such as dexamethasone (Decadron), and hyperosmolar agents, such as mannitol (Osmitrol) and urea (Ureaphil), are essential to combat cerebral edema and inflammation in patients with increased ICP. However, because corticosteroids may hasten the spread of viral infection, they're used with caution where viruses are suspected. Vidarabine or ara-A (Vira-A) specifically combats herpes simplex encephalitis but is ineffective in managing any other viral infections. Treatment for herpes simplex encephalitis typically begins after brain biopsy for tissue specimens but before tests provide virologic confirmation; it is then terminated in those patients who prove not to have this virus.

Pharmacologic treatment of parasitic and fungal infections is specific to the causative pathogen. (See *Managing fungal and parasitic infections.*)

Surgery and supportive measures

Operative management is routinely required for optimal treatment of brain abscesses. It not only supplies specimens for aerobic and anaerobic cultures (spinal fluid cultures usually don't show the organisms within the abscess cavity) but also helps reduce swelling from mass effect.

Supportive measures for other body systems are of paramount importance to treatment. They include maintaining fluid and electrolyte balance; giving symptomatic treatment for fever, headache, seizures, and shock; and holding PO_2 and PCO_2 within normal limits. Hypercapnia and hypoxemia must be prevented, by mechanical ventilation if necessary, since both cause vasodilation, which increases cerebral blood volume and ICP.

NURSING MANAGEMENT

In the patient with neuroinfective disease, changing level of consciousness will probably complicate efforts to secure a complete nursing history and physical assessment.

Early in the illness, the patient may have a shortened attention span and may misinterpret environmental stimuli. He may be disoriented as to time, place, and person. He may have a poor memory, be easily bewildered, and have difficulty following commands. He may be restless, agitated, irritable (because of headache), noisy, and combative. As the illness progresses, level of consciousness deteriorates. The patient may be delusional or appear psychotic. He becomes drowsy, lethargic, and unresponsive except to repeated or vigorous stimulation. Gradually, he becomes unresponsive even to painful stimuli and shows no spontaneous movement.

With the conscious patient, you may need to take the nursing history in several short sessions. You'll have to rely on family and friends to supply missing information.

Managing fungal and parasitic infections

Disorder/organism	Diagnosis	Treatment
Fungal diseases		
Actinomycosis (Actinomyces israelii)	Tissue biopsy for Gram stain (usually reveals causative organism)	Antimicrobial: penicillin, tetracycline (alternative). Steroidal: used with antibiotics
Aspergillosis (Aspergillus fumigatus)	Tissue culture preferred, but biopsy not always possible (fungus often infests vital tissues). CSF, blood, or sputum culture (less reliable). Identification difficult (Aspergillus is a frequent laboratory contaminant)	Antimicrobial: amphotericin B with surgical excision. Steroidal: contraindicated; enhances tissue invasion and fungus dissemination
Blastomycosis (Blastomyces dermatitidis)	Brain biopsy for identification and culture. Ventricular or cisternal fluid analysis	Antimicrobial: amphotericin B. Steroidal: usually avoided
Candidiasis (Candida albicans and C. tropicalis)	Fungus finding in tissue. Fungus identification in CSF or culture. Culture mandatory (species identification cannot be made from direct smears and Candida closely resembles other organisms)	Antimicrobial: amphotericin B alone or combined with 5-fluorocytosine. Steroidal: usually avoided
Coccidioidomycosis (Coccidioides immitis)	Pathogen identification in cerebral tissue or CSF. Culture from same source (less reliable). Serologic tests: IgM precipitant (positive in about 90% of acutely ill patients)	Antimicrobial: systemic and intrathecal amphotericin B. Steroidal: usually avoided
Cryptococcosis (Cryptococcus neoformans)	CSF culture (positive in about 95% of infected patients). Analysis of sera and CSF for antigen and antibody	Antimicrobial: combination therapy with amphotericin B, 5-fluorocytosine, and miconazole. Steroidal: avoided
Histoplasmosis (Histoplasma capsulatum)	Identification of fungus in tissue (especially bone marrow) or isolation in culture	Antimicrobial: amphotericin B. Steroidal: avoided
Parasitic diseases		
Amebiasis (Entamoeba histolytica)	Identification of trophozoites in biopsy specimens from lesions or in CSF serologic tests (indirect hemagglutination antibody, complement-fixation, agar gel differentiation, indirect immunofluorescent antibody)	Antimicrobial: emetine hydrochloride, metronidazole, chloroquine, tetracycline, diiodohydroxyquin, diloxanide furoate, dehydroemetine. Steroidal: contraindicated
Cysticercosis (Taenia solium, porcine tapeworm)	Identification of parasite in nervous tissue, supported by X-ray and immunologic evidence. CT scan for revealing distinct cysts	Antimicrobial: praziquantel. Steroidal: useful to control inflammatory response
Echinococcosis (Taenia echinococcus, canine tapeworm)	Diagnosis dependent on high index of clinical suspicion. Biopsy contraindicated (contamination may imperil operative outcome). Ancillary tests: intradermal, complement-fixation, immunologic panel	Antimicrobial: surgical removal of central nervous system cyst (unilocular cyst); mebendazole (multilocular cysts). Steroidal: helpful in treating cranial nerve palsies from basilar involvement
Schistosomiasis (Schistosoma mansoni, S. haematobium, S. japonicum)	Isolation of ova in stool, urine, brain tissue, or spinal axis tissue. Ancillary tests: complement-fixation, circumoral precipitin, and indirect fluorescent antibody; CT scan for localizing lesion	Antimicrobial: niridazole (Schistosoma haematobium), oxamniquine (S. mansoni, and S. haematobium), praziquantel (S. japonicum). Steroidal: useful adjunct to antimicrobial therapy
Toxoplasmosis (Toxoplasma gondii)	Diagnosis reliant on immunologic tests (particularly rising antibody titers by complement-fixation, Sabin-Feldman dye, or indirect fluorescent antibody). Possible brain biopsy for definitive diagnosis	Antimicrobial: combination of sulfadiazine and pyrimethamine. Steroidal: large doses in acute stages to combat intense inflammatory response; taper quickly since steroids may reactivate latent cystic foci
Trichinosis (Trichinella spiralis)	Larva in blood, CSF, or muscle. Serologic tests (precipitin reaction, indirect fluorescent antibody, complement-fixation, bentonite flocculation, and latex agglutination)	Antimicrobial: thiabendazole. Steroidal: methylprednisolone produces dramatic results

The history: Determine susceptibility

Ask the patient about preexisting problems that increase susceptibility to infectious disease: alcoholism, diabetes mellitus, uremia, cirrhosis, and malnutrition. Ask about recent sore throats, ear infections, coughing or other signs of lung infection, or recent head trauma. Explore any recent history of "dirty" wounds, lacerations, or burns, which could have resulted in tetanus, and ask when the patient last received a tetanus booster. Ask, too, about predisposing conditions that affect the immune system: ischemia, blood dyscrasia, deficient cellular immunity, deficiency or absence of immunoglobulins, long-term corticosteroid therapy, chemotherapy, radiation therapy, prolonged hospitalizations, and prior surgery that interferes with the normal lymph channels. Find out if the patient has had any sexually transmitted diseases, particularly herpes simplex or syphilis.

Keep in mind those patterns of illness that specifically incline toward intracranial infection: penetrating craniocerebral trauma; compound depressed skull fracture; craniotomy; infections of the paranasal sinuses, mastoids, scalp, and face; intrathoracic infections, such as lung abscess and bronchiectasis; congenital heart disease causing left-to-right shunting of blood; recent viral infection or exposure; and a distal chronic septic focus, such as diverticulitis or osteomyelitis. Ask if the patient's ever had tuberculosis or a positive reaction to a skin test. Also consider a history of malaria, histoplasmosis, coccidioidomycosis.

Ask about presenting symptoms to help localize the infection. Try to find out from the patient or family about any abnormal motor function, when it began, what the first symptom was, and whether the dysfunction is worsening. If the patient experienced seizures before admission, ask about onset and progression, what parts of the body were involved, any deviation of the eyes to one side, and any loss of respiratory function or bowel or bladder control.

Consider symptoms that point to increased ICP, but remember that such pressure may rise without any symptoms. Symptoms tend to relate to the location and cause of increased pressure and to the rate of increase. One such cause may be meningitis with purulent exudate, cerebral edema, and hydrocephalus. Ask how long symptoms have been present and if they're growing more severe.

In taking the environmental history, tactfully evaluate the hygienic quality of the patient's living situation, and find out if he lives with pets or near farm animals that may carry parasites. To identify parasitic infections, ask if he's been traveling abroad or to a different region of the country. Ask about his work environment to rule out exposure to other hazards, such as nitrogen mustard or radiation; these may depress bone marrow function, causing agranulocytosis and increased susceptibility to bacterial infection. If symptoms point to botulism, explore the patient's diet history and methods of food preparation, including home canning.

Focus the social history on the patient's family life and support systems. Talk to family members and friends to get health information about your patient, and try to learn their perceptions of the patient's illness. Remember that disorders affecting the brain may scare them into hostile, angry, or guilty reactions, which are counterproductive to the patient.

Physical exam: The systems approach

Begin the physical exam by taking vital signs. Widened pulse pressure, decreased pulse, irregular respirations, and vomiting are symptomatic of brain stem pressure that can lead to herniation, either central or transtentorial (uncal). Key signs and symptoms of such herniation include diminishing level of consciousness, pupillary dilation or constriction with reduced response to light, elevated blood pressure, decreased pulse, widening pulse pressure, changing respiratory function, diminishing sensory function, hemiparesis, hemiplegia, headache, and vomiting. Remember that herniation may also develop in the patient who's not responding to treatment. Thoroughly assess the patient's neurologic status, beginning with level of consciousness. Describe in detail the degree of stimulation needed to rouse the patient and the appropriateness of his verbal responses, avoiding vague labels such as "confused." Precise descriptions will allow others participating in the patient's care to identify subtle changes that could signal deterioration.

Next, assess cranial nerve function and motor activity to help localize the infection. Generalized tonic-clonic seizures may indicate cerebral cortex irritation. Focal seizures, paresis, or paralysis can help pinpoint the affected area. Assess for stiff neck and other signs of meningeal irritation (see *Testing for meningitis*). Ask the patient to flex his neck forward without your help; then attempt to flex his neck yourself. You may find this difficult

Testing for meningitis

Brudzinski's sign

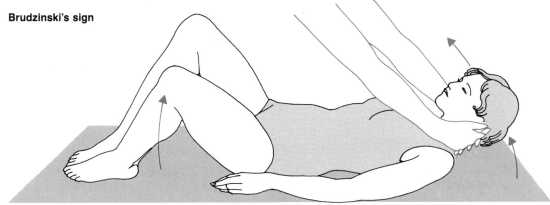

With the patient supine, place your hand behind her neck and bring the head forward to the chest. In meningitis, the patient responds by flexing hips and knees.

Kernig's sign

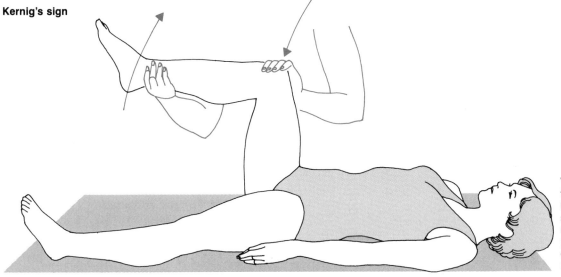

With the patient supine, flex one leg at the hip and knee to 90° and then straighten the knee. In meningitis, the patient experiences pain because of meningeal and spinal root inflammation.

because of spasm in the extensor neck muscles, which may involve back muscles and may be severe enough to cause opisthotonos. Remember that forced flexion will produce severe pain.

Look for other signs of bacterial meningitis. Headache, usually the initial symptom, tends to be severe, probably because of irritation of pain-sensitive dura and traction on related vascular structures. Photophobia, too, is a common sign although the pathophysiology is unclear. Fever may rise to 103° F. (39.5° C.) or sometimes higher and may remain high throughout the course of the illness. In terminal stages, it may rise to 105° F. (40.5° C.) or higher because of damage to brain stem centers concerned with temperature regulation as a result of increased ICP. Also be sure to examine other body systems to evaluate the disease's secondary effects.

Planning and implementing care

Since increased ICP and its complications usually attend CNS infections, monitoring ICP is a vital aspect of your nursing intervention. This means closely watching the effect of both disease and treatment to quash any ICP increase before it can cause permanent neurologic damage. It also means preventing hypoxia and hypercapnia, both potent vasodilators that can raise ICP.

With a complete assessment and identification of patient problems, you can begin to formulate your nursing diagnoses and determine a care plan. Your plan may include these typical nursing diagnoses:

Potential for cerebral injury related to increased ICP. To maintain normal ICP, elevate the head of the bed 30° at all times unless otherwise ordered. Explain to the patient that neck flexion can obstruct venous return and increase ICP and that acute hip flexion and the prone position can increase intra-abdominal or intrathoracic pressure and interfere with cerebral blood vessel drainage.

Carefully observe and monitor respiration and ventilation to keep PO_2 and PCO_2 in normal ranges. Ask the doctor for specific

Three ways to monitor intracranial pressure

Elevated intracranial pressure (ICP) may cause life-threatening complications in central nervous system infections. Here are three ICP surveillance methods:

Ventricular catheter monitoring, the most direct and accurate method, permits evaluation of brain compliance and drainage of large amounts of cerebrospinal fluid (CSF). It also carries the greatest risk of infection. A small rubber catheter enters the lateral ventricle through a burr hole, and its fluid-filled line connects to a domed transducer and a display monitor. If ICP is elevated, pressure exerted on the in-line fluid depresses the dome's diaphragm.

Subarachnoid screw monitoring carries less risk of infection and tissue damage because the screw doesn't penetrate the cerebrum. Instead, it enters the subarachnoid space, then connects to a transducer as in ventricular catheter monitoring.

Epidural sensor monitoring, the least invasive method with the lowest risk of infection, provides questionable accuracy since it doesn't measure ICP directly from a CSF-filled space. Instead, it uses a fiber-optic sensor placed in the epidural space, with cable connection to a monitor.

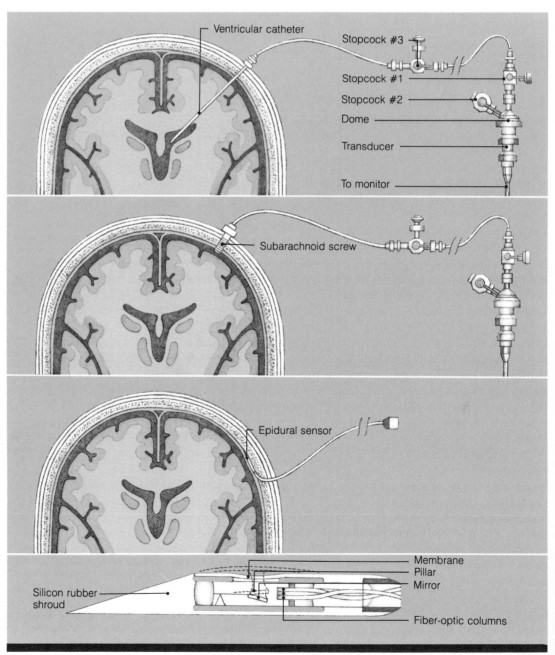

Ventricular catheter

Stopcock #3
Stopcock #1
Stopcock #2
Dome
Transducer
To monitor

Subarachnoid screw

Epidural sensor

Membrane
Pillar
Mirror

Silicon rubber shroud

Fiber-optic columns

instructions on suctioning and coughing because these may dangerously increase ICP.

Continuously monitor ICP for changes. (See *Three ways to monitor intracranial pressure*.) If ICP increases, begin necessary medical treatment as ordered. This may include osmotic diuretics or corticosteroids to reduce cerebral edema and ICP and fluid restriction to decrease extracellular fluids. To avoid complications of drug therapy, you should be aware of the possibility of specific drug interactions, paradoxical responses, and toxic or adverse effects. Your interventions have succeeded if the patient's ICP, serum electrolyte levels, and level of consciousness remain or return to normal.

Potential for alteration in cerebral oxygen demand related to fever. Prevent hypoxia by assessing body temperature at least every 4 hours. Administer antipyretics, as ordered (commonly acetaminophen since aspirin can increase metabolism). Keep room temperature comfortable, remove excess clothing and bedding, and administer tepid baths when the patient is feverish. If ordered, use a hypothermia blanket to reduce temperature. Administer chlorpromazine (Thorazine), if ordered, to control shivering, and appropriate antibiotics to maintain therapeutic blood level and to control infection. Your interventions have succeeded if the patient's temperature remains or returns to normal.

Potential for nosocomial infection. To prevent nosocomial infection, check your institution's infection control policy and take appropriate measures. These measures may range from simple handwashing to enteric precautions or even strict or reverse isolation.

Explain infection control measures to the patient and his family, and stress the importance of their cooperation. Consider your interventions successful if the patient remains free of further infection and his family and the hospital staff do not contract his infection.

Alteration in comfort: Headache and photophobia related to increased intracranial pressure or meningeal irritation. Make the patient more comfortable by elevating the head of the bed 30° to help decrease ICP. Keep the room dark and quiet to reduce external stimuli. Administer ordered analgesics to help relieve pain. Ask the patient which activities provoke or worsen his headache, and help him define factors other than drugs that relieve it. Your interventions have succeeded if the patient is pain-free or as comfortable as possible.

Alteration in comfort: Hyperirritability in response to environmental stimuli related to meningeal irritation. Help the patient tolerate environmental stimuli by keeping the room dark and quiet. Speak to him quietly as you approach to avoid startling him. Provide uninterrupted rest periods by coordinating care around times when the patient is awake and by counseling family members to limit visits to appropriate times. Discourage radio, television, and newspapers. Explain these measures to the patient and his family. Administer ordered sedatives if the patient is restless. Your interventions have succeeded if the patient rests comfortably and his family understands the need for reduced stimulation.

Potential for injury related to seizure activity. Guard the patient's safety during possible seizures by instituting prior precautions: Keep the bed in a low position with the side rails up and padded; keep an oral or nasal airway taped to the head of the bed and a suction setup available at bedside to prevent aspiration of secretions. Carefully observe, record, and report any suspicious seizure-like movements. Administer anticonvulsant medication (commonly phenytoin, phenobarbital, or diazepam), as ordered, to maintain therapeutic blood levels. Your interventions have succeeded if the patient suffers no seizures or sustains no seizure-related injury.

Ineffectual family coping related to patient's poor condition. Give the family emotional support by discussing their perceptions of the patient's illness. Support positive coping mechanisms, and assist family members in communicating effectively among themselves and with the patient. Give them any information they need about hospital and community resources. Allow them to express their fears and anger. Reinforce their openness with nonjudgmental interactions and emphasize that such feelings are normal. Your interventions have succeeded if the family demonstrates effective coping mechanisms.

A final word

You have a vital role to play in all aspects of managing neuroinfective disease—a role that ranges from prevention of disease to restoration of health and function. Your astute observation and timely counseling can help the patient at risk avoid infection. Your skillful care during acute infection can return the infected patient to optimum health and reduce mortality. And your teaching, patience, and concern can enable the patient and his family to cope with permanent sequelae.

Points to remember

- Neuroinfective diseases can be caused by bacteria, viruses, parasites, or fungi.
- These diseases most commonly affect the meninges.
- Bacterial parameningeal infection occurs secondary to adjacent infection of the teeth, mastoids, sinuses, scalp, face, skull, or vertebrae.
- Treatment for viral infections must be generally supportive because no effective antimicrobial treatment is yet available for most viruses.
- Nursing care includes careful monitoring of intracranial pressure to prevent serious complications of central nervous system infections.

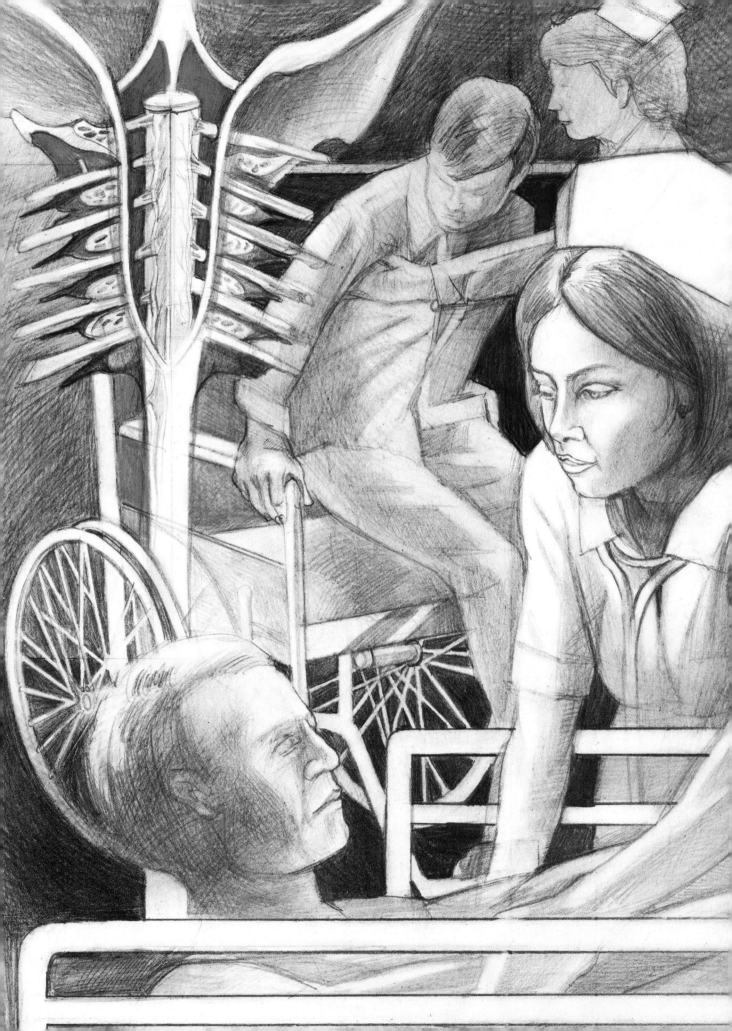

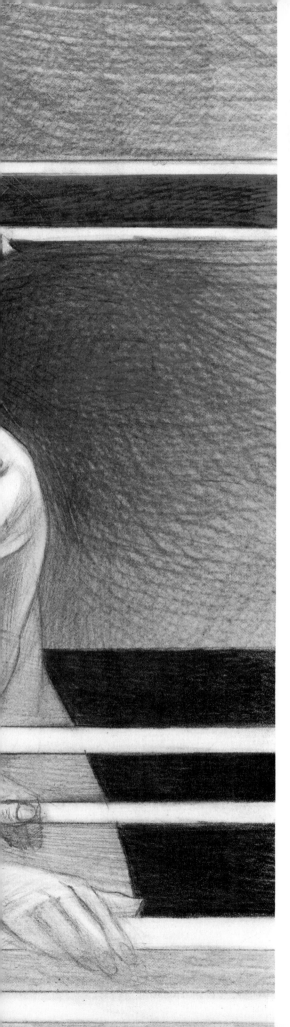

DISORDERS OF NERVE TRANSMISSION

7 MANAGING DEGENERATIVE DISEASES

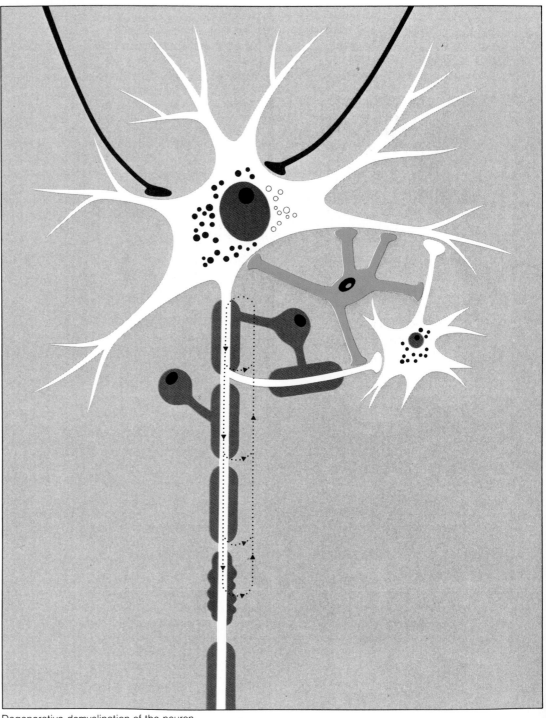

Degenerative demyelination of the neuron

Managing any of the progressively disabling degenerative diseases is undoubtedly among your most frustrating tasks. Whether you call the disease Alzheimer's, Tay-Sachs, or Werdnig-Hoffman, the prognosis is similarly grim. Treatment has little effect on the relentlessly progressive loss of neurons. However subtle the initial signs of neurologic impairment may be, they inevitably become not just obvious but devastating. You can't change this grim prognosis, but you can improve the quality of the patient's life, however short it may be. Most importantly, you can help him maintain his independence as long as possible, which supports his sense of dignity and control. You can also educate the patient and his family about the disease, which helps them prepare for and face each progressive change. Effective teaching begins with your understanding of the underlying pathology.

PATHOPHYSIOLOGY

Although the degenerative diseases produce similarly devastating—and eventually fatal—neuronal loss, they affect different areas of the central nervous system (CNS) and vary in onset, progression, and incidence (see *Clinical characteristics in neurologic degeneration,* pages 90 and 91).

Multiple sclerosis (MS), a disease notorious for its unpredictable exacerbations and remissions, involves sporadic, patchy demyelination of the white matter of the brain and spinal cord. Onset occurs between ages 19 and 30. Rapid progression of the disease may disable the patient by early adulthood or cause death within months of onset. However, 70% of patients lead active, productive lives with prolonged remissions. The disease affects women to men in a ratio of 3:2; whites to blacks, 5:1. Between 100,000 and 200,000 cases are reported annually in the United States.

Amyotrophic lateral sclerosis (ALS), also known as Lou Gehrig's disease, involves degeneration of the anterior horn cells of the spinal cord, motor nuclei of the cortex, and the corticospinal tract. Onset occurs between ages 20 and 70, and the disease is typically fatal within 2 to 3 years, usually a result of aspiration pneumonia or respiratory failure. ALS affects 3 persons in every 100,000, striking men about four times more often than women and whites more often than blacks. In about 10% of patients, ALS is inherited as an autosomal dominant trait.

Parkinson's disease (paralysis agitans) involves degeneration of the basal ganglia, particularly the substantia nigra and corpus striatum. It's associated with deficiency of dopamine, a neurotransmitter required for control of posture, support, and voluntary motion. Onset occurs between ages 40 and 60. The disease affects 100 to 150 persons in every 100,000 and typically strikes men more often than women.

Huntington's chorea involves degeneration of the cerebral cortex and basal ganglia. Like Parkinson's, it's associated with deficiency of a neurotransmitter—gamma-aminobutyric acid (GABA). Onset occurs between ages 20 and 50, and the disease is typically fatal within 15 years. Transmitted as an autosomal dominant trait, Huntington's chorea strikes men as often as women and affects approximately 6 persons in every 100,000.

Alzheimer's disease involves degeneration of the cerebral cortex, especially the frontal lobe, and is characterized by neurofibrillary tangles and senile plaques. This disease typically strikes women more often than men. In the United States, it afflicts about 500,000 persons over age 65. Onset occurs near age 50, and the disease may linger for 10 to 15 years before causing death.

The most common lipid storage disease, *Tay-Sachs disease* (amaurotic familial idiocy, or GM_2 gangliosidosis) results from deficiency of hexosaminidase A, an enzyme necessary for metabolism of gangliosides, water-soluble glycolipids found primarily in CNS tissue. Without this enzyme, accumulating lipids distend and ultimately destroy neuronal cells. This autosomal recessive disorder is quite rare, appearing in fewer than 100 births per year in the United States. However, it strikes persons of Ashkenazic (eastern European) Jewish origin, about 10 times more often than the general population, occurring once in approximately 3,600 births. About 4% of the Ashkenazic Jewish population are heterozygous carriers of the defective gene. The disease typically appears between ages 3 and 6 months and is fatal before age 5. It strikes males as often as females.

Werdnig-Hoffman disease, a lower motor neuron disease transmitted as a recessive trait, involves degeneration of anterior horn cells and cranial motor nuclei. Onset typically occurs before age 1, often in utero. The disease strikes males as often as females and is generally fatal within 4 years.

(continued on page 92)

Clinical characteristics in neurologic degeneration

Alzheimer's disease

Disease process
Slowly progressive neuronal atrophy of the cerebral cortex, especially the frontal lobe, characterized by neurofibrillary tangles and senile plaques

Signs and symptoms
In early disease, behavior changes, myoclonic jerks, memory loss, poor judgment, restlessness, anomia or aphasia, and muscle rigidity; in advanced disease, severe dementia and incontinence

Parkinson's disease

Disease process
Slowly progressive degeneration of basal ganglia, particularly the substantia nigra and corpus striatum, with deficiency of the neurotransmitter dopamine

Signs and symptoms
In early disease, tremor at rest, bradykinesia, masklike expression, fatigue, muscle rigidity, pill-rolling tremor, loss of natural ambulation movements; in advanced disease, severe muscle rigidity, dysphagia, drooling, and severe tremor

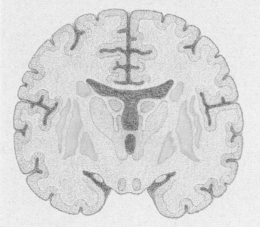

Werdnig-Hoffman disease

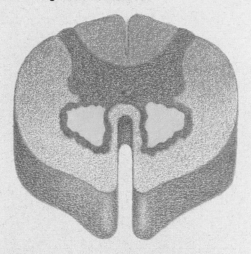

Disease process
Rapidly progressive degeneration of anterior horn cells and cranial motor nuclei

Signs and symptoms
In early disease, flaccid weakness of trunk and leg muscles and shoulder and pelvic girdles, yet mentally alert; in advanced disease, flaccid paralysis

Tay-Sachs disease

Disease process
Rapidly progressive degeneration of cerebral cortex and retina due to accumulation of lipids (lipid storage disease) associated with deficiency of the enzyme hexosaminidase A

Signs and symptoms
In early disease, cherry-red macula, decreased interest in surroundings, startle response to noise, poor vision, generalized muscle weakness, and seizures; in advanced disease, spastic quadriplegia, decerebrate rigidity, and blindness

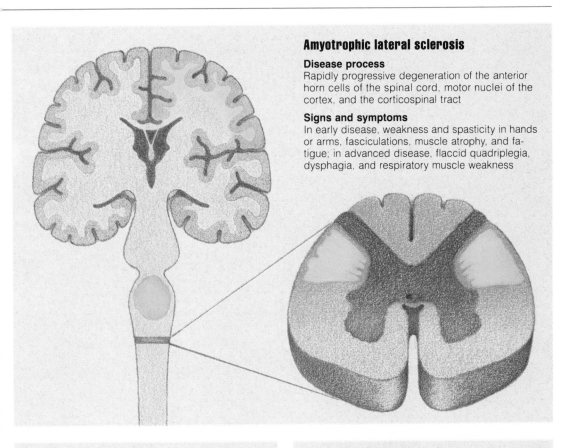

Amyotrophic lateral sclerosis

Disease process
Rapidly progressive degeneration of the anterior horn cells of the spinal cord, motor nuclei of the cortex, and the corticospinal tract

Signs and symptoms
In early disease, weakness and spasticity in hands or arms, fasciculations, muscle atrophy, and fatigue; in advanced disease, flaccid quadriplegia, dysphagia, and respiratory muscle weakness

Multiple sclerosis

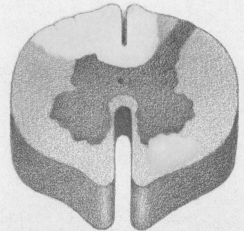

Disease process
Sporadic, patchy demyelination of the white matter of the brain and spinal cord, marked by unpredictable exacerbations and remissions

Signs and symptoms
In early disease, paresthesias, diplopia, nystagmus, central scotoma, impaired motor and sensory function, poor coordination, and, occasionally, seizures; in advanced disease, dementia, blindness, ataxia, incontinence, and spastic paraplegia

Huntington's chorea

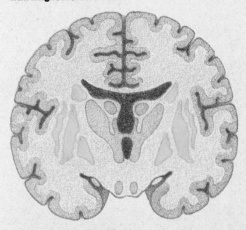

Disease process
Progressive degeneration of the cerebral cortex and basal ganglia with deficiency of the neurotransmitter gamma-aminobutyric acid

Signs and symptoms
In early disease, chorea, "dancing" walk, poor balance, and personality changes; in advanced disease, severe dementia, dysphagia, severe choreoathetosis, incontinence, and respiratory ataxia

Histologic signs of cell body degeneration

Various histologic signs may mark degeneration of the neuron's cell body. In acute cell body degeneration, such signs appear 6 to 12 hours after cellular injury. Ischemic changes include atrophy of the cell body and disintegration of Nissl bodies. Eosinophilia of the cytoplasm and a shrunken, hyperchromatic nucleus are also characteristic. In central chromatolysis, the cell body swells, and the flattened nucleus is displaced to the periphery of the cell. Nissl bodies also appear only at the cell's periphery. Typically, these changes represent the reaction of the cell body to an axonal lesion. Whether the cell completely degenerates or recovers depends on the severity of the axonal lesion. Progressive degeneration eventually causes vacuolation within the cell body, and the cytoplasm disintegrates. Glial cells phagocytose the remaining debris.

In chronic cell body degeneration, atrophy is the distinguishing characteristic. Basophilia of the cytoplasm is also present, and the nucleus appears shrunken and stains more intensely. During cell death, neurofilaments may become thick and tangled, producing the characteristic neurofibrillary tangles of Alzheimer's disease. In diseases like Tay-Sachs, abnormal accumulation of lipids within the cytoplasm eventually causes cell death. Dead cells that haven't undergone phagocytosis may absorb calcium and iron on their membranes.

Mechanisms of neuronal loss

The progressive neuronal loss that characterizes these diseases may result from primary degeneration of the neuron's cell body (see *Histologic signs of cell body degeneration*) or from demyelination. Unfortunately, what triggers cell body degeneration or demyelination often remains unclear. Possible causes of neuronal loss include trauma, genetic defect, exposure to a viral or toxic agent, or autoimmune response.

Demyelination. This process involves destruction of the myelin sheath surrounding the axon (see *Demyelination: Stripping the axon's insulating sheath*). In the central nervous system, the myelin sheath consists of tight spirals of oligodendrocytes, which swell easily in response to toxic or metabolic changes. Breakdown of the myelin sheath releases free fat and triggers a local inflammation marked by accumulation of lymphocytes. Glial cells proliferate and carry out phagocytosis, replacing the myelin with a distinct fibrous plaque. This plaque impairs conduction along the nerve fiber from one node of Ranvier to the next.

Demyelination varies in severity. In moderate demyelination, impulse conduction slows; in severe demyelination, it stops completely. Total demyelination allows degeneration of the axon itself. However, if the demyelinating process stops, regeneration of a new axon is possible from the cell body or the remaining proximal segment of the axon. Nevertheless, the regenerated axon typically fails to restore contact with the innervated structure, resulting in loss of function. Within 24 to 48 hours after relentless demyelination begins, the neuron's cell body also shows degenerative changes. In 12 days, the cytoplasm has a ground-glass appearance, except at the periphery. Whether from cell body degeneration or demyelination, neuronal loss ultimately depletes neurotransmitter receptor sites and neurotransmitters, impairing function. For example, deficiency of the neurotransmitter dopamine in Parkinson's disease results in tremors and muscle rigidity. Deficiency of GABA in Huntington's chorea results in involuntary choreoathetosis.

MEDICAL MANAGEMENT

Competent management of degenerative disease begins with accurate diagnosis, which typically involves excluding treatable disorders that may mimic degenerative disease. Unfortunately, no specific test can diagnose degenerative disease, so a series of tests is usually necessary.

What diagnostic tests reveal

Various tests help establish diagnosis in degenerative disease (see *Diagnostic testing in degenerative disease,* pages 94 and 95). Blood tests reveal enzyme deficiency and byproducts of muscle breakdown and atrophy. However, X-rays are consistently normal since degenerative disease spares the bony structures. Myelograms are likewise normal, eliminating spinal cord compression as the cause of muscle weakness. When disease involves cerebral degeneration, computerized tomography (CT) scan reveals cerebral atrophy and symmetrically enlarged ventricles. Brain or muscle biopsy may reveal characteristic degenerative cell changes. Evoked potential tests of visual, sensory, or auditory pathways may uncover slowed responses indicative of neuronal involvement. Electromyogram tests confirm abnormal muscle contraction in motor neuron disease. Genetic screening for Tay-Sachs disease identifies carriers with decreased blood levels of hexosaminidase A and affected fetuses through amniocentesis. Widespread screening for Huntington's chorea will also soon be possible. A new test, still used only in research, identifies the genetic marker for Huntington's chorea on chromosome 4 in samples of skin, blood, and other tissues of affected individuals or in fetal cells obtained by amniocentesis.

Supportive treatment

Unfortunately, treatment offers no cure for degenerative disease. Instead it aims to preserve the patient's functional ability for as long as possible and to ease his symptoms. Supportive measures include a nutritious, well-balanced diet, suitable rest and exercise, prompt treatment of infection, and generous emotional support.

Physical therapy helps maintain the patient's muscle strength and joint mobility. Assistive devices like braces, splints, or elastic bandages provide stability for weak and spastic muscle. In advanced disease, canes, walkers, or wheelchairs may be necessary for safe mobility. *Occupational therapy* helps the patient effectively manage activities of daily living. Recommending assistive devices for eating, walking, and other activities promotes independence. Therapy also explores alternative employment possibilities to prepare for worsening disability. *Drug therapy* helps control specific symptoms. Anticonvulsants prevent or reduce the frequency or severity of seizures and myoclonic movement. Antidepressants treat and help prevent recurrent depression associated with serious illness or dementia. Antipsychotics lessen irritability and modify confused thought processes characteristic of dementia. Dopamine depleters and GABA-mimetic drugs help control involuntary movement, such as tremors and chorea, in Huntington's chorea. Anticholinergics, antihistamines, antiviral compounds, ergot alkaloids, and GABA-transaminase inhibitors ease muscle rigidity and increase strength. Research into the effects of GABA-degrading enzymes and monoamine oxidase-B inhibitors, which prevent dopamine breakdown, is also currently under way.

Treatment for MS includes high-dose adrenocorticotropic hormone to reduce inflammation and ease symptoms during exacerbations of the disease and diazepam, dantrolene, and baclofen control spasticity. Experimental treatments, such as hyperbaric oxygenation, intensive immunosuppression, administration of synthetic polypeptides (Copolymer I), plasmapheresis, diet therapy with linoleic acid, and intrathecal interferon, have all produced some success, but none are yet recommended for general use.

Surgery is another treatment option for some degenerative diseases. Stereotaxic surgery temporarily relieves unilateral tremors and rigidity in Parkinson's disease. This procedure involves procaine injection, freezing, or electrocoagulation to the globus pallidus or the ventrolateral nucleus of the thalamus. It's typically reserved for young and healthy patients who are mentally sound.

NURSING MANAGEMENT
Caring for the patient with a degenerative disease can be distressing, whether you've practiced nursing for 1 year or 20. After all, you'll see the patient gradually deteriorate, mentally or physically, or both. But you mustn't overlook how much you can do to help the patient and his family. Helping begins with skillful assessment to identify changes in the patient's motor, sensory, or cognitive function that interfere with daily living.

Gather assessment data first
Begin nursing assessment with the patient history. Obtain the history from the patient or from his parents if the patient's an infant or a young child. Always view family and friends

Demyelination: Stripping the axon's insulating sheath

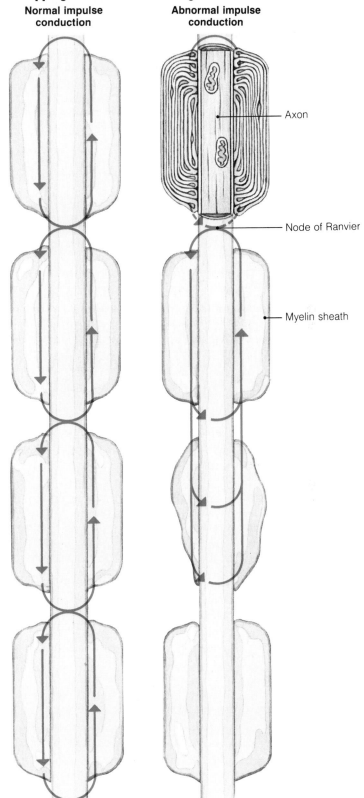

Normal impulse conduction

Abnormal impulse conduction

Axon

Node of Ranvier

Myelin sheath

Because of its high electrical resistance and low capacitance, myelin serves as an ideal insulator, efficiently conducting the action potential from one node of Ranvier to the next. Demyelination, or damage of the myelin sheath, impairs conduction, causing partial loss or dispersion of the action potential.

Diagnostic testing in degenerative disease

Alzheimer's	ALS	Huntington's	Parkinson's	MS
X-rays Normal	**X-rays** Normal	**X-rays** Normal	**X-rays** Normal	**X-rays** Normal
Myelography Normal	**Myelography** Normal	**Cerebrospinal fluid** Decreased gamma-aminobutyric acid	**Cerebrospinal fluid** Normal or decreased dopamine and its metabolites	**Myelography** Normal or enlarged spinal cord possible
Cerebrospinal fluid Normal	**Cerebrospinal fluid** Normal	**CT scan** Ventricular dilation	**CT scan** Ventricular dilation possible with diffuse cortical atrophy	**Cerebrospinal fluid** Myelin, basic protein fractions, oligoclonal bands, increased IgG in 66% of cases, slight increase in white cells
CT scan Symmetrically enlarged ventricles with widening of cortical sulci	**CT scan** Normal	**Blood studies** Normal	**Electromyography** Normal	**CT scan** Increased tissue density of white matter
Blood studies Normal	**Electromyography** Fibrillation potentials and a decreased number of motor units; nerve conduction normal	**Urine studies** Normal	**Blood studies** Normal	**Visual-evoked potentials** Abnormal in about 94% of cases
Urine studies Normal	**Blood studies** Creatine phosphokinase (CPK) normal or slightly increased	**EEG** Loss and slowing of alpha activity	**Urine studies** Normal	**Electromyography** Abnormal in advanced stages
Brain biopsy Neurofibrillary tangles and plaques with positive fuchsin staining	**Urine studies** Increased creatine Decreased creatinine		**EEG** Diffuse, nonspecific slowing of theta waves	**Blood studies** Normal
EEG Diffuse slowing in advanced disease	**Muscle biopsy** Small, angulated atrophic fibers in groups		**Other studies** Tremor studies, decreased performance in serial measurements of functional activity	**Urine studies** Normal
Other studies Frontal and temporal lobe atrophy on pneumoencephalogram	**Other studies** Decreased strength in serial muscle testing, decreased pulmonary function in pulmonary function tests, decreased swallowing ability on fluoroscopy.			**EEG** 44% to 62% of cases show nonspecific abnormalities
				Other studies Positive electronystagmography, decreased performance in serial measurements of functional activity

as a resource to fill in missing details. Besides a thorough description of the present illness, also explore the patient's medieal history as well as his religious, educational, and social background. Always try to elicit a family history of disease since some degenerative diseases, like Huntington's chorea, are hereditary. During the patient history, be sure to ask the following questions:

About symptoms. When did you first notice symptoms of disease? Describe them in detail. Are your symptoms constant or intermittent? What makes them better or worse? How do they interfere with activities of daily living? Can you bathe and dress yourself? Can you prepare and eat food without difficulty? How do you get about in your home and outside? Find out how the patient adapts to impaired function.

About therapy. Have you received any treatment? Is it helping? Have the patient describe the treatment regimen, including the name, dosage, purpose, and side effects of each drug. Determine how well he adheres to treatment. Also evaluate his understanding of the disease.

About occupation. What is your present job? Describe a typical workday, and tell how your disease interferes with your ability to do it. Can you return to work? Do any special arrangements need to be made?

About family and home life. Are you married or single? How many members are in your family? What are their roles? Try to understand the impact of the patient's disease on his family. For example, is the patient the primary breadwinner? Also note the ages of children in the family. Ask the patient if he lives in a house or an apartment. Is it acces-

Tay Sachs

X-rays
Normal

Myelography
Normal

Cerebrospinal fluid
Increased SGOT, SGPT, LDH

CT scan
Ventricular atrophy with widening of sulci

Blood studies
Increased SGOT, SGPT, LDH, CPK; decreased hexosaminidase A; large azurophilic granules in lymphocyte smears of peripheral blood

Urine studies
Normal

Brain biopsy
Neurons distended with lipids, nucleus at cell periphery, and loss of Nissl bodies

EEG
Abnormal when vision loss occurs

Other studies
Rectal biopsy with abnormal lipid accumulation in neurons of Auerbach's and Meissner's plexus; decreased hexosaminidase A in skin biopsy and tissue cultures of fibroblasts

Werdnig-Hoffman

X-rays
Normal

Myelography
Normal

Cerebrospinal fluid
Normal

Electromyography
Abnormal

Blood studies
Increased SGOT, SGPT, LDH, and CPK

Urine studies
Myoglobinuria, creatine, creatinine

Muscle biopsy
Abnormal

sible? Can he move around in it safely, or do changes need to be made?

About resources. Evaluate the patient's coping resources. Do you have many friends or relatives living nearby? Do you belong to a church or local community group? Do you know how to contact national support organizations, such as the MS society? What specific problems has the disease caused? How do you intend to solve them? The answer to this question will help you evaluate the patient's coping ability.

Perform the physical examination

Begin the physical examination by evaluating the patient's level of consciousness and mental status. Ask him to tell you his name, where he is, and the time of day. Note whether he responds promptly or slowly. Then observe his responses to simple commands, such as "Close your eyes" and "Stick out your tongue." Assess memory by noting his attention span and recall of the immediate, recent, and remote past. Also evaluate his judgment. Can he solve simple problems? When talking with the patient, note the flow of his speech, the quality of his voice, and the organization and clarity of his thoughts. Also observe the patient's emotional responses. Does he appear sad, angry, apathetic, or euphoric? Note whether he becomes agitated easily by questions, noise, or activity.

Because depression so often accompanies degenerative disease, be alert for its presence. Does the patient appear sullen or withdrawn? Does he look his stated age or older? Has he experienced recent weight loss or gain? Suspect depression if he complains of insomnia or difficulty in concentrating or if he shows disinterest in personal hygiene and physical appearance.

Evaluate motor function next. Carefully observe the patient at rest and while performing simple tasks. Are his movements slow or sudden and jerky? Note flaccid, rigid, or atrophied muscles and the presence of tremors or contractures. Do tremors occur at rest or only during motion? Observe gait and posture and note any abnormalities. Watch the patient as he walks a few steps, and check for uneven or absent correlative motion of the arms, a telling sign of Parkinson's disease (see *Parkinson's disease: A characteristic posture and gait,* page 96). Then test the tone and strength of his muscles and his balance and coordination. Because impaired motor function can affect muscles in many body systems, be alert for dysarthria; dysphagia; incontinence; and irregular, shallow, or ataxic respirations. Also ask about changes in appetite, sleep patterns, digestion, and libido, all of which may result from impaired autonomic function.

Assess sensory function. Check the patient for pain, touch, vibration, position, and discrimination sense. Evenly distribute your test stimuli over the patient's body for comprehensive testing. Note whether he perceives each stimulus appropriately and symmetrically. Listen for complaints of unusual sensations, such as tingling, burning, or crawling.

Evaluate the patient's eyes. Test visual acuity with a Snellen chart. Ask about eye strain and blurred or double vision. Then assess eye movements, noting nystagmus or eye deviation. Assess visual fields, noting loss of peripheral vision or scotomata. Closely exam-

Straight talk about the disease

Considering its many unknowns, degenerative disease is likely to frustrate and baffle the patient. That's why teaching the patient about the disease is so important. In fact, better understanding promotes better compliance with therapy. Include the patient's family in teaching because they play a pivotal role in care. Explain what is known about the etiology and course of the disease, using vocabulary the patient and his family can readily understand. Describe how the nervous system changes in disease and the associated effects on personality and motor function. Keep your teaching brief and simple, but allow time for questions. Also provide relevant literature about the disease, and refer the patient to community resources, such as the local MS chapter. Offer hope by noting research efforts to understand and cure the disease.

Next, outline the prescribed medical regimen, including the name, dosage, and purpose of each drug. Also describe significant drug side effects. Stress the importance of correct nutrition and exercise and prompt treatment of complications.

Consider your teaching effective if the patient:
• understands the effects and prognosis of his disease
• knows the name, dosage, purpose, and side effects of each prescribed drug
• adheres to therapy.

Parkinson's disease: A characteristic posture and gait

In Parkinson's disease, the patient typically assumes a stooped position when standing or walking. In advanced disease, he displays a propulsive, shuffling gait with his arms flexed and unswinging, as shown.

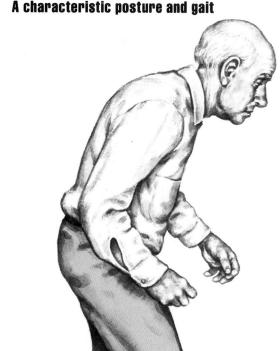

ine each eye. Is the macula cherry red with a white halo? This is a characteristic sign of Tay-Sachs disease. Also be alert for signs of eye irritation—excessive tearing, redness, discharge—and complaints of pain.

Address specific problems

Using data from the history and physical examination, you're ready to address the patient's specific problems through nursing diagnoses.

Among the nursing diagnoses that you're likely to see in degenerative diseases are:

Potential for injury related to muscle weakness or spasticity, sensory impairment, or poor judgment. To prevent injury, evaluate sensory and motor function and mental status daily to identify possible safety hazards. Help the patient ambulate and transfer in and out

of bed, as necessary. Keep the call bell within easy reach, and put side rails up when the patient's in bed. Pad his bed, as necessary, to prevent injury from severe involuntary muscle activity. Apply restraints, as needed, for the confused patient; however, never use *limb* restraints on the patient with Huntington's chorea to avoid broken bones. Outline safety measures, such as safe methods for testing bathwater, for the patient with decreased sensation. Keep the patient's environment clutter-free to prevent falls. Remove sharp objects that may cause injury from the bedside table. Consider your interventions effective if the patient doesn't sustain injury.

Potential for impaired skin integrity related to decreased mobility, impaired sensation, or inadequate nutrition. To prevent decubiti, evaluate the patient's skin every 2 hours for redness or heat. Pay special attention to pressure areas, such as those over bony prominences. Massage these areas frequently to promote circulation. Also carefully observe sacral and perineal hygiene. Wash these areas with mild soap, and lubricate skin with protective ointment. During skin care, also evaluate sensory function. To reduce pressure on the patient's skin, place a water mattress or alternating pressure pad on his bed, and use sheepskin and other protective devices. Also encourage mobility to the fullest extent possible. Help the patient ambulate or transfer from bed to chair, as his condition allows. Instruct him to shift his weight frequently while sitting in the chair. If the patient's bedridden, turn him every 2 hours.

Consider your interventions effective if the patient doesn't develop decubiti.

Alteration in nutrition related to dysphagia, tremors, or chorea. Typically, your goal is to prevent weight loss and aspiration pneumonia. To achieve this goal, first consult the dietitian to determine the patient's ideal daily caloric intake. Also consult the speech pathologist, who will evaluate dysphagia and devise an appropriate feeding program. Before feeding the patient, elevate the head of the bed 90° to ease swallowing and to reduce the risk of aspiration and choking. Offer the dysphagic patient easy-to-swallow pureed or soft foods. Remain with the patient during feeding, as necessary. Check his mouth for residual food after he swallows. Encourage the use of assistive devices, as needed, to promote independence (see *Assistive feeding devices,* page 98). Record the patient's daily caloric intake, and weigh him twice weekly.

Consider your interventions effective if the patient maintains stable, normal weight; demonstrates proper use of assistive devices; eats without choking; shows no evidence of aspiration pneumonia, such as pulmonary congestion, fever, or abnormal respiratory pattern; and meets required daily caloric intake.

Potential for fluid deficit related to decreased mobility, dysphagia, and increased perspiration. To maintain adequate hydration, encourage between 2,000 and 3,000 ml of fluid daily. Keep fluids within easy reach of the patient. Record intake and output, and weigh the patient daily to assess fluid status. Inspect mucous membranes for dryness, and assess skin turgor. To prevent aspiration, elevate the head of the bed to ease swallowing. Auscultate lung fields for congestion every shift.

Consider your interventions effective if the patient maintains normal fluid status and shows no signs of aspiration pneumonia.

Altered urinary elimination related to dementia or decreased mobility, sensation, or sphincter control. Degenerative disease may upset the patient's normal voiding pattern, causing incontinence or retention, and may promote recurrent urinary tract infection. To reestablish a normal voiding pattern, monitor the patient's intake and output. Suggest eliminating fluids after dinner to prevent nocturia. Offer the bedpan or urinal every 2 hours, or assist the patient to the bathroom, as necessary. Perform sterile intermittent catheterization, as ordered. Teach the patient this technique and the details of catheter care, when indicated. Also teach him methods of stimulating urination or ensuring complete bladder emptying, such as Credé's maneuver. Evaluate the color, concentration, odor, and pH of the patient's urine, and be alert for complaints of frequency or burning during urination. Recognize that increased limb spasticity often signals urinary tract infection in patients unable to verbally complain of discomfort. List for the patient other early signs and symptoms of urinary tract infection that require medical attention.

To prevent urinary tract infection, offer cranberry juice and vitamin C, as ordered, to acidify urine and discourage bacterial growth. Have the patient drink 2,000 to 3,000 ml of fluid daily to minimize precipitation of urinary crystals and formation of stones.

Consider your interventions effective if the patient establishes a normal voiding pattern and shows no signs of urinary tract infection.

Alteration in bowel elimination (diarrhea, incontinence, constipation) related to decreased mobility or sensation, inadequate food or fluid intake, or dementia. To establish a normal bowel routine for the patient, begin by monitoring the frequency and type of his bowel movements. Try to anticipate the patient's elimination needs, and offer the bedpan at least every other day. Explain the importance of fluid intake and high-fiber foods to establish regularity and to prevent constipation. Administer a suppository, laxative, or stool softener, as ordered. Assess the patient's abdomen for distention, and watch for nausea and anorexia.

Consider your interventions effective if the patient has a normal bowel movement at least every 2 to 3 days.

Ineffective breathing patterns related to muscle weakness and decreased mobility. Typically, your goals are to promote effective breathing, which maintains adequate oxygenation, and to prevent pneumonia. Assess the patient's lung fields every shift and evaluate respiratory rate, rhythm, and depth every 4 hours. Also note lip and nail-bed color, and evaluate level of consciousness. Teach the patient diaphragmatic and pursed-lip breathing for optimal respiration. Have him cough and deep breathe every 4 hours when he's awake. Perform chest percussion and suction, as needed. Administer oxygen, as ordered.

Consider your interventions effective if the patient uses effective breathing patterns, maintains adequate oxygenation, and has clear lung fields on auscultation.

Impaired mobility related to muscle weakness or rigidity, tremors, or chorea. To maintain mobility as long as possible, perform passive range-of-motion exercises—or, if the patient's condition permits, encourage active range-of-motion exercises—at least three times daily. Show the patient how to safely transfer out of bed, and encourage him to take frequent walks. Teach the patient how to use assistive ambulatory aids, and refer him for physical or occupational therapy, as ordered. Note the effects of drugs on the patient's mobility.

Consider your interventions effective if the patient demonstrates safe mobility at his optimal level, uses assistive devices properly, and understands how the drugs he's taking affect his mobility.

Altered thought process related to dementia. Your nursing goals are to minimize irritability and confusion and to keep the patient oriented

Caring for the patient's family

Supporting the family as they witness the patient's decline is a formidable challenge. Their needs are many, and often you will be the one expected to fill them. Recognize that the patient's disease and its prognosis will affect each family member differently, depending on his personality, relationship to the patient, age, previous experience with illness and death, and religious beliefs. Anticipate the need for genetic counseling when the patient has a known hereditary disease.

Describe what the family should expect at each stage of the disease. For example, assure them that irritability and emotional behavior stem from the patient's disease and aren't intentional. Encourage them to allow the patient to do as much for himself as possible to maintain independence. Also urge them to involve the patient in family life to maintain his sense of value and belonging. Teach the family all aspects of home care, including feeding the patient, caring for his elimination needs, and ensuring his safety.

Throughout the patient's illness, encourage the family not to neglect themselves. The emotional or financial crisis brought on by the patient's illness may severely strain family ties. Don't hesitate to suggest counseling, and encourage them to draw on community resources as well as relatives and friends. Consider your interventions effective if the family:
• verbalizes understanding of the patient's disease
• demonstrates knowledge of at-home care techniques
• displays use of effective coping mechanisms.

Assistive feeding devices

Various devices can help the patient with limited arm mobility to feed himself. Of course, the patient must be able to assume Fowler's or semi-Fowler's position to use these devices properly.

Before introducing the patient to an assistive feeding device, assess his ability to master it. Don't introduce a device the patient can't manage, to avoid discouragement and frustration. If his condition is progressively disabling, encourage the patient to use the device only until his mastery of it falters.

Introduce the assistive device before mealtime, with the patient seated in a normal eating position. Explain its purpose, show the patient how to use it, and encourage him to practice using it.

After meals, wash the assistive device thoroughly and store it in the patient's bedside stand so it doesn't get misplaced. Document the patient's progress, and share breakthroughs with staff and family members to help reinforce the patient's independence. Devices you can use include:

• *Plate guards,* which block food from spilling off the plate, help all patients who have difficulty feeding themselves. Attach the guard to the side of the plate opposite the hand the patient uses to feed himself. Guiding the patient's hand, show him how to push food against the guard to secure it on the utensil. Then have him try again with food of a different consistency. When the patient tires, feed him the rest of the meal. At subsequent meals, encourage the patient to feed himself for progressively longer periods until he can feed himself an entire meal.

• *Long-handled utensils* can help the patient with limited range of elbow and shoulder motion.

• *Utensils with built-up handles* can help the patient with diminished grasp. They are commercially available, but you can easily make them by wrapping tape around the handle of a fork or spoon.

• *Universal cuffs* help the patient with flail hands or diminished grasp. The cuff contains a slot that holds a fork or spoon. Attach it to the hand the patient uses to feed himself. Then place a fork or spoon in the cuff slot. If necessary, bend the utensil to facilitate feedings.

• *Swivel spoons* can help the patient with limited range of forearm motion. They can be used with universal cuffs.

for as long as possible. Evaluate the patient's level of consciousness at least every 8 hours. Orient the patient to person, place, and time, as needed. Assess his memory and attention span. Have him perform short tasks within his attention span to provide stimulation. Keep the patient's environment safe and relatively unchanged since familiarity promotes stability. Minimize noise and other negative stimuli. Supervise the confused patient to ensure his safety. Administer drugs, as ordered.

Consider your interventions effective if the patient remains oriented for as long as possible and sustains no injury due to confusion or poor judgment.

Impaired verbal communication related to dysarthria, muscle weakness, or dementia. Maintaining communication with the patient is crucial because degenerative disease will probably make him feel isolated. When talking with the patient, evaluate the clarity and loudness of his voice and the coherence of his thoughts. Ask the patient several questions that require a one-word or yes/no answer. Note whether he responds slowly or promptly. Assess the patient's reading ability by having him read and interpret a paragraph from a newspaper or magazine. Then dictate a short sentence for him to write. Consult a speech therapist, as necessary, to identify a speech deficit. Encourage the patient to use a language board, pictures, or gestures to compensate for a speech deficit.

Consider your interventions successful if the patient can communicate effectively.

Altered sleep pattern related to depression, anxiety, autonomic disturbance, or dementia. To restore a normal, restful sleep pattern, first establish a regular bedtime. Decrease stimuli 1 hour before bedtime to help the patient relax. Also allow him to express his feelings about the disease or its treatment to relieve anxiety. At bedtime, straighten or change bed linens, as necessary, and fluff the patient's pillow. Then position him comfortably. If he appears distressed, restless, or in pain, provide comfort and reassurance, or give ordered drugs. Be sure the patient's room temperature is comfortable, then dim unit lights and try to minimize noise.

Consider your interventions effective if the patient establishes a normal sleep pattern and obtains adequate rest.

Ineffective patient coping related to progressive loss of function and altered self-image. One of your most important nursing goals in degenerative disease is to maintain the patient's ability to function. Recognize that depression and anxiety can be major obstacles to achieving this goal. In fact, the patient may seriously contemplate suicide because he fears mental and physical deterioration and doesn't want to burden his family or society with his care. So carefully evaluate the patient's emotional response to his disease. Allow him to grieve for the loss of his former life-style. Discuss problems that arise from the disease, and try to help him solve them. Review your care plan with the patient and his family, emphasizing what the patient can do to manage his physical, personal, and social needs. Above all, focus on the patient's strengths, and encourage activities that promote self-esteem and a positive self-image. Help him set realistic goals in light of his disability. Encourage him to pursue vocational goals, and support him in his current occupation, when possible. If the patient has continued difficulty coping, don't hesitate to suggest counseling. Administer drugs, as ordered.

Consider your interventions effective if the patient verbalizes adjustment to his disease, displays a positive self-image, and sets realistic goals for maintaining optimal function.

Self-care deficit related to impaired motor function (muscle weakness and atrophy, tremors, chorea) or dementia. Although you can't restore the patient's lost motor or cognitive function, you can help him care for himself and maintain his independence. Begin by arranging for occupational therapy, as ordered, to identify the patient's specific needs. Then provide and encourage use of assistive devices. Advise the patient to modify his wardrobe for easy dressing, for example, by replacing buttons and shoe laces with Velcro strips. Apply wrist weights to decrease tremors. Space activities to avoid tiring or confusing the patient.

Consider your interventions effective if the patient performs activities of daily living safely and as independently as possible.

Combine skill and compassion

Degenerative neurologic disease typically strikes those in the prime of life, forcing them to accept often difficult life-style changes and, what's most painful, to face their own premature mortality. Effectively caring for such a patient demands all your professional skills in meeting the patient's overwhelming physical needs. More importantly, it demands the generosity to show genuine compassion in positive ways.

Points to remember

• Degenerative neurologic disease is characterized by a relentlessly progressive loss of neurons. Cure is unknown.
• Neuronal loss may result from cell body degeneration or from demyelination.
• No specific diagnostic test can confirm degenerative disease. Instead, diagnosis typically involves systematically excluding other possible causes of signs and symptoms.
• Nursing care aims to maintain the patient's independence for as long as possible, to prevent or manage the many complications of the disease, and to provide comprehensive emotional support for both the patient and his family.

8 MAINTAINING FUNCTION IN MOBILITY DISORDERS

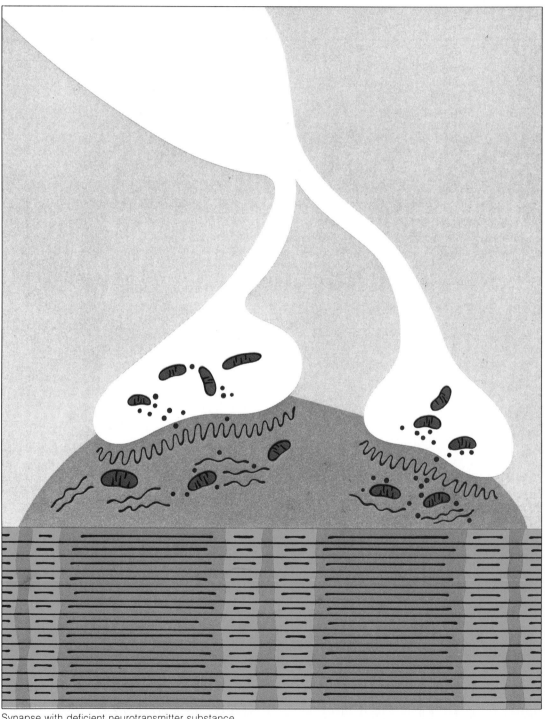

Synapse with deficient neurotransmitter substance

f you've ever cared for patients with disorders affecting mobility, you're familiar with the physical impairments they suffer and the extensive care they may require. In some patients, at some time during the illness, these disorders produce total immobility, which may or may not relent as the acute phase runs its course. With mobility compromised, contractures, decubiti, and cardiopulmonary complications become definite risks that only vigorous and skillful nursing care can prevent.

You also know the importance of emotionally supporting the patient during his adjustment to what's usually a chronic debility and of helping him accept his illness. Perhaps you've helped parents of a child with cerebral palsy or muscular dystrophy overcome guilt feelings and the urge to assume responsibility for a congenital or genetic defect.

Since no therapy has proved completely worthwhile in stemming the effects of these debilitative disorders, the patient's recovery and future mobility level depend largely on your nursing care and emotional support. Knowing all you can about normal muscle control and the aberrant mechanisms that disrupt it will enable you to give the patient the total care he needs and to train his family to continue his care after discharge.

Four major categories

Neuromuscular disorders affecting mobility may be classified as neuromuscular transmission disorders, peripheral acquired neuropathies, genetically determined myopathies, and disorders resulting from damage to an immature central nervous system (CNS). Examples of these major categories follow. Apart from Guillain-Barré syndrome, which usually resolves, all are chronic.

Neuromuscular transmission disorders. Myasthenia gravis (MG), a disorder of neuromuscular transmission that is thought to be autoimmune, results from deactivation of acetylcholine (ACH) receptor sites, which are necessary for normal impulse transmission to the muscle. The disease strikes 2 to 10 persons per 100,000, usually women in their 20s or 30s or men from 40 to 60. MG tends to worsen progressively with occasional remissions. It's fatal for about 5% to 10% of patients because the paralysis progresses to the respiratory muscles and impairs breathing.

Peripheral acquired neuropathies. Guillain-Barré syndrome (GB), also called idiopathic polyneuritis, is considered an autoimmune but postinfectious process that strikes peripheral nerves. A relatively uncommon neuromuscular disorder, it affects men and women equally between the ages of 30 and 50. GB is generally reversible and, with optimal care, shows low mortality; however, about 5% of patients experience recurrence.

Genetically determined myopathies. Muscular dystrophies (MDs) are myopathies inherited as X-linked recessive, autosomal dominant, or autosomal recessive traits. Duchenne type (pseudohypertrophic) MD, the most common form, occurs in 20 to 30 live births per 100,000. Its symptoms appear early, usually beginning between ages 3 and 5, and typically progress to fatal outcome by adolescence. Three less common types—facioscapulohumeral MD, limb-girdle MD, and myotonic dystrophy—have a later onset and a slower progression.

CNS damage disorders. Cerebral palsies (CPs) result from CNS damage, usually related to trauma during labor and delivery or to intrauterine infection. Pinpointing incidence is difficult because causes are chiefly accidental; however, these disorders are not rare. Spastic CP with muscle and mental impairment afflicts about 70% of CP patients; athetoid and ataxic CP are less common. Prognosis varies greatly with the disorder's severity and with the quality of treatment.

PATHOPHYSIOLOGY

Because neuromuscular diseases have various causes—they may be genetic or acquired—they impair mobility through various mechanisms. These mechanisms include dysfunctional transmission, muscle degeneration, and neuronal death in CNS motor pathways.

Dysfunctional transmission

GB and MG both impair the transmission of nerve impulses. Normally, transmission depends on intact myelinated fibers and on normal anatomy and chemical physiology at the myoneural (neuromuscular) junction. In MG, impulse transmission is disrupted at the postsynaptic site.

GB and MG appear to result from an autoimmune response. In GB, this seems to be an autoimmune reaction to myelin that is triggered by a preceding viral infection. In MG, antibodies form against acetylcholine receptor sites in the muscle. In GB, myelin sheaths and sometimes the axons as well deteriorate (see *Nerve degeneration in Guillain-Barré syndrome,* page 102).

Nerve degeneration in Guillain-Barré syndrome

In Guillain-Barré syndrome, the myelin sheath of peripheral nerves and of anterior and posterior roots at spinal segmental levels demyelinate and degenerate. Early in the disease, inflammation and edema occur. Later, patchy demyelination causes Schwann cell loss, leaving a widened node of Ranvier. Since both the dorsal and ventral roots are involved, signs of both sensory and motor impairment appear. These include paresthesias such as numbness, tingling, and burning; and lower motor neuron paralysis with areflexia, caused by degeneration of the motor neuron axon that exits from the spinal cord in the ventral root.

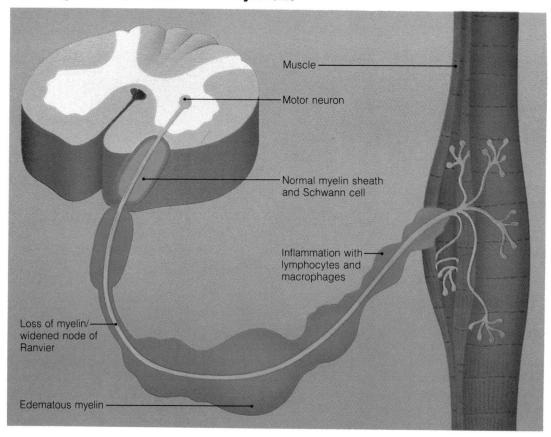

Muscle

Motor neuron

Normal myelin sheath and Schwann cell

Inflammation with lymphocytes and macrophages

Loss of myelin/ widened node of Ranvier

Edematous myelin

Transmission of nerve impulses can be delayed or blocked, even if the myelinated fibers remain intact, because of presynaptic or postsynaptic pathologic changes at the myoneural junction. In MG, these changes are postsynaptic. Antibodies block and destroy ACH receptor sites on the postsynaptic membrane, making less sites available and causing muscle weakness and fatigability. Typically, patients with this condition feel stronger early in the day but notice that their strength wanes as their muscles are used repeatedly.

In GB paralysis and in MG, fatigability causes muscle weakness and impairs mobility. Both diseases affect skeletal and bulbar muscles, causing peripheral limb weakness and weakness or paralysis, or both, in areas controlled by the cranial nerves. Because both diseases can involve respiratory muscles, there is a great danger of respiratory failure. Reduced vital capacity and tidal volume can lead to respiratory distress or arrest. In MG, cardiac distress is secondary to respiratory distress. In GB, cardiac distress is secondary to autonomic nerve fiber involvement. Other autonomic involvement in GB includes blood pressure changes and urinary retention. Neither GB nor MG affect mental capacity.

Muscle degeneration

The fundamental defect in MD is not well understood, but it may be abnormal cell membranes or some type of abnormal cellular metabolism in muscle fibers. The fibers slowly degenerate and waste away, eventually causing severe disability. Buildup of fat cells and fibrous tissue makes these weak muscles look paradoxically large. These degenerative changes develop in individual fibers and small groups of adjacent fibers. (See *Where muscular dystrophies strike,* page 104.)

Motor neuron death

CP results from damage to the brain's motor pathways in utero, during delivery, or shortly after birth. Prenatal causes include maternal infections by viruses, such as rubella, toxoplasmosis, cytomegalic virus, and herpes; adverse conditions that affect the intrauterine fetal environment, such as preeclamptic toxemia, renal disease, maternal diabetes, radiation, malnutrition, and placental insufficiency; and numerous inborn (genetic) metabolism errors. Perinatal problems, such as fetal distress from prolonged labor, complicated delivery, or premature birth, can bring on hypoxia and asphyxia, the most common causes of

CP. Neonatal causes include kernicterus and infections (easily caught in the nursery) that may cause brain damage, such as gram-negative meningitis.

Neuronal death from these insults to the immature CNS causes different types of CP. Changes in the cerebral cortex and subcortical areas cause atrophy and cavitation and affect the patient's mobility in various ways: Spastic CP, the most common form, produces increased muscle tone, hyperreflexia, and weakened limbs (hemiplegia, diplegia); extrapyramidal CP produces athetoid or dystonic limb movements; and ataxic CP produces poor coordination and balance.

Permanent and nonprogressive, CP produces deficits in muscle tone, motor control, coordination, and posture. All forms may be associated with mental retardation and speech impairment. Pathologic involvement varies with the time and extent of brain injury and may become more obvious as the child grows.

MEDICAL MANAGEMENT

A complete neurologic history, including the type of mobility impairment, its onset and progression, a thorough medical and surgical history, and a thorough physical examination, are necessary for differential diagnosis in neurologic disorders. The physical examination includes evaluation of cranial nerve function, reflexes, and sensory function. Diagnosis of CP relies heavily on clinical observation of the disorder's progression and on precise neurologic assessment.

Tests support diagnosis

Specific tests can determine or verify the neurologic diagnosis.

I.V. anticholinesterase. The most reliable test for MG is I.V. injection of an anticholinesterase and evaluation of its response. This test strongly suggests MG when 2 to 10 mg of edrophonium chloride produces improved muscle function within 1 minute, or 2 mg of neostigmine bromide produces improved muscle function within 30 minutes. The effects, however, are transient.

Cerebrospinal fluid (CSF) analysis. Analysis of protein level and pressure in CSF, through a series of lumbar punctures, can help diagnose GB. CSF protein may be normal in the early stages, but it rises as the disease progresses. However, CSF pressure may be elevated even initially in severe cases.

Muscle biopsy. Muscle biopsy showing characteristic muscle fiber changes confirms MD.

Tissue changes in Duchenne type muscular dystrophy

Normal muscle fibers

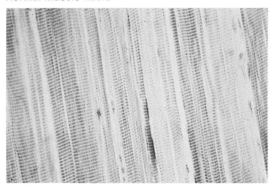

Duchenne type MD

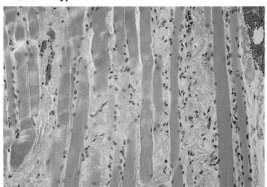

Biopsy of muscle tissue shows changes characteristic of Duchenne type muscular dystrophy (MD). Normal muscle fibers have little connective tissue between them. All are about equal in size, with nuclei at the cells' periphery. In Duchenne type MD, fibers vary in size, connective tissue increases, and nuclei move to the cells' centers.

(See *Tissue changes in Duchenne type muscular dystrophy*.) Electron microscopic studies of muscle biopsy material in MG, depending on the disease's stage, show postsynaptic membrane changes with a reduced number of ACH receptor sites.

Electromyography (EMG). EMG and nerve conduction studies help confirm MG, GB, and MD. In MG, the EMG recording shows a diminishing amplitude of response with repetitive nerve stimulations. In GB, the EMG may show reduced nerve conduction speed. In MD, the EMG recording shows reduced motor unit potential, average duration, low voltage patterns, and fibrillations.

Blood tests. Certain enzyme and antibody titers help diagnose mobility disorders. For example, increased serum creatine phosphokinase (CPK) levels may be noted in Duchenne type MD; even before any overt clinical signs or symptoms, the CPK level may reach a value 100 to 200 times normal. (Normal CPK ranges from 0 to 12 sigma units/ml.) In muscle fiber degeneration, lactic dehydrogenase levels may be elevated, but this effect is nonspecific and usually insignificant in mobility disorders. In MG, acetylcholine receptor antibody titers may be elevated.

Where muscular dystrophies strike

The various muscular dystrophies, all inherited diseases, affect different muscle groups:

Duchenne type muscular dystrophy, inherited in an X-linked recessive gene, initially involves the proximal pelvic girdle muscles. Later, it may affect the muscles of respiration and the myocardium. Fat infiltration into affected muscles causes muscles to appear large, though they are actually weak and atrophic.

Facioscapulohumeral dystrophy, a more slowly progressive disease inherited as an autosomal dominant trait, involves the face, scapula, and upper arm muscles.

Limb-girdle dystrophy, inherited as an autosomal recessive trait, usually begins in the pelvic musculature and spreads to other trunk muscles and the shoulder girdle.

Myotonic dystrophy, inherited as an autosomal dominant trait, affects hands, forearms, feet, and lower legs. Myotonia refers to the muscle's inability to relax, evident in this dystrophy as a handshake that can't let go. Muscles weaken and waste away. Bulbar weakness along with smooth muscle involvement can create swallowing and intestinal motility problems. Involvement of other body systems may result in cataracts, testicular atrophy, and myocardial defects.

In most dystrophies, atrophy and muscle weakness eventually immobilize the patient. In some cases, depending on the type of dystrophy, respiratory and cardiac involvement can be fatal.

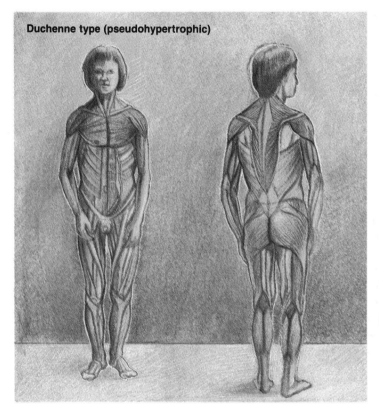

Duchenne type (pseudohypertrophic)

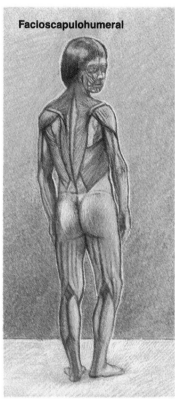

Facioscapulohumeral

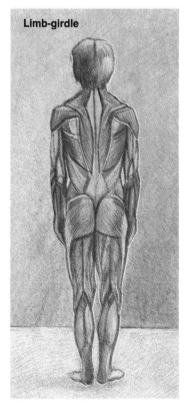

Limb-girdle

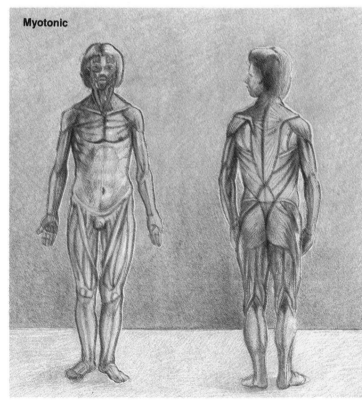

Myotonic

X-ray and computerized tomography. Mediastinum studies may reveal hyperplasia of the thymus or a thymoma, conditions often associated with MG.

Treatment includes physical therapy

Physical therapy is a treatment common to all mobility disorders. In CP and MD, physical therapy begins as soon as the disorder's been identified, to prevent deforming contractures. Passive and active range-of-motion (ROM) exercises help maintain good alignment and positioning. Passive ROM exercises take on particular importance for patients in the acute stages of GB or MG, for, with correct treatment, these patients will recover from their immobilized state and may completely regain their baseline abilities.

Physical therapy, with occupational and speech therapy, won't cure these disorders, but it can help the patient achieve optimal function. Physical therapy usually includes the use of special orthopedic appliances, such as braces and splints, and of self-help devices for feeding and toileting.

Respiratory care. Support for respiratory function ranges from comfort measures to mechanical ventilation. The pulmonary care of patients with MD emphasizes comfort. Maintaining respiratory function may require diaphragmatic breathing, coughing and deep-breathing exercises, postural drainage, and intermittent positive-pressure breathing. MG and GB may progress to the point where intubation and mechanical ventilatory support become necessary. In both diseases, such decompensation of respiratory status can occur rapidly, necessitating prompt and vigorous intervention. Such care should include frequent suctioning and assessment of vital capacity; it may require tracheostomy for prolonged mechanical ventilation.

Drug therapy. Drug therapy is important but isn't curative. Anticholinesterase drugs are the treatment of choice in MG. Oral agents such as neostigmine (Prostigmin) and pyridostigmine (Mestinon) inhibit ACH destruction and allow its accumulation at the synapse relative to the number of receptor sites. This promotes nerve impulse transmission resulting in improved muscle strength. Although this treatment primarily targets motor nerves, it also stimulates autonomic cholinergic fibers, causing side effects such as cramping and diarrhea. Giving anticholinesterase drugs with meals and/or other drugs, such as Lomotil, can offset these side effects. Unfortunately, anticholinesterase drugs become less effective as muscle disease worsens.

Immunosuppressive treatment with corticosteroid therapy is used in MG and GB. In MG, it often serves as an adjunct to anticholinesterase therapy or plasmapheresis, or as a means to eventually improve the patient's strength in preparation for thymectomy. Antacids are given concomitantly to reduce GI side effects; prednisone is given every other day to reduce its cushingoid effects. In GB, prednisone and adrenocorticotropic hormone may help suppress the inflammatory response. However, their use must be selective. Steroids do not necessarily change the course of the disease, and their risks often outweigh their benefits.

Immunosuppressant drugs, such as azathioprine and cyclophosphamide, may prove useful in MG, because of the disorder's underlying autoimmune mechanism. Research in this area continues.

Long-term anticonvulsant therapy helps to control seizures often associated with CP.

Plasmapheresis. This blood-cleansing process is being used more and more frequently in MG and is being investigated in GB. Removing the blood from the body (one unit at a time), separating its components, then replacing the components allows removal of causative antibodies. In MG, plasmapheresis may relieve symptoms for weeks or months, and it's currently used for cases ranging from elective outpatient to the most severe.

Surgical procedures. Surgery is the final choice in treating most mobility disorders. Orthopedic surgery to repair contractures may be necessary in CP and MD. Surgery is often the second treatment of choice in MG. Thymectomy may be recommended in MG in patients with or without tumor because of the thymus gland's role in autoimmune response. In many patients, remission or improvement follows thymectomy, although such remission may not occur for 5 to 10 years.

NURSING MANAGEMENT

Because neuromuscular disorders that affect mobility involve both acute conditions such as GB and chronic conditions such as MG and because effective treatments are so few, maintaining optimal functioning demands vigorous and skillful nursing management.

History points the way

Your nursing assessment relies heavily on a full history and a total physical examination.

Testing for cerebral palsy

Cover a normal 6-month-old infant's face, and he'll pull the cover off with both hands (at right). The infant with cerebral palsy (CP) uses one hand or may be unable to remove the cover at all (below).

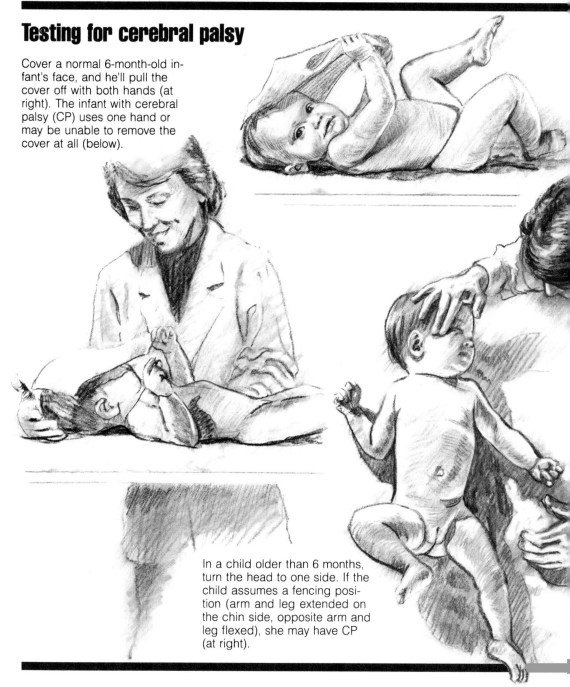

In a child older than 6 months, turn the head to one side. If the child assumes a fencing position (arm and leg extended on the chin side, opposite arm and leg flexed), she may have CP (at right).

Start by asking about the chief complaint. Extraocular muscle weakness, producing ptosis and diplopia, may be the first MG symptom. Slow or abnormal development in a child suggests CP; specific parental complaints may include difficulty in feeding, difficulty in separating the child's legs, and abnormal posturing. Locating areas of muscle weakness helps determine the type of MD.

Next, get a history of the present illness to determine the anatomic site of the symptoms and their onset. Was it sudden, rapid, slow with an intermittent course, or a steadily worsening or improving course? Intermittent muscle weakness with progressive fatigability

that becomes more severe late in the day indicates MG; continuously progressive muscle weakness with muscle atrophy indicates MD. Abrupt onset of flaccid weakness associated with paresthesia, beginning in the lower legs and spreading upward, indicates GB.

Ask about other recent symptoms, illnesses, or significant events to assess the patient's general health. Question the patient closely about any febrile illness, however mild, involving the respiratory or GI tracts, and ask about recent immunizations; these may point to GB. The perinatal history is essential if you suspect CP. Also, get a family history, since hereditary incidence points to MD.

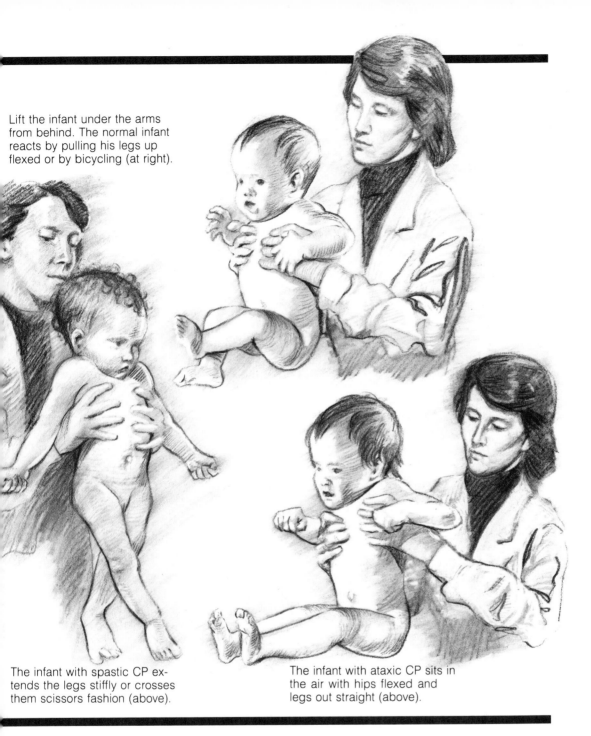

Lift the infant under the arms from behind. The normal infant reacts by pulling his legs up flexed or by bicycling (at right).

The infant with spastic CP extends the legs stiffly or crosses them scissors fashion (above).

The infant with ataxic CP sits in the air with hips flexed and legs out straight (above).

Assess the patient's psychosocial status, his possible reaction to diagnosis, and possible short- or long-term life-style changes. To cope with any of these diseases, the patient must rely heavily on family support and may also require financial assistance. Let him know, also, that community sources of help are available, such as the Visiting Nurse Association, the Muscular Dystrophy Association, and the Myasthenia Gravis Foundation.

Assessment localizes deficits
Physical assessment by inspection, palpation, and auscultation may determine any physical deficits in neuromuscular and cardiopulmo-
nary status. Unilateral or bilateral ptosis, facial weakness, limb weakness, dysphagia, and decreased tidal volume or vital capacity suggest MG. One of the first signs of this disease may be inability to sustain a gaze. These weaknesses combined with areflexia, distal paresthesias, and muscle tenderness on deep palpation suggest GB.

Inability to pucker the mouth to whistle and the absence of facial movements when laughing or crying are early signs of facioscapulohumeral muscular dystrophy. Later signs of varying types of MD include muscle hypertrophy, muscle atrophy, waddling gait, poor postural tone, scapular winging, and inability

Testing for thoracic sensation

In Guillain-Barré syndrome, paralysis moves upward and may ultimately threaten respiratory function. To test for ascending sensory loss, press the patient's skin lightly with your finger or a pin every hour. Start at the iliac crest (T12) and progress to the scapula (T6), noting the level of diminished sensation. If sensation diminishes to T8 or higher, intercostal muscle function and respiration may be impaired. As the disease subsides, sensory and motor weakness progressively recede to the lower thoracic segments, restoring intercostal and respiratory function.

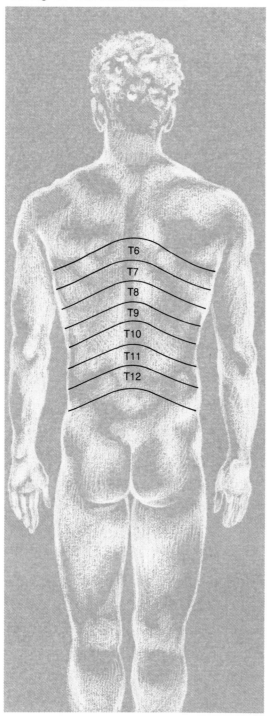

to raise the arms above the head. Auscultation of the heart and lungs may reveal signs of cardiac failure late in the course of Duchenne type MD. In children with MD, motor development is typically delayed.

Spasticity, increased muscle tone, hyperreflexia, hemiplegia or diplegia, and delayed motor development for the child's age typify CP. (See *Testing for cerebral palsy*, pages 106 and 107.)

Nursing diagnoses shape your care plan
With a clear idea of the disorder's progression and the muscle groups involved, you're ready to formulate appropriate nursing diagnoses and goals and to plan supportive interventions. In patients with neuromuscular disorders affecting mobility, your diagnoses commonly will include the following:

Ineffective breathing patterns related to respiratory muscle weakness. Your goals are to provide adequate oxygen to all cells and to prevent respiratory tract infection and atelectasis. To achieve these goals in the patient with MG or GB, assess respiratory status at least every 2 to 4 hours and as needed. Measure vital capacity and tidal volume, auscultate lung fields, and note respiratory rate and depth and use of accessory muscles. Monitor blood gases as ordered. Provide a standby Ambu bag, a respirator, and intubation equipment. If the patient is intubated, suction frequently with precise technique, and attend the patient constantly. In the patient with Duchenne type MD, teach coughing and deep-breathing exercises and diaphragmatic breathing. In any of these disorders, notify the doctor immediately if the patient's status deteriorates. In a patient with GB, to assess ascending thoracic paralysis, test for sensation (see *Testing for thoracic sensation*).

Consider your interventions successful if the patient's PO_2 is adequate, and if he shows no signs of respiratory distress, pulmonary infection, or atelectasis.

Potential for injury related to muscle weakness or spasticity. Your goal is to prevent injury and promote proper use of equipment and body mechanics. To achieve this goal, identify specific risk factors predisposing the patient to injury, and adapt the physical environment to improve safety. Develop safe ways to transfer the patient. Reinforce correct use of equipment. Teach the family proper techniques of body mechanics to lift and move the patient. Consider your interventions successful if the patient remains free of injury.

Impaired mobility related to muscle weakness, atrophy, or nerve degeneration. Your goals are to achieve optimal activity and exercise for the patient, to prevent contractures and complications, and to promote comfort. To achieve them, provide for ROM exercises. Turn and position the patient as necessary, and maintain good body alignment. Give meticulous skin care. Provide for rest periods as needed. Educate the patient and his family about the disease, its cause, symptoms, progression, and specific effects on mobility and life-style. Discuss how best to adapt the home environment and life-style to accommodate the patient's mobility impairment. Also explain the prescribed drug regimen and its possible side effects. For the myasthenic patient, who can expect prolonged therapy with anticholinesterase, warn that overdosage causes a worsening of symptoms and that certain other drugs such as anesthetics, antiarrhythmics, aminoglycoside antibiotics, muscle relaxants, and sedatives may worsen his condition and bring on the need for increased dosage of anticholinesterase.

Consider your interventions successful if the patient is active with limited bed rest, free of decubiti and contractures, and compliant to drug therapy.

Impaired verbal communication related to cranial nerve impairment from muscle weakness or to artificial airway. Your goals are to achieve effective communication, to prevent emotional injury, and to provide for the patient's needs. To achieve these goals, maintain frequent patient contact and anticipate his needs. Reassure him, showing patience and acceptance. Provide alternative communication methods such as writing, simple sign language, a letter board, or a magic slate. Tell the intubated patient that his speech will return when the tube is removed. Help the family explore speech therapy and special education for their child with CP.

Consider your interventions successful if the patient communicates with staff and visitors without stress and indicates that his needs are being met.

Alteration in developmental norms related to CNS impairment at an early age. Your goals are to develop the optimal level of function and to help the patient and his family cope with limitations. To achieve these goals in the patient with CP, assess developmental milestones and review realistic expectations. Have the parents encourage the child to move about on his own and change his position frequently, even if he must be propped up. Have the parents provide much sensory stimulation and help the child develop his speech by distinctly and slowly repeating words. Encourage the child to use his weaker hand by giving him toys too large to handle with just one hand. Reinforce the child's accomplishments and the parents' patience. Give emotional support.

Consider your interventions successful if the parents show their child affection, spend time helping him with developmental exercises, ask appropriate questions about his care, and seek support when necessary.

Alteration in urinary elimination related to poor neuromuscular control. Your goals are to maintain adequate urine output and continence and to prevent infection. For patients on bed rest and those with GB, record urine output at least every 8 hours. Offer the urinal or bedpan every 3 hours, and check for bladder distention as necessary. If necessary, perform and teach the family intermittent catheterization.

Consider your interventions successful if the patient is continent of urine, has no signs of urinary infection or skin breakdown, and if he and his family correctly perform catheterization.

Alteration in bowel function related to immobility and abdominal muscle weakness. Your goal is to maintain regular bowel movements. To achieve this goal, assess the patient's bowel function prior to his illness. Encourage him to drink fluids, if not contraindicated. Limit bed rest as much as possible. Develop a workable bowel movement program, and teach the patient and his family about it.

Consider your interventions successful if the patient is not constipated and understands and follows his bowel regimen.

Alteration in self-concept related to disfigurement, dependence, and psychological stress. Your goals are to help the patient accept himself and his body image, effectively ventilate his feelings, and develop or maintain productive relationships. To achieve these goals, provide an atmosphere of acceptance. Encourage the patient to discuss his feelings and anxieties. Express empathy, reassure the patient, and emphasize his normal characteristics. Explore new coping methods with him. Help him to be as independent as possible, and encourage contact with his peers.

Consider your interventions successful if the patient seems comfortable with himself and others, shows no evidence of withdrawal or denial, verbalizes his feelings of loss and grief, and has a healthy support system.

A final word
Many patients with neuromuscular disorders never completely regain mobility. However, your skillful and dedicated nursing care can help them make the most of residual function and, possibly, return to a relatively normal life-style.

Points to remember

- Disorders affecting mobility can be peripheral nerve function disturbances, neuromuscular transmission dysfunction, muscle disease, or neuronal death in central nervous system motor pathways.
- Myasthenia gravis and Guillain-Barré syndrome appear to be caused by an autoimmune reaction.
- Muscle biopsy confirms muscular dystrophy; I.V. injection of an anticholinesterase drug confirms myasthenia gravis. History and clinical progression diagnose cerebral palsy and Guillain-Barré syndrome.
- In cerebral palsy, the infant lags behind in development and may have a perinatal history of injury.
- Disorders that affect mobility can lead to contractures, decubiti, and respiratory complications.
- Nursing priorities in myasthenia gravis, Guillain-Barré syndrome, and muscular dystrophy are respiratory care and ongoing respiratory status assessment.

9 CONTROLLING SEIZURE DISORDERS

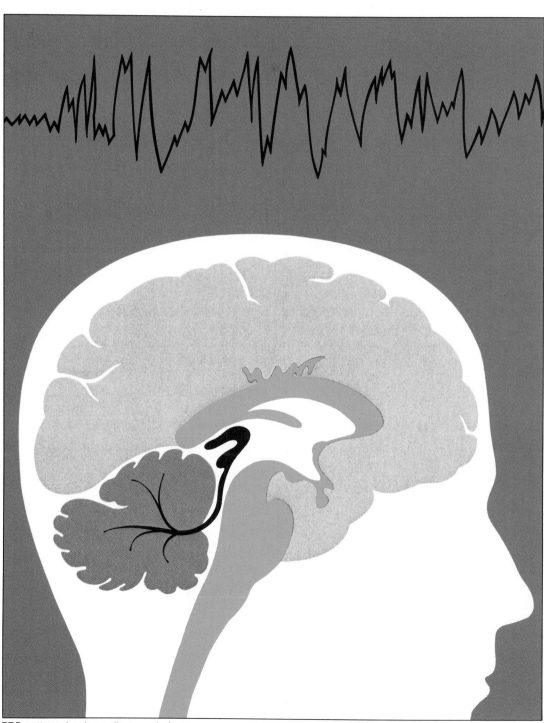

EEG pattern showing epileptogenic focus

Controlling seizures is possible in up to 75% of patients with epilepsy, but it requires prolonged drug therapy, continuing medical follow-up care, and important adjustments in life-style. You can make a pivotal contribution to successful control by helping the patient make necessary psychosocial adjustments and by teaching him how to maintain prolonged drug therapy with the fewest complications. To teach your patient effectively, you must be able to explain what's currently known about epilepsy, its expected impact on daily life, and the measures available to control this often misunderstood disorder.

First, dispel myths

Even after 2,400 recorded years of human experience with epilepsy, ignorant concepts about this disease still abound. So, before you can teach a patient and his family what epilepsy is and what to do about it, you usually need to tell them clearly what it's not. Epilepsy is not a form of insanity or retardation; it's not a reason to feel inferior or unemployable; it's not an impenetrable barrier to achievement; it's not a proven hereditary disease and doesn't tend to get worse with time. Only after you have dispelled these centuries-old prejudices can you expect the patient and his family to hear your teaching.

What is epilepsy?

Epilepsy is not a disease but a symptom, the manifestation of many disease processes. Any repetition of seizure activity, regardless of the interval between seizures, is called epilepsy. Epileptic seizures reflect the paroxysmal, uncontrolled discharge of central nervous system (CNS) neurons leading to neurologic dysfunction. The site of such electrical disturbance determines the seizures' clinical manifestations.

Seizures generally progress through several phases. The first phase (prodromal) may involve mood or behavioral changes. Next may come a sensory warning (aura), which may manifest itself as a "funny feeling"; a peculiar, vile taste or odor; dizziness; headache; spots before the eyes; abdominal pain; or a chill. Clinical manifestation of the aura depends on the cerebral site of epileptic activity and may help localize the seizure's origin. An epileptic cry, resulting from the forceful expulsion of air from the throat, may introduce full seizure activity (ictal phase). The final phase (postictal) is a period of slow recovery, which some-times includes altered levels of consciousness, fatigue, and confusion. (See *Phases of seizure activity*.)

Status epilepticus, a medical emergency, consists of rapidly recurring seizures without intervening periods of physiologic recovery. Most commonly it's triggered by noncompliance with anticonvulsant therapy or by abrupt withdrawal from alcohol or drugs, particularly barbiturates. Status epilepticus is associated with greater morbidity and mortality than simple seizures, but prognosis is good with prompt diagnosis and treatment.

Understanding classification

The most universally accepted system of classifying seizures, the International Classification of Epileptic Seizures, categorizes epileptic activity according to clinical onset. Understanding the classification requires first understanding the cerebral hyperactivity that characterizes seizures.

Electroencephalographic (EEG) recordings in epileptic patients show frequent bursts of cerebral hyperactivity. They may or may not be associated with seizure activity. These bursts of hyperactivity may lead to one of several manifestations. The activity may remain confined to the original focus, it may spread within a localized area, or it may extend to the entire brain. The first two conditions are called partial seizures because the hyperactivity spreads minimally and involves only part of the brain; the epileptic discharges meet with enough resistance to stop the spread. In the third condition, generalized seizure, the hyperactivity spreads to involve the entire brain.

Partial seizures may be simple or complex. Simple partial seizures do not usually impair consciousness. However, complex partial seizures and generalized seizures almost always cause some degree of loss of consciousness.

What causes seizures?

In some patients, epilepsy probably results from an undetermined brain chemistry abnormality, which causes neuronal electrical instability and therefore a low seizure threshold (idiopathic epilepsy); this epilepsy form may show genetic predisposition. Research is currently focusing on biochemical imbalance as a possible cause of some idiopathic seizures.

In other patients, epilepsy results from other diseases or conditions that provoke neuronal irritation or damage. (See *Seizure onset and cause,* page 112.)

Phases of seizure activity

Prodromal. Mood or behavior change that may precede seizure by several hours or days.
Aura. Unusual sound, sight, taste, or smell, warning of impending seizure. Epileptic cry may occur.
Ictal. Seizure activity.
Postictal. After-seizure behavioral changes, lethargy, confusion.

Seizure onset and cause

Age at onset	Usual cause
0 to 2	Congenital defect, anoxia at birth, meningitis, hypocalcemia, hypoglycemia, vitamin B_6 deficiency, phenylketonuria
2 to 10	Anoxia or injury at birth, meningitis, infections, thrombosis of cerebral vessels, idiopathic epilepsy
10 to 18	Idiopathic epilepsy, trauma, meningitis, congenital defects
18 to 35	Idiopathic epilepsy, trauma, tumor, meningitis, withdrawal from alcohol or sedative-hypnotic drugs
35 to 60	Trauma, tumor, vascular disease, meningitis, alcohol or drug withdrawal
Over 60	Vascular disease, tumor, degenerative disease, meningitis

Trauma (head injury) is a major cause of seizures, especially in young adults. Such seizures usually appear within the first year after brain injury; the risk declines to about 10% by the end of the second year. Birth trauma and prenatal or neonatal injury from anoxia, drugs, and infarction also cause later onset of seizures.

Infection may cause seizures for various reasons. An abscess, acting as a space-occupying lesion, may lead to seizure activity by causing local tissue damage. Meningitis and encephalitis may cause seizures as a result of generalized cerebral tissue irritation. Paradoxically, one treatment alternative for these infections—intrathecal instillation of antibiotics—may exaggerate the risk of seizures. Some antibiotics are known to cause local cerebral irritation and may even precipitate seizures.

Cerebrovascular disorders (hemorrhage, thrombosis, embolism) commonly cause seizures in older adults. Arteriovenous malformations and aneurysms may produce hemorrhage or vasospasm that secondarily causes seizures through focal brain irritation. Arteriovenous malformations and hematomas acting as space-occupying lesions may also cause focal cerebral irritation. Cerebral infarction or stroke may result in seizures from irritable foci around dead and damaged tissue areas. Also, some biochemical imbalance associated with tissue damage may alter the seizure threshold in that area.

Intracranial neoplasms may produce seizures through irritation of surrounding tissue.

Metabolic causes are many and are easy to overlook. They may include the expected or idiosyncratic effects of drug therapy; toxins; electrolyte or glucose imbalance; hypoparathyroidism; and vitamin deficiencies. Any of these may interfere with normal metabolic functions and may deprive cerebral tissue of its essential nutrients.

What precipitates seizures?
In epilepsy patients, seizures can be triggered by factors that lower the seizure threshold. (See *Common precipitating factors*.) If the precipitating factor can be identified, such as playing video games, the seizure is called reflex epilepsy. In some patients, none of these factors causes seizures. In others, only specific factors do. Often, combined factors, rather than just one, precipitate seizures. Fatigue, emotional stress, and alcohol consumption or withdrawal together frequently lead to seizure activity.

PATHOPHYSIOLOGY
Seizures result from cerebral irritation produced by excessive firing of neurons that are physically and physiologically abnormal. The triggering mechanism is not well understood, although any chemical or electrical stimulus that depolarizes the neuron tends to produce spontaneous firing. (See *Potential cellular mechanisms in epilepsy,* page 114.)

Cellular activity leading to seizures begins with excitation and depolarization of certain hypersensitive neurons that form the epileptogenic focus. After a brief period of protective hyperpolarization, the cell again depolarizes. Rapidly accelerating, this depolarization sets off a paroxysmal discharge that prolongs membrane depolarization, alters synaptic transmission, and precipitates a seizure. During a seizure, the neuronal discharge rate can reach 1,000 firings/second.

Cellular activity after a seizure sustains membrane hyperpolarization. Depleted cells in the epileptogenic focus stop firing, slowly reducing the firing of peripheral cells, and resting membrane potential slowly returns.

Seizure metabolism
The intense cellular activity during a seizure places a tremendous energy demand on the brain and may lead to secondary and permanent neurologic injury. During a seizure, production of adenosine triphosphate (ATP), the

chief energy source for the brain, increases by 250% to fuel the cellular sodium and potassium pumps, synthesize neurotransmitter substances, and transmit nerve impulses. Simultaneously, cerebral blood flow also increases by 250% to facilitate carbon dioxide removal and meet a 60% rise in demand for oxygen. Normal cerebral blood flow can meet such unusual metabolic demand for glucose and other nutrients as long as hypoxemia, hypoglycemia, or cardiac irregularities don't develop. However, seizures that include skeletal muscle contractions can bring on hypoxemia and hypoglycemia through increased metabolic activity. Under these conditions, available oxygen and glucose may be inadequate to supply the brain; then energy debts follow markedly diminished ATP and rising lactate levels. This usually causes cellular exhaustion and injury.

Clinical manifestations

Whether a patient exhibits motor and/or sensory manifestations in one body part, several, or most depends on the area of the brain subject to paroxysmal discharge.

Simple partial seizures. *Simple motor seizures,* both focal and jacksonian, begin in the motor cortex of the frontal lobe. Clinical manifestations depend on the specific area of irritative focus (see *Where simple motor seizures strike,* page 115). Since a large part of the motor cortex controls face and hand movements, it follows that most motor seizures begin in these areas. A focal motor seizure confines itself to the irritative focal area, such as the hand. A jacksonian seizure is a focal motor seizure with a "marching" spread of activity to adjacent areas. It may start in the fingers, then expand to the hand, arm, face, or entire side of the body. The activity appears to march along the body part as the focus involves adjacent areas of the cortex.

In motor seizures, convulsive activity is usually clonic, beginning with slow, repetitive jerking that may increase in intensity. It may last from 5 seconds to several minutes. During the postictal phase of a focal seizure, a temporary paralysis (Todd's paralysis) may affect the body part experiencing seizure activity. Such paralysis may last from a few minutes up to 24 hours.

Complex partial seizures. These are most often associated with alterations in the level of consciousness. One of the most common types is psychomotor (temporal lobe) epilepsy. Here, the irritative focus occurs in the tem-

poral lobe and possibly the limbic system. Clinical manifestations include automatisms (lip smacking, chewing, swallowing, grimacing, or patting or picking movements of the hands) and sometimes outbursts of rage and violence. Various sensory experiences, including olfactory, visual, and auditory hallucinations, often precede the automatisms. The patient may appear wild-eyed and speak in jumbled, repetitive phrases. Psychomotor seizures may last from 30 seconds to several minutes and are usually followed by postictal confusion. Afterward, the patient doesn't remember any of the events, including the rage attacks.

Generalized seizures. *Absence (petit mal) seizures* affect 6% to 12% of children with seizures, but they also occur in adults. Usually, the onset occurs between ages 4 and 12. Clinical manifestations include brief altered levels of consciousness (absences) lasting from 5 to 30 seconds. The patient stares and may occasionally blink his eyelids. Usually, absence seizures produce no prodrome, aura, or postictal state, and the patient resumes normal activity after it passes. Such fleeting seizures can happen 100 or more times a day. They can cause a school-age child to develop lapses in concentration and a shortened attention span that may cause him to be mislabeled as learning disabled. Fortunately, absence seizures can be controlled with drug therapy, allowing normal participation in school. Moreover, these seizures tend to disappear entirely by age 20 in 50% to 70% of these patients. But some children with absence seizures later develop generalized tonic-clonic (grand mal) epilepsy, most often between ages 10 and 13.

Generalized tonic-clonic seizures. These occur commonly and at all ages. Typically, they're associated with a prodrome or aura, or both. These seizures begin suddenly and are marked by an abrupt loss of consciousness with tonic muscle spasms and an epileptic cry. The patient falls at the onset of the tonic phase, which lasts about 1 minute and is characterized by apnea and cyanosis. The clonic phase then follows, as the patient shows rapid, synchronous muscle jerking and hyperventilation. He may also show simultaneous tongue and lip biting, bladder and bowel incontinence, hypertension, pupillary dilation, tachycardia, sweating, and heavy salivation that looks like foaming at the mouth. Most tonic-clonic seizures last 2 to 5 minutes. Immediately after the clonic phase, the patient

Common precipitating factors
Nontherapeutic drug levels
Drug withdrawal
Noncompliance
Alteration of drug regimen

Physiologic stress
Fatigue
Lack of sleep
Hypoglycemia
Alcohol intake
Water intoxication
Febrile states
Constipation
Certain odors
Certain musical rhythms (steady, pounding beat)
Loud noises
Startle or fright
Menstruation/pregnancy
Flashing lights (TV, video games, strobe lights)

Emotional stress

Potential cellular mechanisms in epilepsy

At the glial cell
Failure to keep
extracellular K+ down

At the dendrite
Potassium leak,
abnormal excitability
from injury

In the cell body
Abnormal membrane →
defect in K+ pumping;
mechanical deformation
(depolarization)

At the synapse
Repetitive after-
discharge following
stimulation; abnormal
'reverse activation' back
across synapse

experiences postictal fatigue, confusion, memory loss, muscle weakness, and irritability. Full recovery may take a few minutes or several hours.

MEDICAL MANAGEMENT
Diagnosis of epilepsy can be difficult and requires a series of steps. The first step is to determine whether the symptoms are in fact seizures or some other disorder that mimics seizures. After true seizures are confirmed, a continued diagnostic investigation must identify their clinical type, any precipitating factors, and localizing features. This leads to the third step, an effort to discover the cause, which is often obscure. For example, post-traumatic epilepsy may be difficult to identify because it may not manifest itself for as long as 2 years after injury. After these three steps, evaluation of the patient's and his family's responses to the seizures, their support systems, and coping mechanisms is also needed to help the patient control seizures.

Because epilepsy is a dynamic disorder and may be associated at different times with various disease processes, its diagnosis should be equally dynamic. Information gained from one seizure episode may not apply to succeeding episodes; auras, manifestations, and foci may all change. Seizures may also be an early symptom of an occult illness that may not be apparent initially. Thus, individual consideration of each patient's signs, continued follow-up care by a doctor, and prompt reporting of any changes are vital for effective diagnosis and treatment.

History and physical examination
In the diagnostic evaluation of a patient with seizures, a carefully assembled medical and family history and a thorough physical examination can be keys to accurate diagnosis. Along with routine physical assessment, evaluation for specific abnormalities may help further define the seizure disorder. For example, in neonates, measurement of the circumference of the head, auscultation for intracranial bruits, and transillumination of the head may reveal hydrocephalus, arteriovenous malformations, or subdural hematomas as the cause of the seizures. Observation of infants and children for developmental achievements may provide a clue to the source of seizures. So may skin lesions, which may point to a specific disorder; for example, seizures with facial hemangioma indicate Sturge-Weber syndrome. Thorough examination of the optic

Where simple motor seizures strike

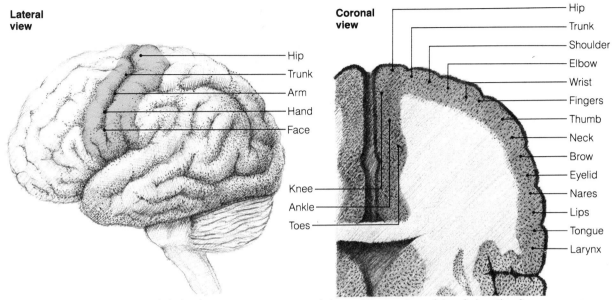

Lateral view

- Hip
- Trunk
- Arm
- Hand
- Face
- Knee
- Ankle
- Toes

Coronal view

- Hip
- Trunk
- Shoulder
- Elbow
- Wrist
- Fingers
- Thumb
- Neck
- Brow
- Eyelid
- Nares
- Lips
- Tongue
- Larynx

The motor cortex site where an irritative focus occurs decides a seizure's signs and symptoms. Lateral and coronal views of the cerebrum (above) show the sites that control motor activity in contralateral body parts.

fundi can supply important clues to nervous system disorders; it may, for example, reveal a cherry-red macula, a sign of Tay-Sachs disease. Detection of cardiovascular disease, blood dyscrasias, neoplastic diseases, metabolic disorders, liver or renal disease, and any sign of increased intracranial pressure offers significant evidence for a possible cause of seizures.

Diagnostic tests

Recognizing the many possible secondary causes for seizures and initiating treatment to avoid irreversible brain damage form an essential part of seizure diagnosis and care. Thus, a general workup to rule out hypoglycemia, hyponatremia, renal disease, sickle cell anemia, and other metabolic disturbances includes a complete blood count, urinalysis, blood glucose and electrolyte levels, and blood chemistry assays. A drug screen may be ordered if abuse is suspected. When meningitis is suspected, a lumbar puncture supplies cerebrospinal fluid (CSF) for culture and sensitivity tests to identify the pathogen. Yellow or bloody CSF may indicate subarachnoid hemorrhage as the cause of seizures.

Neuroradiologic procedures. Plain skull X-rays may show evidence of a calcified pineal body, asymmetries secondary to trauma, or erosion of the dorsum sellae, all of which can cause seizures.

Computerized tomography (CT) scan helps evaluate ventricle size, cortical atrophy, hem-

orrhage, or tumor and shows temporal horn atrophy that characterizes psychomotor epilepsy. Because of the increased availability of CT scan, this test is gradually replacing radionuclide brain scans and pneumoencephalogram.

Radionuclide brain scans are sometimes done to detect arteriovenous malformations, vascular tumors, or subdural hematomas, all potential causes of seizures. If CSF obstruction is suspected, a *pneumoencephalogram* may be done. *Cerebral arteriography* can help detect vascular abnormalities as the cause of seizures. This test is performed when a CT scan fails to define a suspected structural or vascular lesion.

Electroencephalography. The principal screening test for documenting and classifying clinical seizures, EEG should be done on all patients with suspected seizures. Routine EEG detects paroxysmal dysrhythmias, which verify the diagnosis. (See *EEG patterns in epilepsy,* page 117.)

Other ancillary measures may be used to activate or enhance abnormal EEG patterns. Hyperventilation may elicit absence seizures. Sleep may clearly define temporal lobe abnormalities in psychomotor epilepsy. Nasopharyngeal leads may give better tracings of mesial temporal lobe activity. Simple strobe light or auditory stimulation may evoke sensory seizures. Deliberate seizure induction by injecting epileptogenic drugs may help determine the origin of focal seizures.

New frontiers in seizure control

Research in many areas is beginning to provide promising methods for seizure identification and control. Among new methods, positron emission tomography (PET) scans are now being applied to seizure diagnosis. These scans can help show both cerebral blood flow and metabolism. With further refinements, PET techniques may uncover more knowledge about the etiology and neurochemical aspects of seizures.

Current research on prolonged cerebellar stimulation promises to control seizures by inhibiting cortical epileptogenic discharges. This technique involves surgical placement of a stimulus coil over the superior surface of the cerebellum, a procedure that risks damage to the cerebellum but has provided some promising results.

Another procedure, general or local brain cooling, affects epileptic neurons more than normal neurons and has shown some potential by decreasing seizure frequency. Also, operant conditioning (biofeedback) of certain EEG components has provided some relief in intractable epilepsy.

Prolonged EEG recording increasingly aids epilepsy diagnosis and can be helpful even in outpatients. The patient may wear a headband that carries a transmitter with radiotelemetric capability; the transmission can be displayed on a monitor or oscilloscope. With cable telemetry, the patient can selectively record only ictal events. With the cassette recorder, the patient can be monitored after returning to normal activities. The audiovisual tape EEG, with split screen, allows the doctor to videorecord the patient's clinical appearance concurrently with EEG correlations. This is particularly helpful for recording clinical events during the span of a seizure.

Of course, EEG should be used as an adjunct to clinical evaluation because a patient with known clinical seizures may have a normal EEG, and an abnormal EEG may not always indicate seizures.

Treatment

Treatment of epilepsy concerns itself with three major areas: treating or removing causative and precipitating factors, controlling seizures with antiepileptic drugs, and recognizing and managing the physical and emotional problems associated with epilepsy.

In many patients with intracranial tumors, hematomas, vascular abnormalities, abscesses, CNS infections, dietary deficiencies, drug abuse, or metabolic or endocrine dysfunction, the treatment or removal of these causes eliminates the seizures. In about half the patients with meningioma, removing the tumor relieves the seizures; the others must seek seizure control through drug therapy.

Anticonvulsant therapy. The objective of anticonvulsant treatment is complete freedom from seizures without adverse drug effects. The first step is selection of a primary seizure type-specific drug for maximum effectiveness. However, with multiple types and causes of seizures, no drug therapy is universally effective, so the degree and type of response to any drug in an individual patient cannot always be predicted.

The primary drug should be used until therapeutic effects or toxic signs appear. The full therapeutic or adverse effects of any oral medication cannot be evaluated until drug metabolism reaches a steady state, usually during an interval of 4 to 5 times the serum half-life of the drug.

Blood levels of the drug should be monitored frequently. If, after a trial period, the primary drug fails to adequately control seizures, a second drug should be added, increasing the dosage slowly until it reaches therapeutic levels. Drug dosage should be changed for one drug at a time to help identify the cause if a patient develops toxicity. Sometimes drug combinations are more effective than any single drug, and withdrawal of one of the drugs may precipitate seizures. Possible drug interactions represent another concern in combination anticonvulsant therapy. Most importantly, anticonvulsant therapy for major motor seizures should never be stopped abruptly since sudden withdrawal risks status epilepticus.

Prophylactic therapy. Preventive drug therapy often continues 1 to 2 years after one documented, generalized tonic-clonic seizure. If a patient has suffered more than one such seizure, prophylaxis may continue for 2 to 3 years. If the patient remains seizure-free during that time, weaning him from medication may be considered. Then, discontinuation of drug therapy should progress slowly, under a doctor's supervision, to prevent withdrawal seizures. If the patient needs lifetime prophylactic therapy, periodic reassessment, continuing patient education and emotional support help prevent noncompliance, a major source of poor control in managing seizures.

Emergency treatment of status epilepticus. Unceasing seizure activity (status epilepticus) may occur with all types of seizures. Status epilepticus represents a life-threatening emergency for patients with generalized tonic-clonic epilepsy because of its potential for anoxia, cardiac dysrhythmias, and systemic lactic acidosis. Managing this emergency effectively requires a routine of care that follows established priorities. (See *Treating status epilepticus,* pages 118 and 119.)

The most important first step in lifesaving care is always airway assessment. The patient with generalized tonic-clonic epilepsy who's experiencing status epilepticus probably will require intubation and ventilation, but a clenched jaw may make this procedure impossible until the seizure is controlled.

Next may come arterial blood gas analysis, to establish baseline respiratory function, and an attempt to identify the cause. The most common cause is abrupt withdrawal from anticonvulsant drugs. Other causes include infections, electrolyte imbalance, and metabolic disturbance. Analysis of blood glucose and electrolyte levels may narrow the possibilities among these causes.

Next comes seizure control. Because this is

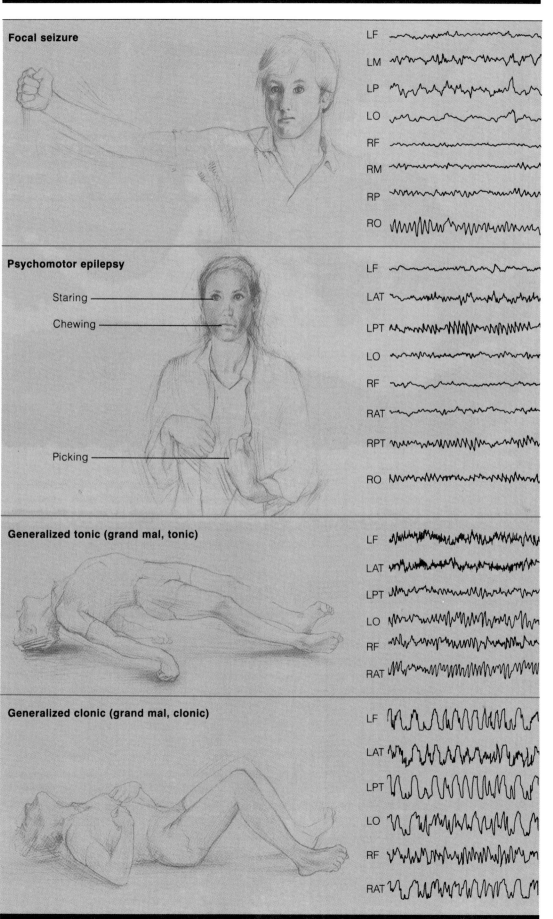

Focal seizure

LF	
LM	
LP	
LO	
RF	
RM	
RP	
RO	

Psychomotor epilepsy

Staring

Chewing

Picking

LF	
LAT	
LPT	
LO	
RF	
RAT	
RPT	
RO	

Generalized tonic (grand mal, tonic)

LF	
LAT	
LPT	
LO	
RF	
RAT	

Generalized clonic (grand mal, clonic)

LF	
LAT	
LPT	
LO	
RF	
RAT	

EEG patterns in epilepsy

By displaying characteristic deviations from normal brain wave patterns, an EEG can identify epilepsy and reveal its type and possibly the epileptogenic focus.

On an abnormal EEG, paroxysmal dysrhythmias may combine with fast and slow waves, suggesting epilepsy. Certain abnormalities characterize specific types of seizures. For example, high-voltage fast spike waves in all leads typify generalized tonic-clonic (grand mal) seizures.

In partial seizures, the EEG may help localize the area where epileptiform discharge originates.

KEY:

LF	left frontal
LM	left medial
LP	left posterior
LO	left occipital
LAT	left anterior temporal
LPT	left posterior temporal
RF	right frontal
RM	right medial
RP	right posterior
RO	right occipital
RAT	right anterior temporal
RPT	right posterior temporal

Treating status epilepticus

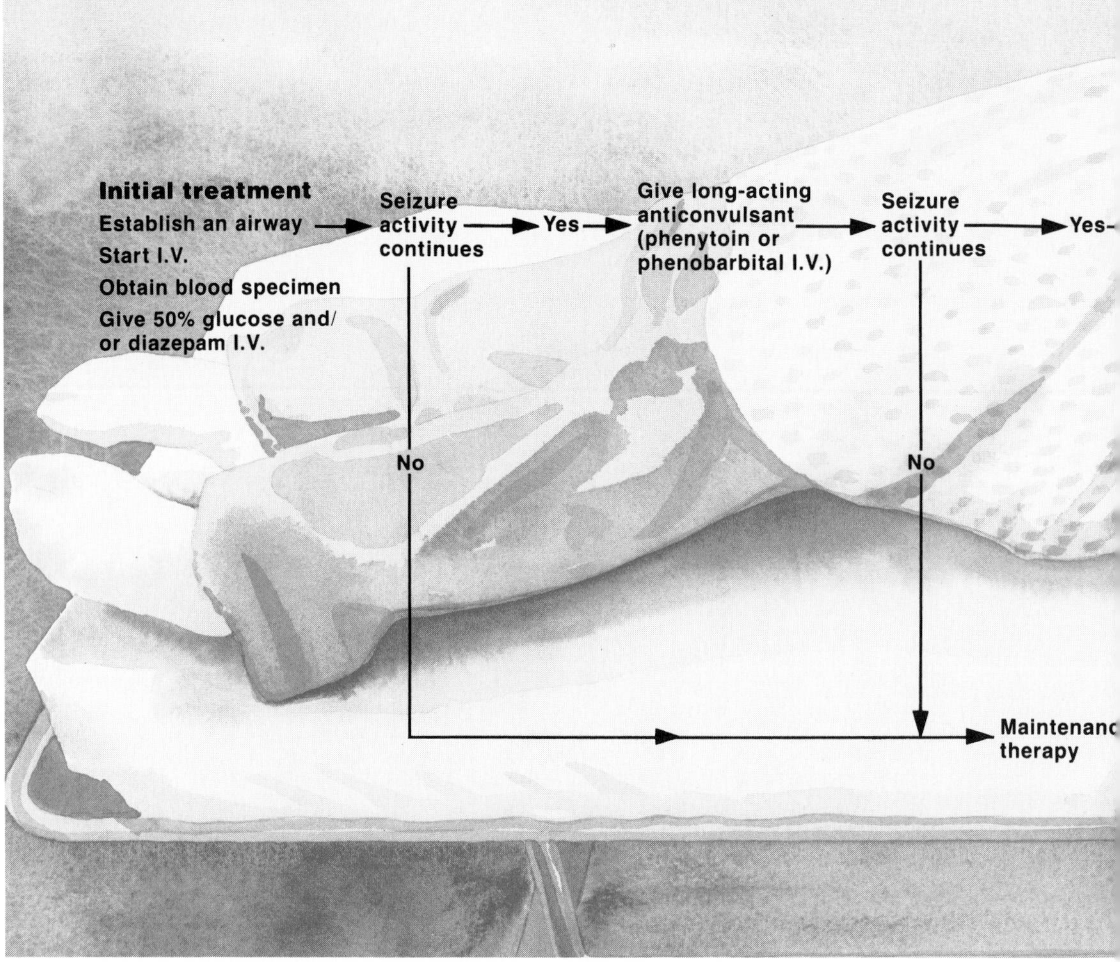

Initial treatment

Establish an airway

Start I.V.

Obtain blood specimen

Give 50% glucose and/ or diazepam I.V.

→ Seizure activity continues → Yes →

Give long-acting anticonvulsant (phenytoin or phenobarbital I.V.)

→ Seizure activity continues → Yes→

No

No

Maintenanc therapy

an emergency, intravenous therapy is the preferred route for administering an anticonvulsant. If the cause has been identified as an electrolyte or metabolic imbalance, therapy may begin with infusion of 50% glucose for hypoglycemia. If no specific treatable cause has been found, the usual preferred therapy is intravenous diazepam (Valium), a fast-acting anticonvulsant with less tendency to produce respiratory depression or hypotension than other anticonvulsants. Because of its short duration of action, diazepam must be followed with a longer-acting anticonvulsant (usually phenytoin [Dilantin]) for maintenance, or seizures will recur in 15 to 30 minutes. Phenobarbital is sometimes used, but it often produces excessive and sometimes undesirable sedation. Thiopental sodium and sometimes paraldehyde may be used to stop seizures abruptly, but these drugs also have potentially dangerous side effects.

Of course, any intravenous anticonvulsant is potentially dangerous and must be carefully administered to the elderly and those with hypertension, heart disease, or cardiac dysrhythmias.

If the status epilepticus doesn't respond to drugs within 60 minutes, general anesthesia and neuromuscular blockade are sometimes considered.

Surgery. Only a small percentage of patients with focal epilepsy require surgery, but most of those can expect complete or nearly complete suppression of seizures. Surgical intervention aims to remove the brain's abnormally discharging areas. However, what appears to be abnormal isn't always the direct cause of seizures; rather, it may lie adjacent to the epileptogenic site and may have been rendered abnormal by the disease process. Many cortical areas can be suppressed with little or no adverse effect, but certain treatments are known to be dangerous. For example, the risk of vasospasm of the middle cerebral artery during surgery has made certain areas of the brain unacceptable for surgical consideration.

The patient must meet certain criteria before surgery's warranted: the seizure focus

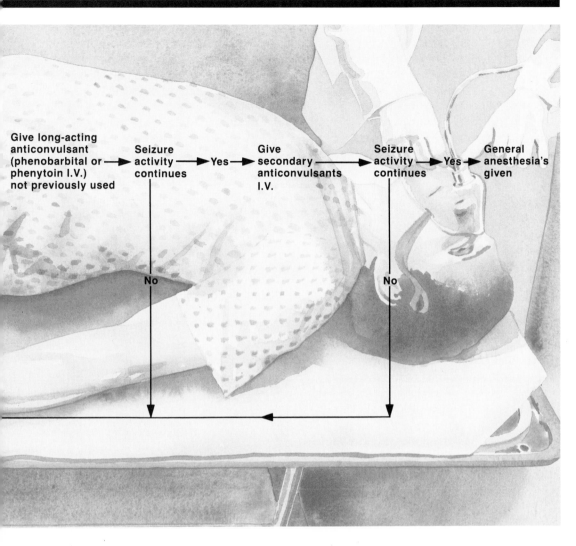

Give long-acting anticonvulsant (phenobarbital or phenytoin I.V.) not previously used → Seizure activity continues → Yes → Give secondary anticonvulsants I.V. → Seizure activity continues → Yes → General anesthesia's given

No

No

must be consistently localized to the same site, a thorough and adequate trial of medical therapy must have been attempted to confirm intractable seizures, and the seizures must have occurred for at least 6 months and must be seriously disabling. Thorough psychiatric assessment should distinguish psychological from physical complaints. In addition, surgery is performed in the hopes of offering the patient significant seizure relief after the minimal risks are weighed against the benefits. In preparation for surgery, the Wada test, intracarotid injection of amobarbital sodium (Amytal Sodium) to temporarily suppress function in one hemisphere, permits evaluation of speech and memory function on the contralateral side. Depth and direct cortical recording and stimulation are now used more frequently for such evaluation.

Surgical intervention may be either resective or stereotaxic. Resective surgery includes temporal lobectomy, which in some cases is being replaced by selective resection of the temporal lobe tip, and cerebral hemispherec-

tomy. About one third of surgical procedures for epilepsy involve the temporal lobes.

Stereotaxic procedures involve inserting a needle through a drill hole in the skull and guiding it under X-ray control to the area targeted as epileptogenic. Small intracerebral lesions can be made at the site to destroy abnormal pathways with minimal risk or adverse effect.

Physical and emotional support. Alcohol abuse, fatigue, emotional unrest, and poor dietary habits are major factors that favor recurrence of seizures. Thus, information on correct use of alcohol, good nutrition, and effective coping techniques forms an important part of seizure management. The epileptic patient needs support and encouragement to live as normal a life as possible.

NURSING MANAGEMENT
Since diagnostic tests and physical findings often prove negative in patients with seizure disorders, having time to elicit a reliable and detailed history is crucial.

Documenting seizure activity

When your patient experiences seizures, carefully observe all phases and record the following information:

Aura: Cry or moan?

Onset pattern: Point of origin?

Activity pattern: Does it spread? Where? How? Motor activities affected?

Seizure duration

Seizure frequency

Postictal pattern: Altered level of consciousness, paralysis, confusion, fatigue?

Consult the patient's family

Because altered levels of consciousness often accompany seizures, rely on the patient's family and other observers to flesh out the patient's descriptions of seizures. Allow adequate time to gather this information, especially the details of seizure activity, since denial and anger are common reactions to these disorders. The patient and his family may need time to confront any facts they've blocked out or forgotten. To help them remember, make your questions as specific as you can.

Explore in depth any history of head trauma, encephalitis, or febrile seizures. Remember that heart disease, diabetes, hypertension, and a family history of neurologic disease may contribute to the seizure disorder. Investigate noncompliance with prescribed treatment, and check for other precipitating factors, such as menses, drug interactions or abuse, physical or emotional stress, and lack of sleep. Get an accurate description of the onset and pattern of seizure activity to help pinpoint where the epileptiform activity originated and spread.

Don't forget that emotional distress can also precipitate seizures in patients with epileptogenic foci and that many myths and fears still surround the patient with seizures. Explore the patient's and his family's responses to this disorder. As soon as you can, get information regarding family life, social life, and school schedules or occupation so you can suggest appropriate resources for assistance.

Establish baseline assessment

Perform a thorough neurologic assessment (as outlined in Chapter 2) and physical assessments specific for seizures. The resulting neurologic baseline will guide your reassessment and evaluation of change during and after future seizures.

If you have an opportunity to witness an actual seizure, try to document your assessment as soon after the event as possible to fully recall the details (see *Documenting seizure activity*). Note the precipitating event, when possible. Was the patient emotionally upset, lacking sleep, watching television, or near flashing lights? Did he mention an aura? In which part of the body did seizure activity begin? Did the signs march? For example, did they start in the fingers and spread to the arm and face?

Describe all visible aspects of seizure activity, including eyelid fluttering, lip smacking, or arm jerking. Note fluctuations in the level of consciousness and how and when these occurred. Observe and record eye movements, pupil size and reaction, and deviation of gaze. Assess and record all physical manifestations, such as bowel or bladder incontinence, tongue and lip biting, apnea, cyanosis, heavy salivation with a foamy appearance, head deviation, falling, and trauma. Record the durations of

Differentiating seizure types

Disorder	Areas involved (focus)
I. Partial seizures (simple)	
A. Focal motor	Motor strip on precentral gyrus in frontal lobe
B. Jacksonian	Motor strip on precentral gyrus in frontal lobe
C. Adversive	Frontal lobe anterior to motor strip
D. Epilepsia partialis continua	Varied
E. Focal sensory	Postcentral gyrus in parietal or occipital lobe
II. Partial seizures (complex)	
Psychomotor	Temporal lobe
III. Generalized seizures	
A. Generalized tonic-clonic (grand mal)	Generalized
B. Absence (petit mal)	Generalized
C. Infantile spasms (salaam, head drop)	Generalized
D. Myoclonic	Generalized
E. Akinetic (drop attacks)	Generalized, with brain stem involvement
IV. Miscellaneous	
Mixed	Frontal, temporal, or occipital focus with generalized spread

both seizure and any postictal state. In the postictal state, carefully assess, monitor, and record any behavior changes, transient hemiplegia, lethargy, receptive or expressive aphasia, and headache. (See *Differentiating seizure types*.)

In status epilepticus, also assess airway and ventilatory status and vital sign changes. Record duration of time between seizures.

Implement your nursing diagnoses

Because seizure disorders involve a dynamic process, you'll continually need to reassess your patient and modify his care plan accordingly. Your plan must be as individual as each seizure to ensure success. At various times in the course of the treatment of epilepsy, you may use the following nursing diagnoses.

Change in consciousness	EEG findings	Impaired capacities
Unilateral: No change in consciousness. Bilateral: Loss of consciousness	Focal waves, slow waves, or spikes	Convulsive movements and temporary disturbance in motor capacity in body part controlled by that brain region
Unilateral: No change in consciousness. Bilateral: Loss of consciousness	Focal waves, slow waves, or spikes	Disturbance in motor capacity. Seizure activity marches along limb or side of body in orderly progression
No loss	Focal waves, slow waves, or spikes	Disturbance in behavior and motor capacity. Head and eyes turn away from focal region; may develop into generalized seizure
No loss	Focal waves, slow waves, or spikes	Form of focal status epilepticus involving a muscle group. May last minutes to weeks with postictal weakness
No loss	Spikes and slow waves over epileptogenic focus in occipital or parietal areas	Subjective sensory experience; may be visual, auditory, olfactory, or somatosensory. Possible "marching" progression
No loss of consciousness; confusion and amnesia	Temporal spikes or slow waves	Hallucinations, dyscognitive states (déjà vu), automatism, and loss of awareness
Loss of consciousness with postictal sleeping	Rapidly repeating spikes in tonic phase; spikes of slow waves in clonic phase	Major tonic muscular contraction followed by longer phase of clonic (jerking) contractions. Possible bowel and bladder control loss, weakness, injury, or learning disorders
Transient losses of consciousness; no postictal state	Spikes and waves, three/second	Interference with conscious response to environment when uncontrolled; possible learning disorders
None; no postictal state	Multiple spikes and slow waves of large amplitude (hypsarrhythmia)	Jackknife, flexor spasms of extremities and head. Severe mental and developmental deficiencies
Possible momentary loss of consciousness followed by confusion	Findings similar to those for infantile spasms	Uncontrollable jerking movements of extremities or entire body
None; no postictal state	Normal to slow background with polyspike or multiple spike waves	Sudden postural tone loss. Possible intellectual, perceptual, and motor impairments
Consistent with type of seizure	Spike, polyspike, or spike-wave patterns with progression of focus to a generalized pattern	Interferences with behavior, learning, or motor functions

Potential for injury related to seizure activity. To prevent injury, begin by instituting seizure precautions at admission to the nursing unit. Keep padded side rails up, and have an oral airway and suction equipment ready for emergency use. Remove potentially harmful objects, such as furniture with sharp corners. Do not allow the patient to smoke in bed. Take rectal rather than oral temperatures. If a seizure occurs, stay with the patient and remain calm. Move harmful objects out of his way. If an aura gives advance warning of a seizure, help the patient lie down to prevent a fall. Guide him gently to avoid his harming himself. Never try to move or restrain a patient during a seizure. You can't stop the seizure, and you may injure the patient by countering the strength of the muscle contraction. If the patient is lying on a hard surface, place a pillow or towel under his head to prevent concussion.

Insert an oral or nasal airway, if possible, to help prevent the patient from biting his tongue and to help him maintain an open airway. If you are outside the hospital setting, insert a folded handkerchief between his teeth. However, never force a clenched jaw open, nor try to insert hard objects, such as a spoon. In either case, you may break teeth, fracture the jaw, or injure soft tissues of the mouth and tongue. Be sure never to insert your fingers into the patient's mouth as he may clench down and sever them.

Your interventions have succeeded if you have prevented or minimized injury to the patient.

Ineffective airway clearance related to seizure activity, preventing swallowing of secretions. To maintain a patent airway and effective breathing patterns to prevent cerebral hypoxia, begin by loosening constricting clothing. Assess breathing pattern and watch for labored respirations, tachypnea, bradypnea, dyspnea, apnea, and cyanosis. Insert an oral or nasal airway, if possible, to prevent aspiration of the tongue and to maintain an open airway. Avoid using a padded tongue blade, which could splinter and cause aspiration of fragments.

Turn the patient to one side to allow the tongue to fall forward and secretions to drain. This is especially important when an oral airway and suctioning equipment are not immediately available. If available, use suction and a suction catheter to help maintain airway patency. Use an Ambu bag, if needed, for manual ventilation. Help in obtaining a specimen for blood gas analysis, if indicated, and give oxygen, if ordered. Help with intubation, which may be necessary, especially in status epilepticus.

Your interventions have been successful if the patient's airway remains patent and if spontaneous respirations and color return to normal within minutes after the seizure ends. You've succeeded in maintaining cerebral oxygenation if the patient resumes his prior level of consciousness and regains normal pupil size and reaction.

Altered level of consciousness related to seizure activity. To help the patient regain his preseizure orientation to reality as soon as possible after a seizure, provide reorientation during the postictal phase.

Your interventions have succeeded if the patient maintains consciousness or regains it as soon as possible after a seizure.

Impaired communication related to seizure activity. To reestablish the patient's preseizure communication level, give slow, simple commands during the postictal phase. Reassure the patient that expressive/receptive aphasia is temporary.

Your interventions have succeeded if the patient is again able to communicate at the preseizure level.

Impaired mobility related to postictal state. To maintain preseizure activity level, assist the patient in daily activities during the postictal phase. Reassure him that any paralysis and immobility are transient. Encourage independence and activity to the extent he can tolerate them. Consider *your interventions* successful if the patient returns to his preseizure mobility level.

Alteration in oral mucous membrane related to anticonvulsant therapy. To prevent gingival membrane damage, suggest frequent mouth rinsing, especially after meals, to help remove food particles and reduce phenytoin concentration in the saliva. Provide or suggest a soft brush to reduce bleeding and the risk of infection from small abrasions. Consider *your interventions* successful if the gingival membrane remains intact.

Patient and family knowledge deficit related to seizure activity. To help the patient and his family understand the disease and the required medical regimen and to enable the family to handle a seizure and identify an emergency situation, teach the patient and his family about seizures and help them identify possible precipitating causes. Explain an aura as a warning sign and help them recognize it as such. Explain the importance of observing and recording seizure activity, its onset, pattern, and duration. Explain physical manifestations, such as staring, chewing, picking, arm jerking, and incontinence, as normal parts of seizure activity. Help family members to establish management priorities for use during a seizure; describe the postictal state and management principles. Teach them about diagnostic procedures, and help with preparations for special procedures, such as a sleep deprivation EEG, angiography, or lumbar puncture. Explain the purpose of anticonvulsant therapy, its desired effects, short- and long-term side effects, dosage schedule, and potential toxicity. Give the patient and his family a written dosage schedule. Encourage good oral hygiene and regular dental care to minimize effects of gum hyperplasia in patients taking anticonvulsants, especially phenytoin.

Encourage monitoring of anticonvulsant blood levels to prevent toxic reaction and ensure effective dosage of anticonvulsant drugs. Suggest practical ways to deal with their common side effects; for example, calamine lotion to relieve itching. Emphasize the importance of strict compliance with drug therapy, including correct timing of medication and meals. Warn the patient about the possible hazards of drowsiness while taking anticonvulsants. Ask him and his family to report side effects, and warn them about possible interactions with other drugs, particularly over-the-counter preparations containing alcohol or caffeine. Explain the possibility of developing status epilepticus as a result of noncompliance; explain what actions the patient's family should take if this emergency occurs.

Explain the importance of good nutrition and suggest consultation with a dietitian or nutritionist for help with planning meals. Explain to women who suffer premenstrual seizures that water and sodium retention may be causative factors, and refer them for dietary help. Encourage the use of multivitamin supplements, if needed.

Explain about seizure recurrence during periods of illness or stress. Give the patient and his family information about surgery as part of the seizure management plan. Let them ask questions and answer them to dispel any myths and fears. Warn against overprotecting the patient, but explain certain modifications in daily living that may be necessary, such as taking showers rather than tub baths and swimming in groups rather than alone because of the danger of drowning during a seizure. Encourage moderate physical exercise and emphasize the need to avoid stress, exhaustion, and contact sports.

Consider *your interventions* successful if the patient and his family understand epilepsy and its treatment plan; if they comply with the care plan and integrate it into their lifestyle; and if family members can care for the patient during a seizure, can identify emergencies, and know what actions to take.

Altered self-concept related to seizure activity. To help the patient develop and sustain a positive attitude and maintain his family and other relationships, talk honestly with the patient about persistent social myths and fears about epilepsy, and prepare him and his family to deal with those views. Explain the possible social stigmas that may affect work and schooling. Offer to provide information to the teachers of school-age patients concerning seizures and management. Discuss the patient's view of himself in relation to his seizures. Determine their effects on his daily living. Provide employment referral if job retraining is necessary. Tell the patient about state and local laws concerning driver's licenses and other legal matters. Encourage genetic counseling for couples who want to have children and make them aware of the risks of anticonvulsant therapy during pregnancy. Refer the patient and his family to a local chapter of the Epilepsy Foundation of America, based in Washington, D.C., for support and patient education materials. If necessary, refer the patient and/or his family to a neuropsychologist for counseling. *Your interventions* have succeeded if the patient maintains his family role and other relationships and if he can identify and use resources to help him live a productive life.

Promote lifelong adjustment
The seizure patient usually faces a lifelong disorder requiring extended drug therapy. At each stage of life, he'll be called on to explain the nature and treatment of his seizures to friends, classmates, teachers, employers, and colleagues and to persuade them that he's capable despite this disorder. Your teaching and support can make his own adaptation easier and his teaching of others convincing. Your efforts to inform him about epilepsy, to dispel myths, and to bolster his self-esteem can play a central part in his understanding and willingness to adhere to therapy and to lead a full life.

Points to remember

- Approximately 2 to 4 million people in the United States suffer from epilepsy.
- In all but a few instances, drug therapy can control seizure activity—reducing frequency or severity—but cannot cure it.
- The EEG remains the primary diagnostic tool.
- A detailed history and thorough neurologic assessment can help pinpoint the epileptogenic focus.
- People with epilepsy can live productive, happy lives.

10 PROMOTING REHABILITATION IN CORD LESIONS

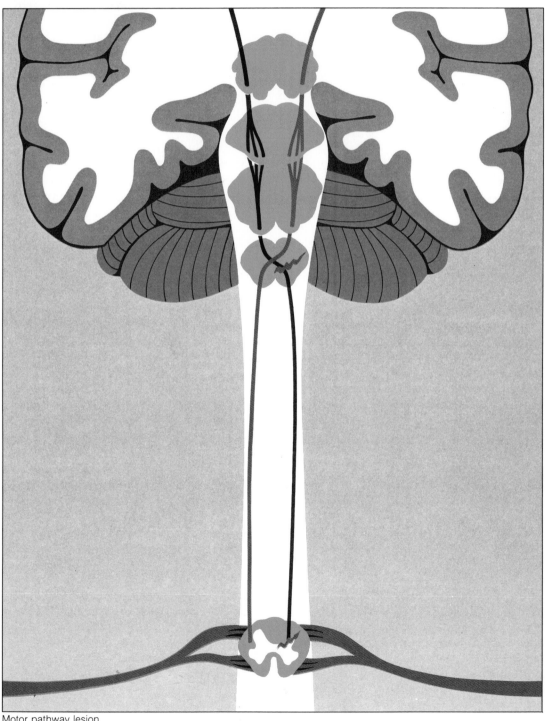

Motor pathway lesion

The total, round-the-clock care that's necessary for patients with spinal cord injury can challenge your nursing skills as severely as the injury threatens to overwhelm these patients' bodies. If you feel less than confident when dealing with such patients, this chapter can help you to understand and master the unusually demanding physical and psychological care that can help them survive with optimal function.

Categories and causes

Spinal cord lesions can be classified into three major categories—trauma, tumors, and congenital defects. (See *Spinal cord lesions,* pages 126 and 127.) Trauma includes flexion, extension, and rotational injuries to the vertebral column resulting in spinal cord damage. Tumors include benign and malignant tumors and are classified according to location. Congenital defects include syringomyelia and spina bifida and may vary in severity.

Trauma. Spinal cord trauma, especially cervical trauma, may cause immediate death, but about 7,000 to 10,000 new cord-injured patients per year survive the initial injury. Most of these patients are males between ages 15 and 30; about half are quadriplegic, and half are paraplegic. These patients face lengthy, difficult, and costly rehabilitation, which may or may not help them regain independence.

Tumors. Spinal cord tumor usually strikes patients between ages 20 and 60, affecting males and females equally. Usually, spinal cord tumor is histologically benign and occurs at the thoracic level.

Congenital defects. Some variant of spina bifida (spina bifida occulta, meningocele, myelocele, myelomeningocele), a congenital neural tube defect, occurs in approximately 2.5% of live births. Myelomeningocele, a severe form of spina bifida, occurs in one or two of every 1,000 live births. Occasionally, spina bifida is associated with syringomyelia, a condition marked by a fluid-filled cavity (syrinx) within the spinal cord.

PATHOPHYSIOLOGY

Spinal cord lesions impair nerve impulse transmission by permanently destroying cellular portions of the spinal cord, as spinal cord tissue doesn't regenerate. They lead to varying degrees of dysfunction, depending on the cause, the degree of transection (complete or incomplete), the location of the lesion (lower or upper motor neuron), and the level (C1 to S4) of spinal cord injury.

Trauma, tumors, and congenital defects

Spinal trauma causes transection when a foreign object or a displaced vertebral bone penetrates the cord. Such transection may be incomplete or complete. Its resulting deficits vary accordingly.

A spinal cord tumor, even when it grows slowly, eventually consumes space in the vertebral column and compresses the cord. Such compression impinges on spinal nerve roots, destroys spinal cord tracts, interferes with blood supply, and obstructs cerebrospinal fluid (CSF) circulation. As the tumor grows, edema and the expanding tumor mass cause further cord compression, resulting in progressive sensory and motor impairment, severe pain, and possible sphincter dysfunctions.

Contusion causes microscopic hemorrhage into the cord, leading to compression. Usually, cord transection doesn't occur and neurologic deficit is transient, but the swelling and hemorrhage can cause permanent deficit.

Different congenital defects cause different pathology. In syringomyelia, progressive spinal cord tissue cavitation usually arises from a congenital defect that causes formation of one or more progressively expanding, fluid-filled cystic cavities. First, dilatation affects the central gray matter of the cervical spinal cord, disrupting crossing pain and temperature fibers. Next, posterior and anterior horn involvement cause segmental weakness.

Spina bifida, a fairly common congenital defect from incomplete vertebral closure, varies greatly in severity from an occult type (without protrusion of spinal cord or meninges and with few clinical signs) to a totally open spine (with displacement and malformation of meninges, spinal cord, and nerve roots). In the common cystic form, a skin-covered sac containing meninges (meningocele), spinal cord (myelocele), or both (myelomeningocele) protrudes through a congenital spine opening. The severity of impairment depends on the degree of nerve involvement. Spina bifida involving cord or lumbosacral nerve roots causes varying degrees of paralysis below the lesion; in severe cases, it causes sensory and motor loss.

Effects of cord transection

Complete transection of the cord causes permanent loss below the lesion of all voluntary *(continued on page 128)*

Spinal cord lesions

Traumatic lesions

Burst injury

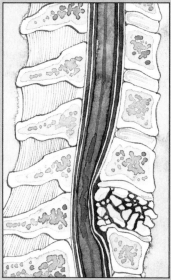

Automobile accident or any direct force which is great enough to shatter the vertebral body, causing bone chips to injure cord.

Compression injury

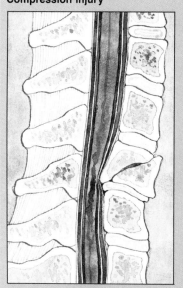

Accidents from diving, surfing, or trampolining, causing vertical blow to head. Resulting dislocation injures the cord.

Flexion injury
Anterior

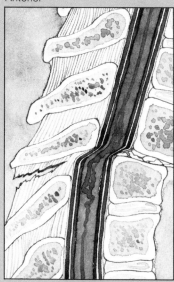

Automobile accidents, generally head-on collisions; falls in which the back of the head receives the force of impact, causing hyperflexion of the neck

Flexion-rotation injury

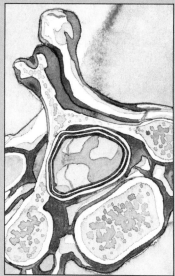

Automobile accidents, falls, or accidents during contact sports or skiing that cause deformation injuries in which spinal cord–supporting structures cannot accommodate movement

Hyperextension injury

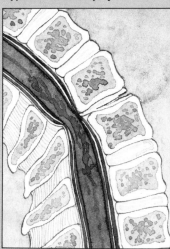

Falls causing backward thrust of the head or rear-end automobile collisions causing acceleration injuries in which sudden, forceful impact and forward movement hyperextend the neck

Penetrating injury

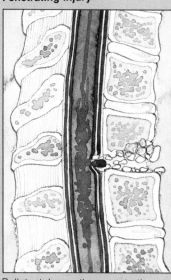

Bullet, stab, or other penetrating wound that causes damage to spinal cord tissue and blood vessels

Tumors

Extradural tumors

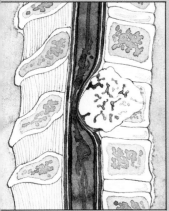

Metastatic or cause unknown. Tumors arise in vertebrae, extradural space, or paraspinal area.

Intradural extramedullary tumors

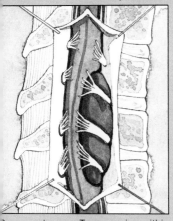

Cause unknown. Tumors arise within or under the dura mater.

Intradural intramedullary tumors

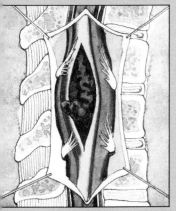

Cause unknown. Tumors arise within the spinal cord.

Congenital defects

Spina bifida

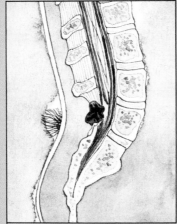

Spina bifida occulta

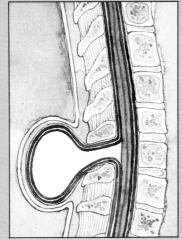

Meningocele

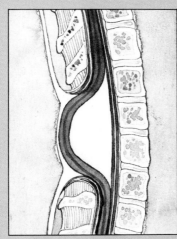

Myelocele

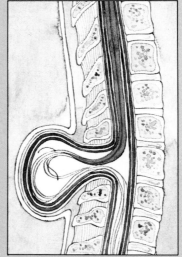

Myelomeningocele

In all types of spina bifida, the neural tube fails to close in first month of gestation. Cause unknown, but may be associated with viruses, radiation, environmental factors, and genetics

Syringomyelia
(Abnormal liquid-filled cavities in the spinal cord)

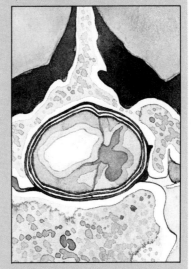

Cause unknown, but associated with other congenital defects, intramedullary tumors, and trauma

Herniated intervertebral disk

The intervertebral disk is made up of a gelatinous substance, which fills the space between each vertebral body. This space, the nucleus pulposus, is surrounded by the anulus fibrosus. Degeneration, trauma (accidents, strain), or congenital predisposition can cause the nucleus pulposus to herniate through the anulus fibrosus.

Cervical herniation causes pain in the neck, shoulders, arms and head; paresthesia and numbness in the arms; and muscle weakness. *Lumbar herniation* causes low back pain; sensory impairment; pain radiating to the buttocks, thighs, calves, and ankles; muscle weakness; and tendon reflexes.

Herniated intervertebral disk is confirmed by plain films, myelography, and electromyography. For cervical herniation, immobilization with a cervical collar is necessary. For both types of herniation, treatment may include traction to relieve pressure on nerve roots, bed rest to reduce inflammation and edema in soft tissue and to relieve pressure on nerve roots, drug therapy to treat symptoms, and surgery to remove the herniated disk and relieve pressure. Drug therapy includes muscle relaxants to increase range of spinal motion, anti-inflammatory agents to treat the inflammatory response, and analgesics to control pain and discomfort.

When caring for a patient with herniated intervertebral disk, make sure he maintains bed rest and traction, and give him medications as ordered. Postoperatively, teach him to strengthen abdominal muscles and flexors of the spine, and teach him good body mechanics.

motor and sensory function and temporary loss (spinal shock)—lasting from weeks to months—of reflex, autonomic, bladder, bowel, and sexual function.

Spinal shock may result from any process that cuts off neuronal discharges from higher centers and abruptly stops normal impulse firing, causing immediate flaccid paralysis and loss of all sensation, reflex activity, and autonomic functions below the lesion. Its physiologic effects include loss of vasomotor tone, which lowers blood pressure; loss of thermoregulation; intestinal peristalsis; bladder sphincter contraction; detrusor muscle atony; bowel distention; and reflex erection in males.

As spinal shock resolves, spinal neurons slowly regain excitability, so reflex activity and autonomic control may return; voluntary motor and sensory function will not. Sometimes, as flaccid paralysis subsides, isolated cord segments develop excessive reflex activity, causing spastic paralysis. (See *Levels of spinal cord innervation,* page 130.)

Incomplete transection causes loss of some sensory and/or motor function below the lesion, depending on whether the ascending or descending tracts are severed. Ascending tracts control sensory function; descending tracts, motor function. Obviously, incomplete transection allows a much better prognosis for the return of normal function than complete transection.

Upper and lower motor neuron lesions
Remember, spinal cord lesions do not always cause complete transection. Signs result from the interruption of specific pathways in the cord that are affected. Spinal shock may occur in both, but later physical findings differ in upper motor neuron and lower motor neuron lesions. In an upper motor neuron lesion, the interruption of innervation is in the descending motor pathway. Above the lesion normal function occurs; below the lesion voluntary movement is lost, but reflex activity is seen in muscles with intact reflex arcs. This means, clinically, that spastic paralysis is present with little muscle atrophy. Dysreflexia is common.

In patients with lower motor neuron lesions, the damage is to the anterior horn cells of the spinal cord or the spinal roots, resulting in flaccid paralysis and muscle atrophy.

Level of injury determines effects
Spinal cord injuries most often involve the fifth, sixth, and seventh cervical, the twelfth thoracic, and the first lumbar vertebrae, where

greater range of mobility increases vulnerability to injury. Injury at C2 or C3 is usually rapidly fatal. Injury above C4 causes respiratory impairment and paralysis of all extremities. Any cord lesion above T6 disrupts sympathetic control, causing vasodilation, hypotension, and sometimes compromised cardiac output. And since the parasympathetic system remains intact through the vagus nerve, bradycardia occurs. A lesion above T1 also interrupts intercostal (T1 to T6) and diaphragmatic (C4 and C5) innervation, causing difficult, deep inspiration; progressive hypoventilation; atelectasis; respiratory fatigue; and eventual respiratory arrest. (See *Levels of spinal cord innervation,* page 130.)

After spinal shock resolves, a lesion above T6 usually causes dysreflexia. The dysreflexia results from uninhibited sympathetic discharges elicited by noxious stimuli, such as a distended bladder or rectum or a pressure area on the skin. These discharges cause reflex stimulation of the sympathetic system, which, because the lesion has interrupted nerve impulse transmission, cannot be mediated by higher nervous system centers. Reflex stimulation causes pelvic visceral spasm, which, in turn, causes vasoconstriction below the lesion and hypertension. Compounding this problem, unopposed parasympathetic innervation depresses the heart rate, creating severe bradycardia.

Effects of impaired blood supply
The spinal cord depends on an adequate blood supply to provide oxygen and nutrition for its cells. When edema, hemorrhage, or nerve fiber compression compromises blood supply, secondary damage destroys myelin and axons; myelomalacia—abnormal spinal cord softening and necrosis—follows. Eventually, phagocytosis disposes of the debris resulting from tissue breakdown. These secondary reactions are considered the primary causes of spinal cord degeneration at the site of injury. Secondary reactions to cord injury are now considered reversible if correctly treated within 4 to 6 hours after injury. If the cord has not been completely transected, prompt and vigorous treatment may prevent partial function loss from becoming complete and permanent.

MEDICAL MANAGEMENT
Correct treatment of spinal cord injury must begin—in the case of trauma—at the scene of the accident because incorrect first aid can aggravate and increase permanent neurologic

loss. After emergency first aid, repeated evaluation of neurologic status, emphasizing function distal to the injury, is necessary. A graded scale is used to evaluate the strength of each muscle group and reflex, and a standard dermatome reference is used to test sensory function. Such evaluation often reveals multiple sensory, motor, and reflex abnormalities. Regular and frequent follow-up exams evaluate any improvement or deterioration that necessitates changes in treatment.

Tests pinpoint location and cause

Diagnostic tests typically include plain X-rays, tomography, computerized tomography (CT) scan, myelography, electromyography, and evoked potentials.

Plain X-rays. These films determine the position of vertebrae and any displacement or fracture that may be impinging on the cord. Plain films are particularly helpful in defining bone injury. Films of the pelvis and lower extremities may show hidden fractures in anesthetic areas below the lesion.

Tomography. Because this test shows vertebral dimension, it can clarify questionable plain X-ray results.

CT scan. This test defines the extent of cord injury by tumor, bone, blood, CSF, a foreign object, edema, or softened tissue better than plain X-rays and tomography.

Myelography. A spinal cord lesion may block the dye used in myelography, allowing visualization of the affected area. With spinal cord tumor or herniated intervertebral disks, this test shows partial or complete CSF block.

Electromyography/Evoked potentials. These tests define the segmental level of spinal cord lesions by measuring electrical conduction. Peripheral nerves are stimulated, and resultant muscle response is measured and recorded at various spinal levels.

Treatment to improve function

Treatment goals are to stop cord damage progression and to preserve or improve residual neurologic function. Treatment may include traction, surgery, immobilization, radiation therapy, drugs, and, in some centers, hypothermia to inhibit the progression of injury. After surgery and/or traction achieves vertebral column alignment or decompression, immobilization is the key. Physical and occupational therapy are given daily.

Traction. Cervical traction—Gardner-Wells or Crutchfield tongs or halo fixation—realigns vertebrae displaced through trauma. (See *Common types of traction,* page 132.) Thoracic and lumbar lesions sometimes need extensive traction. A halo device can be used along with Steinmann's pins in both femurs, which are connected to the halo by adjustable rods. Opposing traction may be applied to the halo and femoral pins. Later, when the patient is ready to ambulate, a body cast or jacket connected to the halo maintains spinal alignment and stabilization. Along with traction for cervical, thoracic, or lumbar lesions, a Stryker frame or a Roto Rest bed should be used to strengthen spinal stability.

Surgery. Some doctors believe early surgical intervention allows for better alignment, early mobilization, and shorter recovery; others consider it unnecessary. But surgery is common for certain kinds of trauma, tumor, and congenital defects.

• *To remove bone fragments or penetrating foreign object.* After traumatic injury leaves bone fragments in the spinal cord or after a penetrating wound, surgery is necessary to remove the fragments or foreign object and to prevent further damage to the cord.

• *To relieve compression.* With cord compression or progressive neurologic deficit, laminectomy allows for decompression and fusion with bone grafts or synthetic materials. Fusion stabilizes the vertebral column and protects the spinal cord. To increase stability of thoracic or lumbar areas, steel rods (Harrington, Luque) may be placed along the vertebral column.

• *To excise tumors.* Most tumors require decompression laminectomy, but intradural extramedullary tumors are excised under an operative microscope. Such surgery is extremely delicate, as the spinal cord can be easily damaged. Extradural tumors may require surgery as well as other treatment.

• *To reduce CSF pressure.* For syringomyelia, decompression by draining the spinal cord can reduce CSF pressure and temporarily relieve symptoms. Decompression is achieved by occluding the upper end of the central canal, opening the spinal cord cavity, using a ventriculosubarachnoid shunt, or unroofing the spinal cord.

• *To correct herniation.* In myelomeningocele, surgery reduces the protruding meninges and spinal cord and closes the sac. After surgery, the degree of residual neurologic deficit varies according to the severity of the original herniation. Surgery is rarely required for the types of spina bifida that don't herniate the meninges or spinal cord.

Levels of spinal cord innervation

This lateral view of the spinal cord shows the level of origin for the nerves supplying the limbs, diaphragm, intercostal muscles, sympathetic outflow, bladder, bowel, and external genitalia. A complete transection above T1 causes quadriplegia; below, paraplegia.

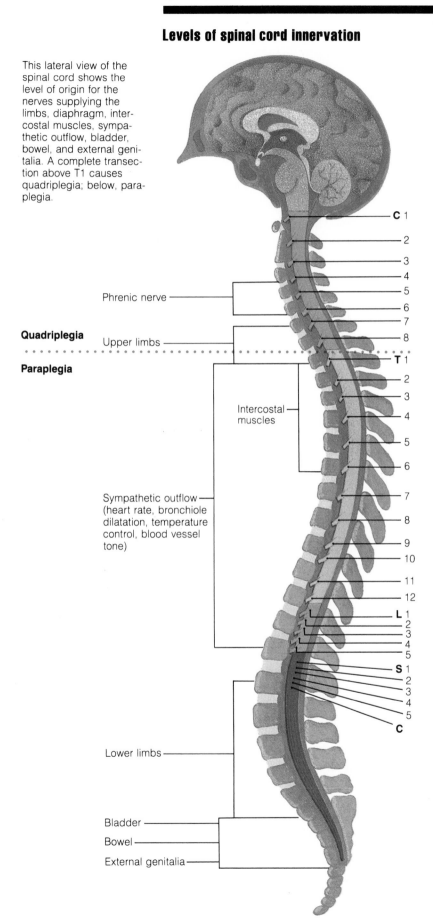

Phrenic nerve

Quadriplegia

Upper limbs

Paraplegia

Intercostal muscles

Sympathetic outflow (heart rate, bronchiole dilatation, temperature control, blood vessel tone)

Lower limbs

Bladder
Bowel
External genitalia

C 1
2
3
4
5
6
7
8
T 1
2
3
4
5
6
7
8
9
10
11
12
L 1
2
3
4
5
S 1
2
3
4
5
C

Immobilization. To prevent vertebral column instability and to aid healing, vertebral alignment should be followed by immobilization, with duration varying according to the injury's severity. Complete bed rest may be needed for 1 to 6 weeks, followed by about 6 months of limited ambulation using immobilization devices. To maintain cervical immobilization when the patient is moved, his neck must be stabilized. Cervical immobilization devices include hard and soft cervical collars, sandbags along the sides of the head and neck, and the already-mentioned halo traction with jacket. Thoracic stabilization devices include braces and corsets.

Drug therapy. Therapy to reverse secondary reactions to spinal cord injury may include an anti-inflammatory (dexamethasone); an osmotic diuretic (mannitol) to reduce edema; and a plasma expander, such as dextran, to support capillary blood flow within the cord. Cimetidine and antacids are often given with dexamethasone to reduce gastric acid secretion and prevent stress ulcers.

Antineoplastics may sometimes be used to treat spinal cord tumors, depending on tumor type and location. After spinal cord injury, if sympathetic outflow is compromised, a vasopressor (dopamine) may be needed. Atropine or another cholinergic blocker can relieve bradycardia from unopposed parasympathetic stimulation. A muscle relaxant (baclofen) can relieve muscle spasms that occur after spinal shock resolves. Subcutaneous heparin may prevent deep vein thrombosis.

Radiation. This therapy, along with other therapies, can treat malignant tumors involving the spinal cord. Radiation is specific to tumor type, size, and invasiveness. Usually, therapy consists of 3,000 to 4,000 rads in divided doses over a 5- to 6-week period. Radiation may cause myelopathy—progressive spinal cord necrosis with symptoms of sensory loss, motor weakness, and sphincter disturbances—6 months to 1 year after treatment.

NURSING MANAGEMENT
Because spinal cord lesions affect so many systems at once, developing and carrying out an appropriate nursing plan challenges all your nursing skills from assessment to evaluation. But effective supportive care is possible however severe the injury. Overall, your goals are to achieve the highest possible rehabilitation level and to prevent further injury by continual assessment and reevaluation.

Guidelines for assessing level of a spinal cord lesion

Ask the patient to...	Observe this body part and test sensation with light touch, pinprick, and position	Cord level associated with motion	Cord level associated with sensation
Shrug his shoulders; take a deep breath (diaphragm should descend, causing abdomen to bulge)	Shoulder, chest, and abdomen	C3 to C5	C4
Bend his elbow	Elbow	C5	Radial side C6 Ulnar side T1
Bend his wrist up	Wrist	C6	C6 (thumb side of wrist)
Oppose his thumb to each fingertip; make a fist	Thumb First two digits Little finger	C8 to T1	C6 C7 T1
Tighten his abdomen	Abdomen Pubis Navel Nipple line	T5 to T12	L1 T10 T4
Flex his hip	Hips	L1 to L3	L2
Straighten his leg	Knees	L2 to L4	L3
Bend and straighten his toes	Toes	L5, S1, and S2	L5
Tighten his sphincter muscle around your finger	Perineum	S2 to S4	S5

Patient history first

To help define the lesion type and site, record the patient's account of his injury or illness. If injury is the cause, try to get a description from a witness, including any vehicle or weapon involved, the patient's position when the injury was sustained, and any positioning that relieves or aggravates symptoms.

Try to get the patient to pinpoint his chief complaints. The most common ones are pain and paresthesia of the back and legs, followed by motor losses. Find out how quickly his complaint developed. For example, a slow-growing tumor causes insidious changes.

Next, take the patient's medical and surgical history. Does he have arthritis of the spine, congenital deformities, or a history of cancer? Has he had previous injury or surgery to the back? Does he have a family history of malignancy or lower back pain? Also, ask if he uses alcohol, is taking any drugs, or smokes.

During the patient history, provide initial support and reassurance to begin developing rapport. Try to understand his support systems and coping mechanisms. Does he have a family or significant others he can call on? How independent/dependent is he? Can he verbalize his feelings and fears? How does his illness affect his job status or life-style?

If the patient has slowly developing symptoms, defining sexual dysfunction can help define the lesion. Usually, a patient with a spinal cord lesion lacks genital sensation and can't achieve orgasm during intercourse. A male patient with an upper motor neuron lesion (S2 to S4) can usually achieve erection but can't ejaculate; a male patient with a complete lower motor neuron lesion at the same level can't achieve erection.

Conduct a physical examination

If you suspect a cervical lesion, test respiratory status and the cervical area (C1 to C4 control diaphragmatic innervation). Assess respiratory rate and quality, and breath sounds. At first, the patient with a cervical lesion can compensate for loss of breathing musculature and maintain adequate ventilation. But, eventually, he develops atelectasis secondary to hypoventilation. If ventilation is adequate, begin a detailed neurologic check.

Assess sensory and motor functions, including the extremities. (See *Guidelines for assessing level of a spinal cord lesion.*) Check for hyperactive deep tendon reflexes and positive Babinski's reflexes indicating spinal cord com-

Common types of traction

Halo fixation with jacket

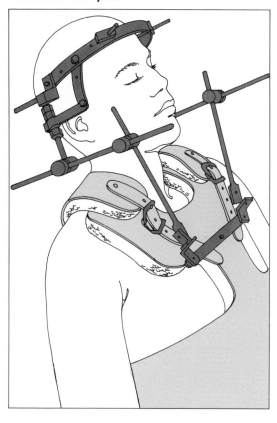

Gardner-Wells tongs

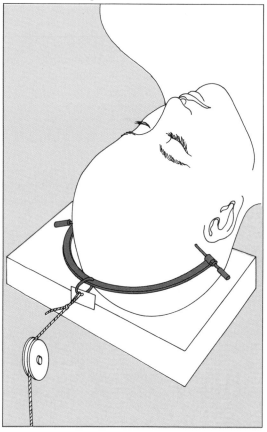

pression and upper motor neuron lesion. Slowly growing tumors and intervertebral disk disease may compress nerve roots and cause depressed tendon reflexes at that particular root level.

Check the extremities, using gravity, resistance, pinprick, and touch. Since lesions don't always produce equal bilateral involvement, test each side of the body. For example, Brown-Séquard syndrome affects half of the spinal cord, causing unilateral loss of motor function on the same side, loss of pain sense on the opposite side, spastic muscle tone with an upper motor neuron lesion, and flaccid muscle tone with a lower motor neuron lesion. (Brown-Séquard syndrome results from a partial cord lesion that transects or compresses only half of the cord.)

Perform cardiovascular assessment in a patient with a spinal cord lesion high enough to affect sympathetic outflow and in any patient who shows spinal shock. Measure blood pressure and pulse and heart rate. Watch for hypotension due to vasodilation and blood pooling in the lower extremities. Elevating the patient's head may cause sudden hypotension for which he cannot compensate. Also watch for bradycardia from unopposed vagal influence. When you take the patient's pulse, consider his pulse rate before injury. The spinal cord–injured patient is often young and athletic, so his pulse rate before injury may have been 50 to 60 beats/minute. After injury, his rate may drop to 30 to 40 beats/minute.

Begin GI assessment by listening for bowel sounds. Spinal shock and S2-to-S4 lesions interfere with peristalsis and sphincter control. This causes absent bowel sounds, ileus, and gastric dilatation, which can adversely affect breathing. Lower motor neuron lesions can permanently destroy normal bowel function. Also assess all nasogastric drainage and stools for occult blood. Ulcers may result from a stress response to spinal cord lesion or treatment with steroids.

Assess the genitourinary system. A spinal cord lesion above S2 to S4 causes neurogenic bladder and loss of voluntary control. A lower motor neuron lesion with spinal shock causes loss of reflex emptying. Check for signs of loss of reflex emptying—bladder distention and overflow incontinence. Since the loss of reflex emptying predisposes to bladder infection, assess urine color, clarity, and odor.

Develop nursing diagnoses

Since spinal cord lesions involve long-term

treatment and potentially serious complications, continually reevaluate your diagnoses and modify your care plan accordingly.

Altered respiratory status related to loss of phrenic nerve stimulation and/or intercostal stimulation. Your goal is to achieve and maintain effective lung ventilation and adequate body tissue oxygenation. Auscultate the lungs for atelectasis and secretion pooling. If the patient can't cough or deep breathe, suction him. To avoid hypoxia, give supplemental oxygen before, during, and after suctioning. To prevent vagal stimulation, perform suctioning gently and briefly. To prevent further cervical damage, the patient may also need mechanical ventilation via tracheostomy. To reduce the risk of infection, use aseptic technique during suctioning and tracheostomy care.

A quadriplegic who has lost phrenic function may permanently depend on mechanical ventilation unless phrenic pacing is used. Before phrenic pacing, explain routine preoperative and postoperative care. The doctor orders the pacing schedule and the amplitude setting, but you must watch for fatigue and inadequate oxygenation, which could force discontinuation of pacing.

To enhance pacemaker effect, place the patient in semi-Fowler's position. If he wants to drink during phrenic pacing, always begin by giving him only one small sip to make sure he isn't prone to aspiration. Also help him cough and deep breathe to prevent pooling of secretions in the lungs.

Even the patient who can maintain adequate ventilation independently may need assistance with coughing. To add volume to coughing, place both your hands below his diaphragm and push upward when he exhales. Your hand movement replaces paralyzed abdominal muscles. If the patient needs aggressive chest physiotherapy, avoid placing him in positions that could pressure the diaphragm and abdominal contents and further compromise breathing. Consider your care effective if the patient achieves adequate ventilation.

Impaired mobility related to voluntary motor deficits. Your goals are to maintain and promote limb movement, to prevent muscle atrophy and contractures, and to promote safety. Prepare to meet these goals by attending inservice programs on alignment, traction devices, and operation of special beds.

Continually assess motor function as spinal shock and edema resolve. Alert the doctor to any changes. Perform range-of-motion exercises several times a day on all paralyzed extremities. This maintains muscle tone and prevents venous stasis in the lower extremities. Also, to prevent venous stasis, apply elastic stockings to the legs.

To prevent frozen shoulder contracture, position the patient's arms at 90° angles to his sides several times a day for 1 to 2 hours. Full range of motion may not be possible in a patient confined to traction. Instead, logroll such a patient often, making sure to maintain body alignment. (See *How to position a paralyzed patient to lie on his side,* page 134.) You may need another nurse to help you.

Check traction setups every shift to make sure frames are secure, pulleys are correctly aligned, and weights are hanging free. If the patient is in skeletal traction, check insertion sites every shift for drainage, swelling, or redness. Daily, cleanse insertion sites; apply a bactericidal ointment; and apply a fresh sterile dressing. If the patient is in a body cast, make sure the cast isn't too tight. Check for redness, swelling, and skin breakdown around edges. Give routine skin care and pad pressure points.

Take special care to protect the patient from falling out of bed. Always keep side rails up except when you are giving direct care. Use Stryker frames and Roto Rest beds correctly and with safety belts secured.

Make sure the paralyzed patient has some way to call for help, such as a sensitive call bell. A quadriplegic patient on a mechanical ventilator may need constant surveillance.

Encourage and support the patient's efforts in occupational and physical therapy. Check his vital signs before and after therapy to avoid excessive fatigue. Before getting any quadriplegic patient out of bed, watch for orthostatic hypotension—a possible result of compromised sympathetic vascular control.

Teach the patient and his caretakers methods of transferring from a bed to a wheelchair and from a wheelchair to a car. Emphasize the use of good body mechanics for the caretakers and proper alignment for the patient.

Your interventions are effective if the patient has no contractures and little muscle atrophy, if proper alignment is maintained and injury is avoided, and if all his physical needs are met and he can call for help as needed.

Altered sensory function related to sensory tract destruction by spinal cord lesion and reduced environmental stimuli. Your goals are to maintain optimal sensory function and to prevent injury. To achieve this, continually

Nursing care for an infant with spina bifida

An infant with spina bifida requires specialized nursing care to prevent contractures, decubiti, local and urinary tract infections, and other complications; and family teaching and support.
• Prevent local infection by cleansing the defect gently with sterile saline solution. Then cover it with sterile dressings moistened with sterile saline solution.
• Prevent skin breakdown by placing sheepskin under the infant.
• Hold and cuddle the infant, but make sure not to apply pressure to the defect. When you return him to his crib, position him on his abdomen to prevent contamination of the defect with urine or feces.
• Measure head circumference daily, and watch for signs of hydrocephalus and meningeal irritation, such as fever or nuchal rigidity.
• Minimize contractures with passive range-of-motion exercises.
• Monitor intake and output. To prevent urinary tract infection, perform Credé's maneuver every 2 hours during the day and once during the night.
• Teach parents how to recognize early signs of complications, such as distended scalp veins from hydrocephalus; to credé the bladder regularly; to prevent bowel obstruction; and to recognize lagging development early. Refer parents for genetic counseling. Also, teach parents that folic acid during the first 3 months of pregnancy may prevent spina bifida.

How to position a paralyzed patient to lie on his side

Adjust pulley position to maintain proper traction angle. To maintain this angle, move the pulley each time you turn the patient.

Use pillow to support back.

Use pillow to maintain ankles at 90°.

Use foam wedge under side of face to avoid weight of head on tongs.

Use an axillary pillow to protect lower arm from body weight.

Use drawsheet for easy turning.

Use pillows between knees and ankles to relieve pressure against skin.

Use egg-crate mattress to prevent decubiti.

test and record sensory function and limitations. Notify the doctor of any changes.

Make sure a patient who is confined to bed doesn't become sensorially deprived. Position him so he can see any activity on the unit, and talk to him frequently. If available, give him prism glasses so he can see around him while on the Stryker frame. Advise him of his limitations, and protect him from bodily harm he can't feel. When you position him, make sure he's not lying on his arm or on any object. Along with sensory loss, the patient may sustain autonomic disturbances that interfere with temperature regulation and are aggravated by heat and cold. So regulate the room temperature, make sure he is adequately covered, and eliminate drafts. Advise the ambulatory patient to be extremely careful with hot water, heating pads, or very cold weather.

After successful interventions, sensory functioning is preserved, the patient remains oriented and aware of his environment, the patient and those taking care of him are aware of his limitations, and the patient's body temperature remains normal.

Altered urination related to loss of bladder innervation. Your goals are to achieve regularly predicted bladder emptying and to prevent infection. Begin bladder retraining immediately after the acute phase.

Throughout training, use aseptic technique during catheterization to prevent infection. Teach the patient and his family to use aseptic technique as well. Try to distribute the patient's fluid intake evenly to equalize bladder filling between catheterizations and, if necessary, restrict fluid to 1,800 ml every 24 hours.

Begin bladder training in the patient with

upper motor neuron lesion by performing intermittent catheterization every 4 hours. Obtain urine volumes of less than 500 ml at each catheterization. If you obtain more than 500 ml, schedule catheterization once every 3 hours.

Soon, though the patient will still be unable to perceive the need to void, he should be able to void by reflex after light thigh stroking or pulling of pubic hair. Initially, catheterize after voiding for residual urine. If you obtain more than 100 ml, delay training for a day. Eventually, the patient can become continent after careful bladder training.

A patient with a lower motor neuron lesion cannot reflex void. However, since his sphincter is flaccid, he can relieve himself using Credé's maneuver. Have him press inward and downward on the abdomen, starting at the umbilicus and moving down to the pubis. If he can't move his arms, perform this maneuver for him. After he voids, catheterize for residual urine. Since the sphincter is flaccid, you should get no more than 50 ml. Otherwise, check for residual urine each time he voids until residual urine is less than 50 ml.

Teach the patient and his family to watch for signs of urinary tract infection (cloudy, foul-smelling urine; fever; flank pain). Also teach them signs of autonomic dysreflexia (rising blood pressure, slow pulse, headache, profuse sweating) caused by bladder distention. After successful bladder training, the patient should be continent and free of infection.

Alteration in bowel elimination related to loss of innervation to the bowel and rectum. Your goal is to have the patient have a bowel movement every 1 to 3 days without using an enema. Bowel training works in most spinal cord patients because large bowel innervation is independent of spinal cord lesion.

First, assess bowel function. Prior to his lesion, how often did the patient have a bowel movement? Was it in the morning or evening? What types of food has he been eating?

Give Colace twice daily, as ordered, to soften the stool. To initiate bowel movement, insert a Dulcolax suppository approximately ½ hour after breakfast or supper. The doctor may vary this schedule according to the patient's past bowel schedule. Before inserting the suppository, insert your finger in the patient's rectum to stimulate reflex emptying. After you insert the suppository, help the patient to the commode. To maintain a successful bowel program, the patient may need to change his diet. He should follow a well-balanced diet high in roughage, and he should avoid foods that cause diarrhea or constipation. Also, teach him signs and symptoms of autonomic dysreflexia, which can interfere with bowel control. After successful training, the patient should move his bowels every 1 to 3 days without using an enema.

Impaired skin integrity related to bed rest and immobility. Your goal is to prevent skin breakdown. Reposition the paralyzed patient every 2 hours. Frequently massage pressure points. Protect these points with tincture of benzoin or commercial skin preparations and lamb's wool or foam padding. To prevent breakdown from exposure to urine or feces, maintain meticulous skin care around the perineum. If the patient needs long-term bed rest, use a special mattress.

Teach the paralyzed patient and/or his caretaker to relieve pressure from anesthetic areas by shifting the patient's weight every 30 to 60 minutes. A paraplegic can shift his weight by lifting his body off the chair with his arms. A quadriplegic must be tilted side to side or backwards by a caretaker.

Make sure the patient maintains adequate nutrition because poor nutrition threatens skin integrity and interferes with healing. Because the patient can't eat until paralytic ileus resolves, the patient initially may achieve a catabolic state, breaking down body fat and protein to sustain metabolism and greatly hampering tissue healing. If skin integrity is broken, extensive decubiti can form and cause necrosis and sepsis. To combat this, promote early parenteral nutrition and nutritious feeding supplements, as tolerated and ordered.

Your interventions are successful if pressure points and reddened areas are well protected and if the patient avoids skin breakdown.

Sexual dysfunction related to sensory and motor deficits of spinal cord lesion. Your goal is to help the patient understand sexual changes and develop new ways to gratify sexual needs. The patient with spinal cord injury usually has questions about sexual function. Unfortunately, sexual counseling is often neglected. Be open to questions from both the patient and his partner and be ready to answer these questions correctly. Remember that the female patient also needs advice about birth control. If needed, refer the patient for additional sexual counseling. After teaching, the patient and his partner should understand sexual function and have developed effective ways to gratify sexual needs.

Disturbance in self-concept related to changes in physical function and life-style. Your goal is to help the patient and his family accept and cope with these changes. A diagnosis of spinal cord lesion brings overwhelming feelings of despair or hopelessness, which provokes a cycle of emotional stages similar to those in the dying patient. These stages include initial denial, awareness and anger, adjustment and anxiety, and finally acceptance and reorganization. Help the patient move through each stage by encouraging him to verbalize his feelings, by not being judgmental, by being as honest as possible, by involving him in his care, and by praising his accomplishments.

Support the patient's family and others who are close to him. Make them aware of the stages of grieving the patient will probably experience, and help them work through their own guilt feelings and fears.

You've helped the patient and his family if the patient can verbalize his feelings, if he takes the initiative to learn and to care for himself, and if his family and significant others can express affection and support.

Defining your role

Providing effective nursing care for the patient with a spinal cord lesion hinges on continual, precise neurologic assessment. If you don't know what to look for or if you don't check the patient frequently enough, he may develop a complication that threatens his life or inhibits his chances for optimal recovery. With the right care and reassurance, you can help the patient survive and have a better chance to live a meaningful life.

Points to remember

- Spinal cord lesions can be classified into three major categories—traumatic injury, spinal cord tumors, and congenital defects.
- The underlying pathophysiology in spinal cord lesions is interference with vascular supply or direct compression and destruction of nerve fiber tracts.
- Initially, treatment of spinal cord injury involves alignment and stabilization of the vertebral column, using traction, surgery, or immobilization to prevent further spinal cord injury.
- Nursing assessment of sensory and motor function of each body area can help determine the vertebral level of spinal cord lesion.
- A patient with a cervical lesion will be a quadriplegic and may require phrenic nerve pacing from loss of diaphragmatic innervation. A patient with a complete thoracic or lumbar lesion will be a paraplegic but will probably breathe independently. Both types of patients require assistance with mobility.
- Neurogenic bladder, a common spinal cord lesion deficit, requires bladder training, which is usually successful.

11 RELIEVING NEUROLOGIC PAIN SYNDROMES

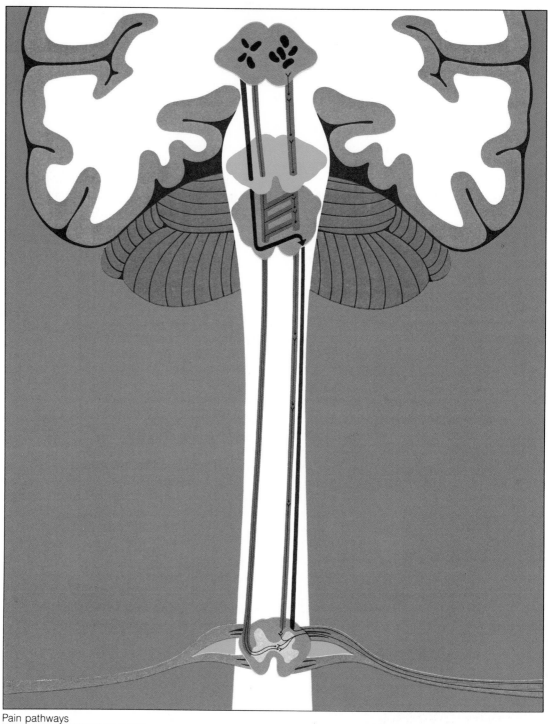

Pain pathways

Managing pain successfully is undeniably one of your most important nursing responsibilities—and sometimes the most difficult to meet. It requires much more of you than simply administering analgesic drugs. It requires considering each patient's unique perception of pain and response to it. It may require skillful counseling and persistent teaching of special pain-control techniques like distraction and deep relaxation. It certainly requires learning all you can about what causes pain disorders and the many ways you can help the patient cope with them.

The universal experience

Pain is part of the universal human experience. Everyone can recognize it, but no one can reliably define it, measure it, or predict its effects in others. We perceive it in others only indirectly through its effects on heart rate, respirations, and behavior.

We know that pain tolerance varies greatly and is significantly influenced by culture, prior pain experience, and personal values. But now, we're beginning to understand the physiologic mechanisms that govern the efficacy of mind-over-matter techniques, such as meditation, yoga, and hypnosis, and to explain the action of common pain-killing drugs and ancient practices, such as acupuncture. We know now that pain may be reduced and even overcome through psychological as well as medical treatments.

PATHOPHYSIOLOGY

Pain is a response to noxious stimuli and often signals an underlying disorder. Acute pain lasts only days or weeks. Usually, it stems from a specific illness or injury and gradually subsides with recovery. Chronic pain, however, may last for months or years, may have no obvious cause, and may involve both physiologic and psychological factors. Moreover, it exerts a profound influence; more than one third of Americans endure recurrent or persistent pain.

Common causes and manifestations

Pain commonly results from inflammation, distention, traction, ischemia, displacement, dilatation, hemorrhage, contraction, or pulsation of blood vessels, neural structures, skin, muscles, or the viscera. This pain may surface as headaches, trigeminal neuralgia, peripheral neuralgia, causalgia, phantom limb pain, or low back pain. (See *Common pain disorders: Causes and precipitating factors,* page 138.)

Headaches. The three common types of chronic headaches are migraine (vascular), cluster (vascular), and tension. *Migraine headaches* produce intense, unilateral, throbbing pain, but the pain may spread to frontal and temporal regions or to the opposite side of the head. Migraines occur more frequently in women. They last the longest of the chronic headaches, from several hours to a day or two. (See *What happens in migraine vascular headache.*)

Cluster headaches occur more commonly in men. Unilateral piercing pain strikes the orbital region, often with associated nasal drainage and ocular irritation. These headaches last anywhere from 10 minutes to 2 hours and recur for a number of days, then remit for long periods.

Tension headaches, also called muscle contraction headaches, produce generalized, steady pain or aching in the occipital and neck regions. They occur in all age-groups, occur equally in men and women, vary in intensity, and may persist for weeks to months.

Trigeminal neuralgia. Also known as tic douloureux, this pain syndrome is localized to the distribution of the fifth cranial nerve region. Most common in older adults, it typically becomes more intense in the spring and fall. Minimal stimulation from talking, chewing, brushing teeth, or face washing produces sharp, excruciating pain in the mouth, gums, lips, nose, cheeks, and chin. Bursts of pain last seconds to minutes and occur in clusters.

Neuralgia, causalgia, and phantom limb pain. These neurologic syndromes involve peripheral nerve injury. Neuralgic pain, severe and unrelenting, results from peripheral nerve degeneration and involves a limb or the trunk. Causalgia, a burning pain sensation in a limb, usually persists about 6 months after a traumatic partial nerve injury, such as from an accident or a combat wound. The pain often flares up, intermittently becoming more acute. Permanent phantom limb pain, as opposed to phantom limb sensation, occurs in 5% to 10% of amputees. The pain may resemble that felt in the arm or leg before amputation, may spread to other body areas, and may persist for years.

Low back pain. As many as 80% of patients with low back pain—a common, poorly understood pain disorder of musculoskeletal

What happens in migraine vascular headache

First phase (prodrome)
• Intracranial artery vasoconstriction, causing cerebral and retinal hypoperfusion
• Increased platelet aggregation and release of serotonin
• Aura—visual, sensory, or motor disturbance.

Second phase
• Vasodilation and distention of intra- and extracranial arteries, causing pulsation—throbbing pain
• Edema of the vessel walls containing bradykinin—may lower pain threshold
• Increased sodium levels—facial edema, swollen fingers, abdominal distention, weight gain, oliguria
• Nausea, vomiting, anorexia.

Third phase
• Vessel rigidity—steady, excruciating ache
• Sustained neck and scalp muscle contraction—persistent tension and pain after attack.

Common pain disorders: Causes and precipitating factors

Migraine headaches: Related to menstruation, oral contraceptives. May be triggered by chocolate, cheese, and other foods containing tyramines; alcohol; monosodium glutamate; sodium nitrate and nitrites; stress; fatigue; inappropriate diet; hypoglycemia; bright lights; noise; vasodilating drugs

Cluster headaches: Triggered by alcohol, emotional stress, and overwork; nitroglycerin

Tension headaches: Associated with depression, anxiety, tension

Trigeminal neuralgia: Caused by disease processes of the fifth cranial nerve or by multiple sclerosis. Aggravated by stimulation of the area (talking, eating, touching face, putting on lipstick, brushing teeth)

Causalgia: Caused by damage to peripheral nerves, often from high-velocity missile injuries such as gunshot wounds. Triggered by friction from clothing, limb movement, heat, noise, emotional stress

Peripheral neuralgia: Caused by damage to peripheral nerves from viral infections, diabetes mellitus, poor circulation, vitamin deficiencies, and ingestion of toxic substances. Aggravated by friction from clothing, noise, emotional stress

Phantom limb pain: Caused by a loss of nervous input from an amputated limb. May be triggered by touching other sensitized body areas, urination, defecation, emotional stress

Low back pain: Caused by many musculoskeletal and systemic conditions, such as neoplasms; trauma; congenital, inflammatory, circulatory, or metabolic disorders; and psychogenic causes. Predisposing factors include obesity, inactivity, and poor body mechanics.

origin—have no evident organic or structural basis for the pain. The sharp or aching pain commonly radiates down either leg along the path of the sciatic nerve and may immobilize the patient. It afflicts mainly adults, especially the elderly.

Pain theories throughout history

In ancient times, pain was regarded as a supernatural intrusion. Later, Aristotle described pain in more physiologic terms as a sensation and considered the heart the vital organ that perceived pain.

Specificity theory. In 1644, Descartes suggested the specificity theory: that specific pain receptors in the skin directly transmit their pain messages to the brain. In 1842, Müller refined this theory by asserting that sensory nerves carry pain information from the skin to the central nervous system (CNS), and that the quality of sensation depends on the part of the brain activated. In 1895, von Frey observed, under the microscope, free nerve endings widely distributed over the skin and concluded that these nerve endings are the receptors for pain, touch, and temperature sensation, with each sensation projected to a specific brain center.

Later scientists identified two types of pain fibers, the smaller-diameter type A fibers called A-delta and the very small-diameter type C fibers, both with relatively slow conduction properties. They demonstrated that the anterolateral part of the spinal cord and the spinothalamic tract were components of the pain pathway. The fibers transmit pain impulses through the dorsal root ganglia to neurons in the dorsal horn of gray matter. Reflex withdrawal may be carried out through motor (efferent) fibers to skeletal muscles that immediately withdraw from the stimulus. Other pain impulses cross to the opposite side of the cord and ascend the spinothalamic tract to the brain. The impulses are relayed from the thalamus via the thalamocortical tracts to the sensory cortex.

The specificity theory proved to have significant limitations. Many neurosurgical procedures to alleviate pain sensation by destroying a part of the pain pathway failed to relieve pain or reduced pain only briefly. Also, the specificity theory cannot explain such phenomena as phantom limb pain, referred pain, pain after exposure to a light touch or other usually benign stimuli, and pain that persists long after the pain stimulus has been removed.

Pattern theory. This theory evolved directly from difficulties encountered in the specificity theory. According to the pattern theory, pain results from intense peripheral stimulation, which produces a nerve impulse pattern in the dorsal horn of the spinal cord. These impulses are then relayed to the CNS, where they are interpreted as pain.

The pattern theory provides possible explanations for neuralgias, causalgias, and phantom limb pain. Initial injury or amputation of an arm or leg is believed to trigger abnormal firing of neurons, which continue their activity in a cyclic pattern. In the brain, this neural activity is perceived as pain despite the fact that a stimulus no longer exists.

Problems with the pattern theory include the disunity among its various components, and its failure to explain pain that recurs after surgical interruption of the pain pathway at the spinal cord level and pain differences after exposure to different stimulation intensities (for example, a pinprick versus a cut).

Affect theory. In 1894, Marshall described pain as emotions that affect all sensory events and many individual experiences, such as the pain associated with grieving. In its pure form, the affect theory totally ignores a physiologic basis for pain. However, current theory recognizes affect, or feelings, as one component of the pain experience. Anxiety, fear of the unknown, or lack of support from family and friends can heighten pain, while reducing some of those stresses can ease it.

Gate control theory. In 1965, Melzack and Wall proposed the gate control theory. It incorporates some ideas from the earlier theories while delineating ways that both afferent and efferent input can influence pain perception. This theory now serves as the basis for many clinical interventions to relieve pain. (See *Gate control theory of pain.*)

As an adjunct to the gate control theory, recent research has identified certain receptor sites for opiates such as morphine. These areas are the hypothalamus, which integrates visceral pain; the substantia gelatinosa of the spinal cord, which transmits pain impulses; the midbrain nuclei corresponding to the cranial nerves controlling cough reflex, secretions, and gastric motility; the amygdala of the limbic system, which is concerned with emotional behavior; the area postrema of the periaqueductal gray matter, which is associated with nausea and visceral pain; and the gastrointestinal tract, in general. In contrast, almost no receptor sites appear in the white

Gate control theory of pain

According to the gate control theory proposed by Melzack and Wall, pain results from stimulation of the smaller-diameter type A nerve fibers, called A-delta, and the very small-diameter type C fibers. These sensory (afferent) fibers penetrate the dorsal horn of the spinal cord and terminate within the spinal substantia gelatinosa. When sensory stimulation reaches a critical level, a so-called gate in the substantia gelatinosa opens, allowing nearby T (transmission) cells to project the pain message to the brain. Thus, the small fibers function to enhance pain transmission.

In contrast, large-diameter, type A sensory fibers, called A-beta, function to inhibit pain transmission. Stimulation of these large, fast-conducting afferent fibers opposes the smaller fibers' input and activates the substantia gelatinosa gate to close, thus blocking the pain transmission. In addition, descending (efferent) impulses along various tracts from the brain and brain stem can enhance or reduce pain transmission at the gate. For example, triggering selective brain processes, such as attention, emotions, and memory of pain, can intensify pain by opening the gate.

Unlike earlier pain theories, the gate control theory explains how external methods and cognitive techniques can modulate pain transmission. For example, stimulation of the large A-beta fibers, through massage, heat or cold applications, acupuncture, transcutaneous electrical nerve stimulation, or dorsal column stimulation, can override sensory input and block pain transmission at the gate. Cognitive techniques, such as distraction, biofeedback, cognitive coping, and relaxation training, which operate through the descending fibers, can reduce pain by closing the gate.

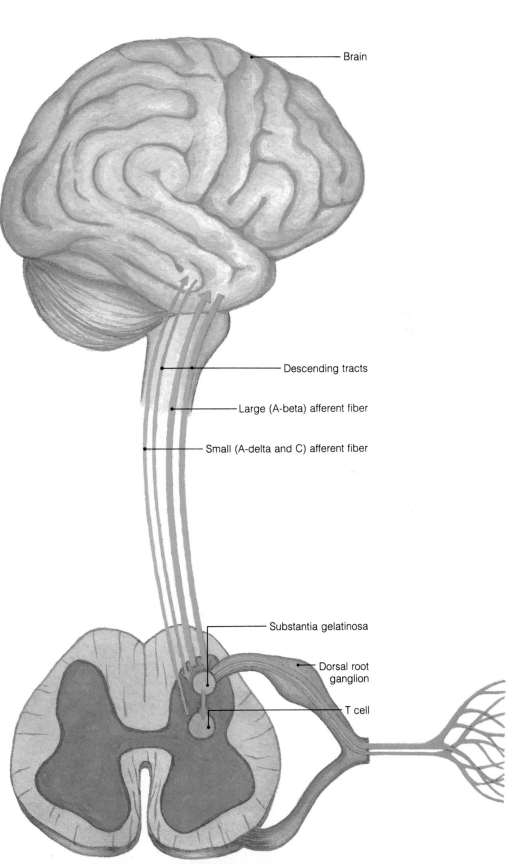

Brain

Descending tracts

Large (A-beta) afferent fiber

Small (A-delta and C) afferent fiber

Substantia gelatinosa

Dorsal root ganglion

T cell

matter of the cerebellum, cerebrum, and spinal cord.

Further research on these receptor sites has uncovered two families of endogenous opiates—endorphins and enkephalins—that modulate pain signals at these sites. They have different biosynthetic pathways, but their actions are similar. (See *How endogenous opiates work.*) The endorphins are concentrated in the pituitary gland, the hypothalamus, and various brain stem areas. Enkephalins are distributed in the brain and spinal cord and also in the adrenal gland and intestines. Endorphin and enkephalin release is activated by noxious stimuli.

The endogenous opiates appear to support the gate control theory on a cellular level, since they alter pain transmission at points in the main pathway identified by the gate control theory. Stimulation of CNS gray matter, known to be rich in endogenous opiates, has relieved otherwise intractable pain. Naloxone (Narcan), an opiate antagonist, also reverses the stimulation effects of endorphins and enkephalins.

These discoveries may help in developing new synthetic analogues for pain relief without morphine's side effects and dependency. Electrical stimulation may also come into wider use as a therapy for intractable pain. Indeed, many methods of pain intervention may prove to relieve pain by stimulating the endogenous opiate system.

MEDICAL MANAGEMENT
Successful pain management demands an individual approach. Since many types of treatment are available and response varies among patients, a search for an effective method may be necessary. Active involvement of the patient and his family in this search is vital.

A complete medical history and physical examination should precede any treatment plan. Establishing such a data base helps the health-care team determine the possible primary causes and impact of coexisting health problems and assists in identifying secondary causes of pain. For example, a patient with low back pain may, in fact, be suffering from

How endogenous opiates work

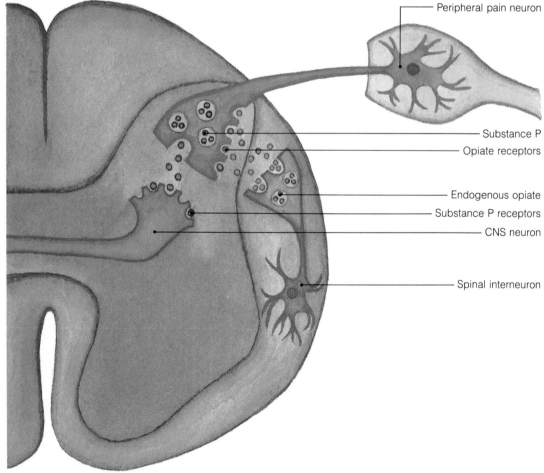

The endogenous opiates—endorphins and enkephalins—reduce pain perception by blocking the release of pain neurotransmitters at opiate receptor sites in the spinal cord. In theory, spinal interneurons synapse with the terminals of peripheral pain fibers and release endogenous opiates, which bind with terminal receptors. This action inhibits the release of substance P, a chemical transmitter, thus reducing the number of incoming pain impulses that can transfer to central nervous system (CNS) neurons for communication to the brain. Morphine and other opiates imitate the blocking effect of endogenous opiates by binding with free opiate receptors on the pain fibers.

Peripheral pain neuron
Substance P
Opiate receptors
Endogenous opiate
Substance P receptors
CNS neuron
Spinal interneuron

renal calculi. Or the patient with headache may have a brain tumor.

The neurologic component of the examination should be carefully considered. However, in some pain disorders, such as trigeminal neuralgia, the neurologic assessment may reveal no abnormalities.

Special diagnostic tests: Eliminating secondary causes

Management of pain syndromes requires various special tests to identify or rule out treatable secondary causes of pain. For example, routine X-ray studies of the affected body parts may determine structural integrity; electrodiagnostic tests, such as electromyography, may evaluate nerve and nerve-muscle conduction function; and computerized tomography (CT) scans or electroencephalography may rule out a brain tumor or seizure disorder. In acute headache not recognized as migraine, a lumbar puncture with cerebrospinal fluid examination may rule out infection or hemorrhage. However, this procedure should be performed with extreme caution in the patient with increased intracranial pressure, since it may precipitate life-threatening brain herniation. Bone scan; CT scan of the spine; myelogram; urinalysis; and blood tests, including complete blood count, serum calcium, and the rheumatoid factor, may be necessary to evaluate back pain.

Treatment: Sometimes frustrating

Trying to identify the most effective treatment for resistant pain syndromes is often a matter of trial and error. Some of the most effective narcotic medications have side effects that prevent their daily use, and some techniques, such as biofeedback, require specialized training and much practice. However, persistent effort to find an effective treatment may pay off with complete relief or at least the reduction of pain to a tolerable level; such effort typically involves interdisciplinary interventions along with vocational and psychological counseling.

Drug therapy. This is generally tried first and may include nonnarcotic analgesics; narcotic analgesics; and drugs with other systemic effects, such as ergot alkaloids, tricyclic antidepressants, and anticonvulsants.

Nonnarcotic analgesics, such as acetylsalicylic acid (aspirin) and acetaminophen (Tylenol), and nonsteroidal anti-inflammatory agents, such as indomethacin (Indocin), are used most frequently. These drugs reduce pain by blocking the synthesis of prostaglandins at the local tissue level.

Narcotic analgesics, of which the prototype is morphine, act centrally to reduce pain by binding with opiate receptor sites. Other narcotics, such as hydromorphone (Dilaudid), meperidine (Demerol), and codeine, have similar analgesic effects but differ in onset and duration of action. Concerns about addiction, tolerance, and physical dependence after narcotic administration are largely unfounded during short-term use for acute pain. However, in chronic use for intractable pain, drug habituation may result.

Ergot alkaloids, such as ergotamine (Gynergen) and methysergide (Sansert), are used to treat and to prevent vascular headaches. In migraine attacks, cerebral artery pulsation and distention are thought to be triggered by changes in vasoactive substances (such as serotonin, tyramine, and prostaglandins). Ergot alkaloids relieve pain through direct vasoconstriction that reduces pulsation. When given at maintenance doses, these drugs also control vascular tone to prevent migraine and cluster headaches. (See *What to tell the patient about taking ergot alkaloids,* page 146.) Propranolol (Inderal), a beta-adrenergic blocking agent, also inhibits vasodilation and has been found effective for migraine prophylaxis. Amitriptyline hydrochloride (Elavil), a tricyclic antidepressant; lithium; and cyproheptadine (Periactin), an antihistamine, are also used to prevent vascular headaches because of their possible effects on serotonin and catecholamines.

Anticonvulsants, especially phenytoin (Dilantin) and carbamazepine (Tegretol), have proved effective in relieving pain from trigeminal neuralgia and central pain syndrome through a depressant effect on the CNS.

Surgery. Many patients, unable to relieve severe pain through conservative treatment, eventually turn to neurosurgical procedures (see *Neurosurgical techniques for treating chronic pain,* page 142). Such procedures interrupt the pain pathway by surgery, phenol or alcohol injections, electrocautery, or radio frequency coagulation.

Physical treatments. Physiologic interventions generally provide relief by inhibiting T-(transmission-) cell function, usually through stimulation of the large, inhibitory type A-beta fibers, which override the smaller pain-conducting fibers. These interventions include massage, heat or cold application, electrical nerve stimulation, acupuncture, and electrical stimulation of acupuncture needles (hyperstimulation).

Transcutaneous electrical nerve stimulation (TENS) involves electrical stimulation of sensory nerves through the skin, creating a tingling sensation. TENS effectively reduces pain in many conditions, such as phantom limb pain, causalgia, cancer, back pain, arthritis, headache, and postoperative incisional pain. (See *Using transcutaneous electrical nerve stimulation [TENS].*) Electrical stimulation of peripheral nerves can also be achieved through percutaneous and permanent implant methods. Dorsal column stimulation achieves pain relief by placement of electrodes into the epidural space of the spinal cord on the dor-

Neurosurgical techniques for treating chronic pain

Technique	Mechanism of action	Limitations
Chemical nerve blocks	Neurolytic agent such as alcohol or phenol destroys fibers, or anesthetic temporarily impedes pain transmission. May be performed to evaluate effectiveness of block before surgical transection. Used for peripheral vascular disease, trigeminal neuralgia, causalgia, and cancer.	May be difficult to locate specific pathway to interrupt. May cause numbness and paresthesias or transient urine retention, paresis, or headache. Pain relief may last only weeks or months.
Neurectomy	Obliterates pain transmission pathways through excision of the peripheral nerve.	May fail to relieve pain. Provides limited, temporary analgesia.
Rhizotomy	Blocks nerve transmission through transection of nerve root between dorsal root ganglion and cord. Also done via percutaneous route to destroy type C fibers. Often used for trigeminal neuralgia and head and neck cancer pain.	Requires transection of several roots. Obliterates all sensation, though sensation may slowly come back with pain or severe paresthesias. If bilateral, may cause postural hypotension. If at a lower body level, may cause bowel, bladder, and sexual dysfunction.
Sympathectomy	Impedes transmission along sympathetic afferent nerve pathways through pharmacologic block or surgical transection. Used for causalgia, phantom limb pain, and pain due to vascular disorders.	May cause autonomic dysfunction. May fail to relieve pain.
Cordotomy	Interrupts ascending spinothalamic tract by surgical transection (laminectomy) or by percutaneous diathermy or radiothermy coagulation. Erases pain and temperature sensation below level of interruption and on opposite side of body but doesn't impair motor function. Used most effectively for cancer pain in legs and trunk.	Must be bilateral if pain is midline. Sensation may slowly come back with pain and paresthesias. Complications include leg weakness, urine retention, and sexual dysfunction in the male.
Intrathecal injection	Selectively destroys small nerve fibers by injecting alcohol hypertonic saline solution or other neurolytic agent into cerebrospinal fluid around spinal rootlets and dorsal horn. Used for malignancies, midline pain, and visceral pain.	Difficult to regulate location of injected agent even with tilt table, fluoroscopic control, postprocedure aspiration of agent, and use of multiple needles.
Cranial stereotaxic surgery	Destroys pain perception pathway in the brain through radiothermy coagulation or freezing after stimulation localizes the site by producing pain. Procedure performed in conscious patient using a model brain for reference and radiology with contrast media to highlight landmarks.	Complex procedure requiring special training and involving intraoperative X-ray study. Difficult to locate exact point to ablate because of variance in anatomic locations. Pain tends to return within months, so use is reserved for patients with poor prognosis.
Thalamotomy	Diminishes pain perception by interfering with transmission of impulses through the medial nuclei of the thalamus. Used for central pain syndromes or for intractable pain.	Usually reserved for the terminally ill. May cause ataxia and hemiparesis. Pain tends to recur.
Cingulotomy	Alters affective response to pain or relieves cancer pain in head and neck through interruption of portions of cingulum (frontal white matter). Removes suffering quality of pain, although mechanism is unclear.	Usually must be bilateral. Reserved for patients with strong psychogenic component to pain.
Lobotomy	Alters motivational-affective response to pain through destruction or excision of frontal lobe.	Last resort for intractable pain. May cause personality changes.

Using transcutaneous electrical nerve stimulation (TENS)

To ensure that the patient benefits from TENS, first support him in the decision to try this method of chronic pain relief. Then help the patient apply, regulate, and care for the TENS unit properly, as described below.
• Encourage him to rent the TENS unit for several months before buying the expensive equipment because pain relief may be transient.
• Assist him in finding electrode placement for optimal pain relief. Try placing electrodes directly over the painful area, along the nerve pathways, or at points along the same dermatome as the pain.
• Apply conductive gel to each electrode; then place the electrodes and secure them with tape around all sides.
• Turn on the unit and increase the wave amplitude (intensity) until the patient perceives a tingling sensation.
• Set the amplitude, rate, and pulse width at prescribed settings; then increase or decrease these controls, depending on what the patient finds most comfortable.
• Monitor the patient for muscle twitching, which indicates excessive stimulation.
• Remove the electrodes between uses or at least once a day if treatments are frequent. Wash the electrodes and the patient's skin with soap and water to remove gel, perspiration, and dead skin cells. Inspect skin for redness and irritation. Let skin dry thoroughly and apply a soothing skin preparation, if available. Reapply the freshly gelled electrodes in the same spots unless redness persists after skin care.
• Show the patient how to attach the TENS unit to clothing.
• Have the patient express his feelings about wearing the unit throughout the day.

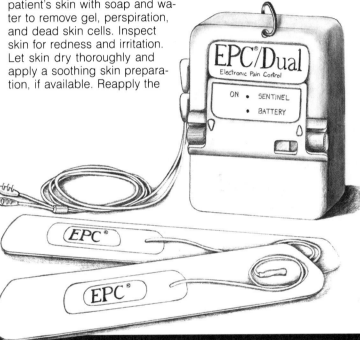

sal column surface, either percutaneously or through laminectomy. With these methods, patients control electrical stimulation by use of an external transmitter.

Acupuncture, an ancient Chinese therapy, is based on the belief that energy flows through the body along specific pathways called meridians and that pain results when this energy flow is blocked. Selective stimulation at specific sites along these meridians, through insertion of needles into tissue, is believed to restore energy flow and produce analgesia or anesthesia in the body parts along that meridian. Acupuncture may relieve pain by stimulating nerve fibers that can close the gate in the gate control theory of pain.

In hyperstimulation, the intensity of stimulation, rather than the specific site of stimulation, affords pain relief. An electric current may be passed between acupuncture needles, or the needles may be twirled, to create greater afferent input.

Psychological treatments. Cognitive processes have long been known to influence the pain experience. Psychological interventions, such as behavior modification, distraction, biofeedback, hypnosis, and cognitive coping skills, aim to reduce the anxiety and fear that often accompany pain and heighten its perception. (See *Controlling chronic pain,* page 144.)

Behavior modification is based on the premise that individuals with chronic pain learn a certain set of negative behaviors, such as whining, grimacing, and avoiding work and strenuous activity. These behaviors earn extra attention and privileges from friends and family, which in turn reinforce them. Behavior modification techniques reinforce positive behaviors, such as decreased use of analgesic drugs, and teach the patient's family and friends alternative ways to interact with the patient.

Biofeedback, especially useful against pain

Controlling chronic pain

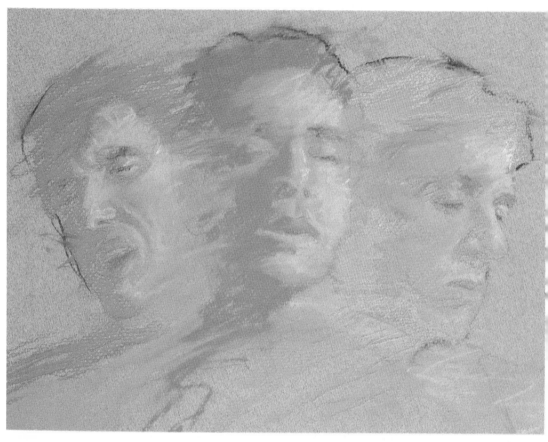

You can help the patient reduce physical pain levels through psychological controls, such as distraction, deep relaxation, and biofeedback. Indispensable to these and similar methods are the support and encouragement you give the patient to increase his sense of control over pain.

Distraction
Visual, auditory, or mental distraction eases brief episodes of pain.
• Have the patient recount an interesting experience.
• Suggest that he turn on the radio or a favorite cassette tape when pain begins. Have him close his eyes and concentrate on listening, raising or lowering the volume as his pain increases or subsides. Or have him sing, silently or aloud, as he taps out the song's rhythm.
• Teach the patient to do deep breathing exercises. Have him stare at an object and slowly inhale and exhale as you count out a comfortable rhythm for him. Tell him to focus attention on the movement of his breath or on any restful image; then let him take over the count. Provide greater distraction by having the patient massage his arm or abdomen as he breathes.

Relaxation
For enduring pain, deep relaxation techniques, such as meditation, yoga, and self-hypnosis, can reduce anxiety, muscle tension, fatigue, and pain.
• If your patient doesn't already practice one of these techniques, begin with a simple, natural method, such as sighing, yawning, or concentrating on a pleasant mental image.
• Next, introduce deep breathing exercises. As the patient breathes rhythmically, have him concentrate on the rise and fall of his abdomen. Tell him that he's relaxing more with each deep breath, and note that he may feel weightless, pulsating, tingling, or heavy sensations.
• Tell him to mentally transport himself to a pleasant location and to notice the details of sight, sound, smell, taste, and touch.
• Then, on a count of three, instruct him to wake up relaxed and alert or to fall asleep. With practice, your patient can lead himself through this exercise.

Biofeedback
This training uses electromyography, electrocardiography, or a thermistor to demonstrate the effectiveness of relaxation practices. Through an auditory or visual display during a relaxation practice, it shows the patient that he can voluntarily reduce autonomic processes, such as heart and respiration rate, blood pressure, body temperature, and muscle tension.

associated with tension, increases the patient's control over pain by enhancing his control over physiologic processes. Like behavior modification, biofeedback requires extensive training and motivation, and may fail when the patient leaves the reinforcing atmosphere of a hospital or pain clinic.

Relaxation therapy shows the patient ways to achieve musculoskeletal relaxation through deep breathing and muscle exercises.

Hypnosis induces a deep trance to provide relaxation and relief of anxiety. Posthypnotic suggestion later maintains these effects.

Cognitive coping skills require that the patient first gain some knowledge of the painful event or experience, then undergo a training period in which he learns techniques for coping with the pain. These techniques are commonly used in preoperative teaching and prepared childbirth.

Continuing research

The search for more effective pain relief methods continues. Current investigations are exploring ways to increase stimulation of endogenous opiate production and to perfect continuous delivery of morphine through a reservoir implant for cancer pain. Also being studied is the effect of placebos and their relation to the endogenous opiate system.

Neurosurgical investigations are evaluating the effectiveness of glycerol injection into subarachnoid spaces for trigeminal neuralgia and creation of multiple electrolytic lesions in the spinal cord's dorsal root entry zone for spinal cord injury and neuralgia. Pharmacologic investigations continue to search for new analgesic agents and new analgesic uses for agents known for other specific effects. For example, calcium channel blockers like verapamil are being evaluated for potential vasoconstrictive actions in migraine prophylaxis. Some investigations are exploring the effects of therapeutic touch, a holistic discipline somewhat related to acupuncture.

NURSING MANAGEMENT

Because reactions to pain and to attempts to control it are so variable and so personal, your interactions with the patient can make a critical contribution to management of chronic pain. You see him daily and directly monitor his response to treatment and his need for further measures. Your support and encouragement often represent the motivating factor in the patient's efforts to cope with and surmount his pain.

Evaluate the patient's pain reaction

Of course, you'll begin your assessment with a full history and a careful interview to define the patient's own perception of his pain and its causes. Ask about the pain's duration to identify the problem as chronic or acute. Ask about its characteristics, location, intensity, quality, and pattern of onset. Also have the patient describe any physical or psychological factors that precipitate pain. Inquire about a history of injuries—such as falls, spinal cord injuries, amputations, and gunshot wounds— or diseases—such as diabetes mellitus—that cause neuropathy. Obtain a family history of related conditions, such as headaches and back pain, because migraines and musculoskeletal disorders may be hereditary. Also, a family history of pain syndromes tells you about familial influence on the patient's reaction to pain. Remember, too, that ethnic and sociocultural factors may influence pain perception and responses to it.

The patient's response to pain is important in assessing the total pain experience. Is anxiety evident? Evaluate the anxiety level and the patient's anticipation of the painful event, since anxiety produces muscle tension, which increases the pain.

Find out about previous forms of therapy, use of analgesic drugs, and medical or surgical management, as well as the patient's past coping mechanisms, to identify successful approaches precisely.

Obtain a psychosocial assessment because chronic pain significantly affects interpersonal relationships to a degree that directly corresponds to the level of pain. Ask the patient to describe his typical day to gauge life-style changes; a patient with chronic pain tends to spend less and less time in social and recreational activities. Observe the patient's behavior for a manipulative attitude, anger, or depression. Assess his dependence on the secondary gains he obtains from his illness.

Assess severity of pain

Examine the patient to evaluate his general health as well as the symptoms associated with pain. Observe facial expression, posture, movement, and position changes. Obtain baseline vital signs to assess changes during a pain episode. Observe and palpate for evidence of injury, deformities, or contractures affecting body parts. Assess for reflexes; sensory changes, such as paresthesia; and motor dysfunction, such as incontinence. However, remember that a patient with chronic pain

What to tell the patient about taking ergot alkaloids

• Store the drug in a light-resistant container.
• Keep this drug handy at all times, since it's most effective when taken at the first sign of headache.
• Take the drug immediately after onset of the first symptoms. In classic migraines, the prodromal stage is marked by an aura; in common migraines, by lethargy, malaise, irritability, and inability to work.
• Usual dosage is one or two tablets (1 mg each) at the onset and another every 30 minutes until headache subsides (to a maximum of 6 mg per attack and 10 mg per week).
• Sublingual tablets or intramuscular injection may give faster relief. Rectal suppositories are available to relieve migraine associated with nausea and vomiting.
• Do not exceed prescribed dosage. Be alert for signs of ergot toxicity, such as a daily headache or pain, pallor, or coldness of the extremities.

may adjust to the experience and exhibit few, if any, overt symptoms.

You may find a pain assessment questionnaire, such as the McGill-Melzack Questionnaire, useful for obtaining information. Completing this questionnaire with the patient can enhance a trusting and therapeutic relationship. This completed form can also serve as a data base for the entire health-care team so they need not question him repeatedly about his pain. This technique gives the patient fewer opportunities for negative behaviors, such as complaining and seeking sympathy.

Intervene to improve coping

Remember that any nursing-care plan you set up for the patient in pain needs the active participation of your patient and his family for success, so try to involve them in every stage. Use all the data you've gathered to formulate relevant nursing diagnoses, set goals, and plan appropriate interventions like the following:

Alteration in comfort related to pain. To make the patient more comfortable, administer medication as ordered and according to your assessment of the pain; consult with the doctor about prescribed medication whenever necessary. Remember that your attitude toward the patient's pain can profoundly influence the doctor's orders, particularly *p.r.n.* orders, so strive for an objective, nonjudgmental approach. Don't let societal values dictate your behavior or persuade you to favor the quiet, cooperative patient over the one who requests more than the usual amount of pain medication. Your fear of potential drug addiction, tolerance, or dependence may lead you to discourage medication; as a result, the doctor may prescribe inadequate doses. Although placebos should be avoided, express the belief that pain will be relieved when you administer one. Placebos may have a biochemical effect on the body that actually relieves acute and chronic pain. Recognize that they may also cause adverse side effects.

If pain analgesics have been ordered p.r.n., frequently assess the patient's need, and administer them before the pain becomes so severe that it cannot be relieved. You may want to give analgesics on a routine, round-the-clock basis to allay the patient's fears that the pain will be allowed to get out of control. Evaluate the response to a particular drug schedule and adjust the schedule as necessary. Always involve the patient in adjusting the schedule so that you may attain the most

effective program. Educate him about his pain relief program according to his level of understanding; include information about drugs as well as other treatment methods.

If neurosurgical treatment becomes necessary, inform the patient about the surgery he faces and what he should expect. You may not be able to evaluate the extent of pain relief for several days after surgery, but be alert immediately for complications—increased intracranial pressure, respiratory depression, motor weakness, bowel and bladder incontinence, sensory loss, and hypotension. Keep the patient on bed rest as ordered, usually for 24 to 48 hours postoperatively.

Your interventions have succeeded if the patient's pain is controlled with minimal use of narcotics.

Anxiety related to anticipation of pain. To control anxiety, teach the patient to watch for its signs, including restlessness, irritability, inattentiveness, fatigue, and uneasiness. Explain that anxiety may intensify pain. Help the patient identify stressful situations that may initiate or aggravate his pain. Then teach or arrange instruction in stress-reducing techniques, such as biofeedback, self-hypnosis, relaxation therapy, or cognitive coping skills. Provide the opportunity to practice any effective technique in a comfortable position and a quiet place without interruptions. Don't overlook the opportunity to relieve anxiety simply by spending some time listening and talking to the patient. You may find this especially effective in managing the patient who's perceived as demanding.

Your interventions have succeeded if the patient's daily anxiety level diminishes; if he performs relaxation techniques before, during, and after pain episodes; and if his fear of pain and the frequency and intensity of pain episodes decrease.

Inadequate sleep related to pain. To help the patient get adequate sleep at night and lessen his fatigue during the day, first remind him that fatigue can intensify perception of pain and even trigger pain episodes. Help the patient plan his day with sufficient and varied activities, because insomnia may result from inadequate physical activity during the day. Poor sleep patterns may also result from a noisy, uncomfortable environment. Make sure the sleeping place is quiet and comfortable. Position the patient comfortably with good body alignment, and cushion any painful areas.

Provide some tips on getting to sleep: The

patient should use the bed only for sleeping and lie down only when tired. If sleep does not come within 20 minutes, he should get up and do something else. Relaxation techniques may help induce sleep.

If simpler measures fail, sedative drugs may be necessary to provide adequate rest. However, don't give sedatives routinely since they disrupt the sleep cycle; the patient may then sleep an adequate number of hours but wake up tired. Certain other drugs, such as amitriptyline hydrochloride (Elavil), have been reported to reduce pain and promote sleep in patients with chronic pain.

Consider your interventions successful if the patient is getting 8 hours or an appropriate amount of continuous sleep at night and suffers no drowsiness during the day.

Poor coping mechanisms related to chronic pain. To improve coping mechanisms, be alert for maladaptive behavior, such as focusing all attention on pain. Watch for any alteration in family members' roles as each member adapts to additional responsibilities. Observe the patient's interaction with friends and family members to evaluate coping mechanisms, and assess the patient's and the family's readiness to change. Guide the patient in behavior modification, but remember that its success depends on the patient's insight and the enthusiastic support of family members. By establishing good rapport with the patient, you may support his motivation and ability to follow prescribed treatment. Assist the patient in any physical or cognitive diversionary activity that reduces pain perception. Teach the patient to focus awareness on any stimulus other than the pain. If necessary, use such distractions as counting items, singing, exercise, or interacting with others. Try to plan diversionary strategies that make use of the patient's special interests.

Consider your interventions successful if you and the patient have identified adaptive and maladaptive coping mechanisms and if the patient carries out behavior modification and distraction techniques with progressive control of pain and a reduced toll on family members.

Impaired ability to perform activities of daily living. To increase the patient's exercise tolerance and participation in daily activities, determine how much activity the patient can sustain before he suffers pain and fatigue. Encourage appropriate activities, but set the required limit below his tolerance level at first to ensure successful completion. Gradually increase the activity quota as the patient's endurance improves. You may wish to implement this program with token rewards, such as television time or a weekend pass. Preset the goal he must achieve to earn the reward, and raise the goal as the activity becomes easier. Ensure that the entire health-care staff interacts appropriately with the patient. This may involve providing written guidelines for other members of the staff.

Consider your interventions successful if the patient shows independence and interest in carrying out daily activities and gradually increases his tolerance for exercise.

Knowledge deficit about measures to prevent chronic pain. Begin a program of instruction to help the patient understand and practice preventive health-care measures, decrease pain frequency and intensity, and prevent further disability. Assess the patient's level of understanding and knowledge concerning general health and his own disorder. Begin teaching general measures to promote health and specific measures to prevent pain. Recommend adequate sleep, exercise, and good diet. If the patient has lost weight because of his chronic pain, teach him that inadequate dietary intake can reduce resistance to disease; explain which foods may aggravate his pain. If he has gained weight from inactivity, teach him that the added weight puts stress on the musculoskeletal system and may intensify his pain or cause muscle and joint dysfunction.

Teach a patient with musculoskeletal pain proper body alignment and good body mechanics. Advise him to do back-strengthening exercises; to wear medium-heel, soft-soled shoes; and to sleep on a firm mattress. Explore ways to restructure the patient's lifestyle and environment to decrease daily stress. Counsel the patient who's prone to migraines and causalgia to avoid exposure to irritating environmental factors, such as loud noise and bright lights.

Consider your interventions successful if the patient begins practicing appropriate dietary, sleep, and exercise patterns and self-care measures for his pain disorder.

A final word

Helping the patient with chronic, sometimes intractable, pain can represent a major nursing challenge. It's a challenge you can meet successfully if you're willing to work with the patient in a positive, persistent, and compassionate way.

Points to remember

- Pain is a subjective experience; patients with similar pain disorders may perceive different degrees of pain sensation and respond in different ways.
- The gate control theory of pain involves sensory input from pain nerve endings and descending input from the cerebrum to modulate pain perception.
- Transcutaneous electrical nerve stimulation, a method of cutaneous stimulation, may relieve chronic and, at times, acute pain.
- Nursing management of the patient with pain should incorporate the patient's prior pain experience and previously successful methods of pain relief.
- Alleviating pain may involve changing the patient's behavior. He may need to learn new interpersonal and social skills along with new ways to cope with stress, such as relaxation techniques, biofeedback, or self-hypnosis.

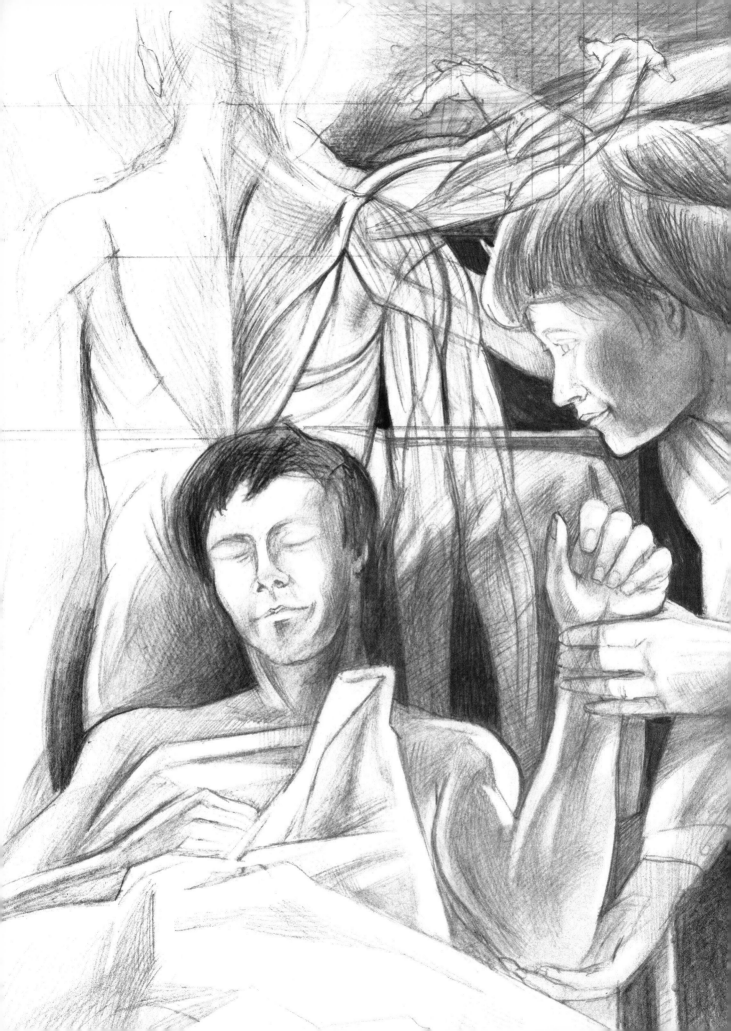

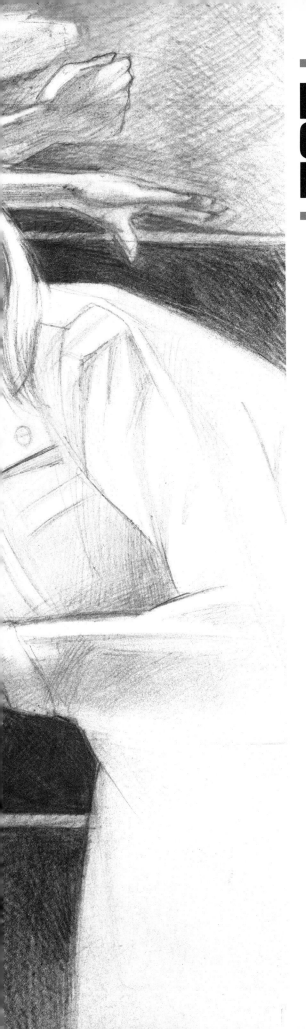

DISORDERS OF CIRCULATION AND METABOLISM

12 COPING WITH CEREBROVASCULAR DEFICIT

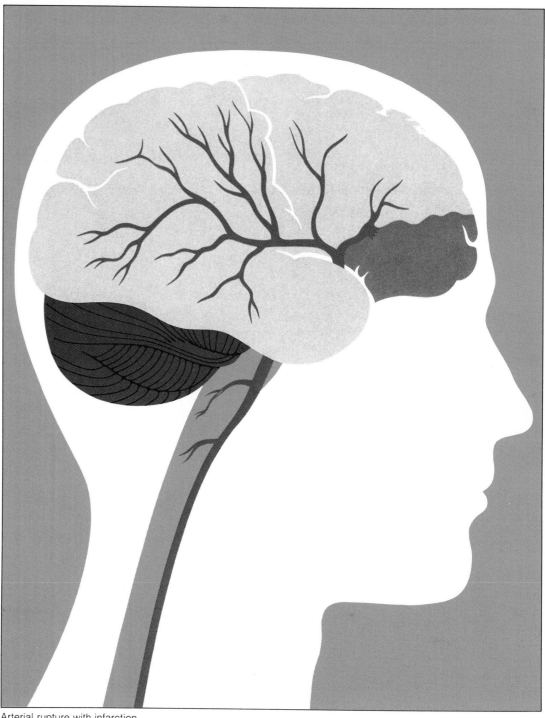

Arterial rupture with infarction

Caring for patients with cerebrovascular disease poses special problems. Not only must you try to ease physical discomfort, but you must also try to dispel some of the confusion and desolation cerebrovascular deficits leave in their wake. A thorough understanding of the mechanisms and consequences of cerebrovascular impairment will help you develop reasonable care plans that can make your task more manageable and this disease less frightening for your patient.

Debilitating disease

Cerebrovascular disease, which includes the condition we commonly call a stroke, follows heart disease and cancer as a major cause of death in the United States and is also one of the major causes of physical disability. Although it occurs in all age ranges, it more commonly affects the elderly, especially men, who already have multiple health problems. It strikes suddenly, sometimes without warning, leaving its victims confused and frightened by their sudden inability to walk, talk, or perform simple tasks. Cerebrovascular disease seldom resolves to complete recovery, usually forcing its victims to endure debilitating neurologic deficits.

Ischemia or hemorrhage

Cerebrovascular disease may be classified as ischemia or hemorrhage. Ischemia indicates decreased blood flow to the brain because of partial or complete arterial occlusion; hemorrhage indicates bleeding into brain tissue from a ruptured artery.

Ischemic types include transient ischemic attack (TIA), a focal neurologic deficit often lasting just minutes and no longer than 24 hours and completely resolving without permanent damage. TIA's focal signs include hemiparesis, unilateral loss of vision, and speech disturbances. Generalized, vague symptoms, such as dizziness, weakness, blurred vision, and blackout spells, usually do not indicate a TIA episode but, rather, nonspecific cerebral ischemia. TIAs may precede strokes and are usually associated with atherosclerotic thrombotic disease.

Ischemic stroke, also known as ischemic cerebrovascular accident, involves a focal neurologic deficit lasting longer than 24 hours and usually resulting in permanent residual impairment. Its cause is commonly cerebral artery occlusion by a thrombus or an embolus. (See *Causes of cerebral embolism*.)

Intracranial hemorrhage includes intracerebral hemorrhage (ICH) and subarachnoid hemorrhage (SAH). ICH involves a focal area of bleeding into brain tissue from a ruptured intracerebral artery most often caused by hypertension. SAH involves bleeding into the subarachnoid space most commonly from a ruptured aneurysm or ruptured arteriovenous malformation (AVM) in a major cerebral artery or branch. (See *Causes of intracranial hemorrhage,* page 152.)

PATHOPHYSIOLOGY

In cerebrovascular disease, either occlusion or rupture of a cerebral artery compromises the brain tissue which that artery supplies. Occlusion interrupts blood flow, producing tissue ischemia and infarction. Rupture permits hemorrhage into brain tissue or surrounding space, which compresses brain tissue and leads to increased intracranial pressure (ICP) and possible herniation.

After occlusion: Ischemic infarction

Interrupted blood flow halts the supply of oxygen, glucose, and other nutrients to the affected brain tissue. If deprivation continues for longer than a few minutes, neurons in the area undergo necrotic changes. If deprivation is severe or prolonged, a large section of the brain becomes infarcted. In the acute phase of a large infarction, changes in permeability of the cell membranes may result in local edema and capillary compression. If the edematous area is large, ICP may rise, threatening herniation of brain tissue. The edema normally peaks in 5 to 7 days and thereafter gradually disappears. When infarction develops, tissue softens, and, gradually, phagocytic removal of necrotic debris forms a cavity.

Atherosclerotic thrombi. The most common underlying factor in ischemia and infarction, atherosclerosis leads to thrombus and embolus formation, which occludes the arteries supplying the brain. Although the causes of atherosclerosis and thrombosis are not completely understood, such conditions as hypertension, aging, and diabetes mellitus are known to produce vascular changes that favor their development.

The formation of a thrombus proceeds in the following sequence. With aging, the innermost layer of the artery thickens; as lipids and fibrous tissue accumulate, they produce elevations or plaques (atheromas), which project into the vessel lumen. Continued accumulation eventually narrows the lumen and alters

Causes of cerebral embolism

Cardiac causes

Dysrhythmias (especially atrial fibrillation)
Myocardial infarction
Valvular disease or prosthesis
Cardiac surgery complications
Mitral valve prolapse
Congenital septal defect with paradoxical embolism

Noncardiac causes

Arterial atherosclerosis
Cerebral artery thrombosis
Trauma to neck vessels
Fat or air embolism
Neck or thoracic surgery complications

Causes of intracranial hemorrhage

Hypertensive intracerebral hemorrhage

Ruptured saccular aneurysm or arteriovenous malformation

Hemorrhagic disorders
  Anticoagulant therapy complications
  Blood dyscrasias
    Aplastic anemia
    Hemophilia
    Hyperfibrinogenemia
    Hyperfibrinolysis
    Leukemia
    Liver disease
    Thrombocytopenic purpura

Septic embolism

Vascular inflammatory disease

Trauma

hemodynamics, hampering blood flow in vessels distal to the stenosis. Frequently, the plaque surfaces become roughened and ulcerated; platelets and fibrin adhere to the roughened surfaces and form a clot (thrombus).

A developing thrombus may eventually occlude the lumen completely, interrupting blood flow to a distal brain area and causing cerebral infarction. In larger vessels, such as the internal carotid or vertebral arteries, thrombus formation is especially likely at branching points where atherosclerotic plaques commonly accumulate. Arterial occlusion often progresses in steps, allowing partial compensation through development of collateral circulation in the vessels that form the circle of Willis. Widespread cerebral artery changes may also occur, especially in the small, penetrating branches of the middle cerebral artery, causing small, deep infarctions (lacunae).

Embolic occlusions. When a fragment of a thrombus travels through the blood vessels to lodge in a cerebral artery, the embolus may cause occlusion, ischemia, and infarction. An embolus may break off from any thrombus, but a cerebral embolus most commonly originates in the heart. Mural thrombosis frequently results from ineffective emptying of blood from the left atrium, as in atrial fibrillation, or from clot formation over a damaged endocardium, as in myocardial infarction (MI). Unlike the slowly developing thrombus that blocks cerebral blood flow gradually, allowing development of collateral vascular pathways, a large embolus can cause sudden, fatal occlusion.

Microemboli, primarily composed of platelets, are commonly believed to cause transient ischemic changes, such as TIAs. Because of their small size and platelet and fibrin composition, they're usually lysed, allowing restoration of blood flow to brain tissue before permanent damage occurs.

After hemorrhage: Intracranial hypertension

In intracranial hemorrhage, blood escaping from a ruptured artery invades brain tissue or surrounding spaces. Compromise of the artery results from a degenerative change in the arterial wall or from a defect, such as an aneurysm or arteriovenous malformation.

Intracerebral hemorrhage. In this type of hemorrhage, escaping blood dissects, displaces, and compresses surrounding brain tissue. If a large volume of blood escapes, rising ICP can cause midline displacement

and herniation. At the same time, hemorrhage also halts the flow of necessary nutrients to brain tissue in the distribution area of the involved vessel.

ICH is most common in patients with hypertension, which causes degeneration of the walls of small, penetrating arteries deep within the cerebral hemispheres or brain stem. These arteries rupture and bleed into brain tissues, resulting in an intracerebral hematoma that compresses the tissue. Depending on the amount lost, blood may also rupture into the ventricles, leak into cerebrospinal fluid (CSF), and compress the brain stem. Massive ICH bleeding often ends in coma and death.

Subarachnoid hemorrhage. This type of hemorrhage results from a cerebral aneurysm, which appears most commonly as a sacular dilation in an artery of the circle of Willis or its major branches, usually at a bifurcation. Such an aneurysm, thought to result from congenital arterial weakness combined with degenerative changes, may rupture with a sudden, high-pressure release of blood into the subarachnoid space, irritating the pain-sensitive meninges and causing severe headache and nuchal rigidity. This may compromise the flow of blood to the brain area supplied by the ruptured vessel and lead to infarction. Vasospasm may also occur, causing tissue ischemia both proximal and distal to the ruptured aneurysm. Besides entering the subarachnoid space, the blood may form an intracerebral hematoma, displacing and compressing surrounding tissue and introducing the complications that can accompany ICH. SAH tends to recur within 7 to 10 days of the initial bleeding, possibly because of the natural lysis of the primary clot.

Another source of SAH is arteriovenous malformation (AVM), a congenital tangle of dilated thin-walled vessels in which blood from the arterial system is shunted directly into the venous system, as in a fistula. Characteristically, an AVM causes no symptoms for many years but may eventually rupture. Because this malformation often lies within cerebral tissue, it causes bleeding into the subarachnoid space and, possibly, into the brain's parenchyma.

Compensatory mechanisms

Two compensatory mechanisms protect the brain during adverse conditions by adjusting blood flow to maintain a constant supply of oxygen and glucose even when arterial pres-

Collateral blood flow and the circle of Willis

An anastomosis of extra-cranial arteries, major intracranial arteries, and the circle of Willis can supply arterial blood to the brain through several routes if one route becomes blocked. Under normal conditions, anterior circulation supplies most of the brain's cerebral hemispheres, and posterior circulation supplies the brain stem, cerebellum, and occipital lobes of the cerebral hemispheres. Four major vessels in the neck—two internal carotids in the anterior circulation and two vertebral arteries that merge into one basilar artery in the posterior circulation—supply blood to the head. These major arteries plus the anterior and posterior cerebral arteries join communicating arteries to form the circle of Willis (see illustration) at the brain's base.

Blood shunts from one part of the brain to another by way of this interconnecting system. For instance, if obstruction in the right internal carotid artery interrupts blood flow to the right cerebral hemisphere, the vertebral/basilar system shunts blood to that hemisphere through the posterior communicating artery or from the left carotid artery through the anterior cerebral artery. Often, such shunting lessens the effect of an occlusive loss of one or more of the major vessels by providing an adequate alternative blood supply.

However, in some individuals, the circle of Willis has congenitally missing arteries or small-diameter arteries with limited capacity to shunt blood where needed. In addition, atherosclerotic changes may affect the vessels' ability to shunt adequate blood.

- Middle cerebral stem
- Anterior communicating artery
- Anterior cerebral artery
- Internal carotid artery
- Posterior communicating artery
- Posterior cerebral artery
- Basilar artery
- Vertebral artery
- Anterior spinal artery

sure is changing. *Collateral circulation* provides alternative pathways for blood flow blocked by an occlusion (see *Collateral blood flow and the circle of Willis*); *autoregulation* maintains cerebral blood circulation at a constant rate.

Autoregulation. To maintain a constant oxygen and glucose supply to brain cells, blood must flow to the brain at a constant rate of about 750 ml/minute. The autoregulation system ensures this constant flow despite arterial pressure changes. It operates through vasodilation or constriction, triggered by serum oxygen and carbon dioxide concentrations and arterial blood pressure. If blood pressure drops or the carbon dioxide level rises, cerebral arteries dilate to allow more blood, and thus more oxygen and glucose, to reach the brain. Conversely, when blood pressure rises, cerebral arteries constrict to keep the flow and pressure constant. This protective mechanism for supplying oxygen and glucose to the brain can fail when overtaxed; for example, when cerebral arteries are severely impaired by atherosclerosis, occlusion, or rupture.

Variable neurologic sequelae

Cerebrovascular impairment can produce variable effects, from mild, transient symptoms to widespread and devastating failure of neurologic function. Most incidents, unfortunately, leave behind permanent deficits that range from mild hand weakness to complete unilateral paralysis and loss of speech. The severity of the residual deficit, the resulting loss of function, and the prognosis all depend on the arterial site of occlusion or rupture and the extent of ischemia or hemorrhage. (See *Sites and signs of neurologic deficits.*)

MEDICAL MANAGEMENT

Successful medical management of ischemic or hemorrhagic cerebrovascular disease attempts to support vital functions, restore cerebral circulation, reduce neurologic deficits, and prevent progression.

When cerebrovascular disease is suspected, a careful patient history should include the time over which the suspected stroke or TIA evolved; ischemic and hemorrhagic strokes usually evolve over minutes or hours, not weeks. The history should also include risk factors, such as hypertension or heart disease, that may complicate treatment. (See *Clinical characteristics of cerebrovascular disease,* page 156.)

The physical examination includes a general assessment of the patient's condition, with special attention to cardiac and circulatory findings since these may suggest a cause. It centers on a complete neurologic examination, with efforts to localize neurologic symptoms to a single arterial distribution.

Diagnosis: Defining site and severity

Diagnostic procedures help define the type of stroke and its possible focus and cause.

Scanning tests. *Computerized tomography (CT) scan* can determine the location and character of a stroke and differentiate it from imitative disorders, such as primary or metastatic tumor or traumatic subdural or epidural hematoma. Since ICH and SAH may appear immediately at the stroke's onset, CT scan identifies hemorrhagic stroke early by contrasting blood and tissue densities.

It may also show distortion of brain structure from large areas of hemorrhagic or edematous compression (mass effect) and, with the use of intravenous contrast dye, large aneurysms and AVMs.

CT scan may not reveal early stages of ischemic stroke unless cerebral edema with mass effect causes structural distortion. The ischemic lesion often can't be detected because it and the surrounding healthy tissue have about the same density immediately after the stroke. However, within a few days, infarction and, later, cavitation often become apparent. In TIAs, CT scan may be negative because TIAs do not involve permanent tissue changes. CT scan may also fail to show lacunar infarctions.

Positron emission tomography (PET) scan makes possible the study of cerebral metabolism and the visualization of cerebral blood flow changes, especially in ischemic stroke.

Magnetic resonance imaging (MRI) allows study of lesions without radiation exposure.

Lumbar puncture. Examining CSF helps diagnose SAH and, occasionally, ICH. In SAH, CSF is grossly bloody and does not clear; in extensive ICH that involves the ventricular system, it may also be bloody. With either type of hemorrhage, CSF pressure is usually elevated. Lumbar puncture is contraindicated if a large lesion or increased ICP is suspected, because of the danger of brain herniation.

Other noninvasive tests. An *electroencephalogram (EEG)* may detect focal slowing in an area of cortical infarction. This may prove especially useful if the results of the initial CT scan were negative. An EEG can differentiate seizure activity, which produces specific dysrhythmias, from stroke.

An *electrocardiogram (EKG)* is a routine procedure to help rule out MI and cardiac dysrhythmias, especially atrial fibrillation. If an intermittent dysrhythmia is suspected, a 24-hour continuous EKG tracing (Holter monitoring) is appropriate.

An *echocardiogram* demonstrates valvular disease or a thrombus on the heart wall or valve, both potential sources of emboli.

Other noninvasive tests serve as preliminary screening for carotid artery disease. They include supraorbital Doppler testing, oculoplethysmography, carotid phonoangiography, and ultrasonic imaging of the carotid arteries in the neck. If these tests show deficits and if lesions are suspected, an angiogram may be performed to provide more precise information.

Invasive tests. Angiography and digital subtraction angiography (DSA) allow visualization of the neck and cerebral arteries to help confirm cerebrovascular disease and to determine the need for medical or surgical intervention.

Angiography. The cerebral angiogram permits evaluation of the arteries for stenosis, plaque formation, and occlusion when surgery is considered after ischemic stroke and TIA. Angiography also precedes corrective surgery on aneurysms and AVMs in SAH and may be necessary for the differential diagnosis of the causes of hemorrhage and infarction. In addition, it evaluates the adequacy of collateral circulation.

Cerebral angiography poses a special risk because it involves introducing a catheter

Sites and signs of neurologic deficits

Anterior circulation— carotid distribution

Middle cerebral artery syndrome

Most common; may be complete or partial (*top illustration*)

• Motor and/or sensory deficits contralateral to hemispheric lesion
• Aphasia (with dominant hemisphere involvement)
• Homonymous hemianopsia
• Neglect of paralyzed side (with nondominant hemisphere involvement)
• Apraxia

Internal carotid syndrome

Resembles middle cerebral artery syndrome; may be complete or partial (*middle illustration*)

• Motor and/or sensory deficits contralateral to lesion
• Altered level of consciousness (with greater hemispheric involvement)
• Aphasia (with dominant hemisphere involvement)
• Neglect
• Apraxia
• Homonymous hemianopsia
• Ipsilateral blindness—usually transient (amaurosis fugax)

Anterior cerebral artery syndrome

Least common; may be complete or partial (*bottom illustration*)

• Motor and/or sensory deficits (more prominent in leg than arm)
• Urinary incontinence
• Flat emotional affect (slowness, lack of spontaneity)

Posterior circulation— vertebral/basilar distribution

Vertebral/basilar artery syndrome

(*Middle illustration*)

• Motor and/or sensory deficits on the same side of the body as lesion or on both sides or in all extremities (quadraparesis)
• Nystagmus
• Vertigo with nausea and vomiting
• Diplopia and lateral and vertical gaze palsies
• Visual field deficits
• Ataxia
• Dysphagia
• Dysarthria
• Coma (large brain stem involvement)

Posterior cerebral artery syndrome

(*Bottom illustration*)

• Visual field deficits—including cortical blindness
• Blindness (if bilateral involvement)
• Sensory loss on one side

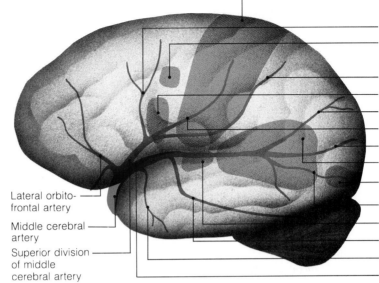

Motor/sensory cortex
Prerolandic artery
Eye/head contraversion area
Anterior parietal artery
Broca's area
Posterior parietal artery
Rolandic artery
Angular artery
Wernicke's area
Visual cortex
Posterior temporal artery
Auditory area
Anterior temporal artery
Temporal polar artery
Inferior division of middle cerebral artery

Lateral orbito-frontal artery
Middle cerebral artery
Superior division of middle cerebral artery

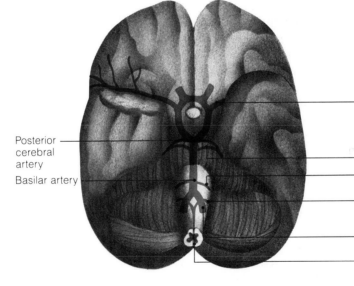

Internal carotid artery
Superior cerebellar artery
Anterior inferior cerebellar artery
Posterior inferior cerebellar artery
Vertebral artery
Anterior spinal artery

Posterior cerebral artery
Basilar artery

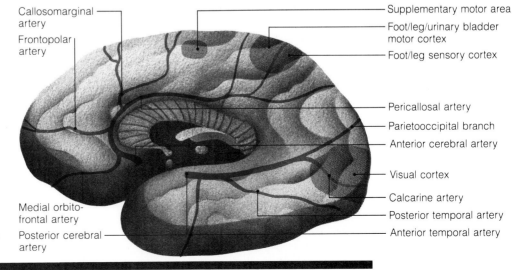

Supplementary motor area
Foot/leg/urinary bladder motor cortex
Foot/leg sensory cortex
Pericallosal artery
Parietooccipital branch
Anterior cerebral artery
Visual cortex
Calcarine artery
Posterior temporal artery
Anterior temporal artery

Callosomarginal artery
Frontopolar artery
Medial orbito-frontal artery
Posterior cerebral artery

Clinical characteristics of cerebrovascular disease

Characteristics	Thrombosis	Embolism	Intracerebral hemorrhage	Subarachnoid hemorrhage
Prodromal warning	Common	No	No	Rare
Onset during sleep	Sometimes	Rare	Rare	Rare
Development	Gradual	Sudden	Gradual or sudden	Sudden
Quick reversal	Possible	Possible	No	Possible
Bloody cerebrospinal fluid	No	Rare	Common	Yes
Coma	Rare	Rare	Common	Common
Decreased consciousness	Rare	Rare	Common	Common
Headache	Rare	Rare	Common	Common
Hypertension	Common	Possible	Nearly always	Common
Nuchal rigidity	No	No	Sometimes	Yes
Vomiting	Rare	Rare	Sometimes	Sometimes

and contrast dye into diseased arteries. In ischemic stroke, such manipulation may dislodge a small embolus or worsen thrombosis. In SAH, it may cause vasospasm or rebleeding, thereby worsening the original neurologic deficit or creating a new one. Thus, cerebral angiography is performed only when easier and safer techniques have failed to define suspected lesions.

Digital subtraction angiography. DSA may be used instead of cerebral angiography to visualize neck vessels and the large vessels of the circle of Willis. Since this procedure usually uses intravenous injection of a large bolus of contrast medium, it's less likely to cause embolism or arterial spasm. In addition, it requires less vascular manipulation than traditional arterial catheterization. DSA may also be performed using arterial injection of contrast dye.

Laboratory tests. Electrolyte profile, complete blood count, tests measuring cholesterol and triglyceride levels, and clotting profile are routinely performed to support diagnosis, guide intervention, and monitor the patient's status.

Electrolyte profile assesses fluid volume and electrolyte balance essential for homeostasis, since overhydration increases ICP.

Complete blood count, especially hemoglobin and hematocrit levels, gives a baseline of the

blood's oxygen-carrying ability. Occasionally, hematocrit reflects a high blood viscosity that may predispose the patient to infarct.

Serum cholesterol and triglycerides are checked for high levels often encountered in patients with atherosclerotic and thrombotic cerebrovascular disease.

Clotting profile, including prothrombin time, partial prothrombin time, platelet count, and fibrinogen value, can rule out clotting abnormalities, particularly in ischemic stroke. It also serves as a baseline for anticoagulant therapy during treatment with heparin.

Treatment to prevent complications and recurrence

Effective management of cerebrovascular disease begins with careful assessment and monitoring of cardiac and respiratory status to ensure adequate function. It also involves drug therapy to prevent worsening of the infarction or hemorrhage or to avoid repeated episodes and may include prophylactic or restorative surgery.

Supportive measures. Because, in the acute phase, especially in hemorrhagic stroke, a stroke victim may be comatose or have a decreased level of consciousness, his ventilation may be endangered. The patient may require supplemental oxygen, an artificial airway, or even intubation and mechanical ventilation.

Hyperventilation is ordered to maintain low arterial CO_2 levels in patients with suspected cerebral edema since high levels may dilate cerebral arteries and increase ICP. The patient should remain on bed rest for several days while receiving carefully monitored I.V. therapy to support blood pressure and enhance cerebral perfusion. In hemorrhage or complex infarction, ICP may be monitored (see Chapter 6).

Drug therapy. In the acute stage of a large ischemic or hemorrhagic stroke, drug therapy may include cortisone and dehydrating agents, administered intravenously if necessary. Dexamethasone may be administered intravenously or intramuscularly concomitantly with mannitol to reduce cerebral edema.

Anticoagulants may be used after TIAs to prevent further episodes or infarction and after thrombosis or embolism to prevent worsening. Heparin is given intravenously for several weeks, followed by warfarin (Coumadin) orally for several months. Aspirin, dipyridamole (Persantine), and sulfinpyrazone (Anturane), as antiplatelet drugs, are prescribed on a long-term basis to reduce platelet adhesiveness and possibly prevent future clots. These anticoagulants and antiplatelet agents should be given only after intracranial hemorrhage has been ruled out and no evidence exists of contraindicating conditions, such as bleeding ulcer or blood dyscrasia.

Antihypertensives may be used in intracranial hemorrhage with severe hypertension to reduce blood pressure gradually. Such therapy should avoid inducing hypotension, which would compromise cerebral perfusion.

Antifibrinolytic agent aminocaproic acid (Amicar) may be given to retard normal clot lysis and prevent rebleeding of a ruptured aneurysm.

Serotonin antagonists, such as reserpine and kanamycin, may be used to try to relieve vasospasm and prevent further ischemic stroke, which may complicate SAH. However, no drug has yet been found that effectively combats vasospasm. Also, vasodilators have not proved effective in treating cerebral ischemia.

Sedatives, such as phenobarbital, may be ordered for SAH.

Surgery. Certain surgical procedures may prevent TIA recurrence, restore impaired circulation, prevent repeated hemorrhage, or relieve pressure to avoid herniation (see *Surgery for cerebrovascular disease,* pages 158 and 159).

Prevention. Risk factors known to increase the probability of stroke include hypertension; atherosclerosis; diabetes mellitus; cardiac disease, including infarction, dysrhythmias, and valvular disease; and polycythemia. In those patients at risk, routine checkups, intermittent diagnostic studies, and prompt and vigorous interventions may prevent stroke.

NURSING MANAGEMENT
Your chief concerns are preventing complications, providing for patient comfort, and helping the patient handle the emotional effects of sudden physical impairment. Understanding what caused the stroke and the patient's prognosis for regaining function enables you to prepare a care plan that will guide the patient through recovery toward rehabilitation.

Clues from the history
Because cerebrovascular incidents may involve altered levels of consciousness and sustained speech and memory deficits, you'll probably need several sessions to complete the patient's history and may have to rely on his family or friends for details. Ask about presenting symptoms, such as headache, vomiting, nuchal rigidity, or loss of consciousness, and their onset. Use the information about headache, nuchal rigidity, and changes in consciousness to classify and grade suspected SAH (see *Classifying subarachnoid hemorrhage,* page 160).

Listen for clues to recurring TIAs. Ask the patient for a detailed description of every incident he remembers. In particular, ask exactly what he was doing when the attack started, whether his head was turned or bent, what the first symptom was, how the deficit evolved, how long the incident lasted, and the number of attacks he's experienced. If the patient has difficulty recalling, ask him to describe the first or the most recent attack, whichever is easier for him to recall.

Evaluate risk factors
In evaluating risk for cerebrovascular incidents, note the patient's age. Ask about hypertension, how long he's had it, what drugs he's taking, and what his prevailing blood pressure level is.

Ask about diabetes or cardiovascular disease and compliance with diet restrictions and drug schedules. Remember that a history of MI, dysrhythmias, or valvular disease caused by rheumatic fever may indicate embolic origin of ischemic stroke. Since pregnancy and the postpartum period increase the

Surgery for cerebrovascular disease

Current surgical interventions in ischemic cerebrovascular disease (transient ischemic attack [TIA] in particular) include carotid endarterectomy and extracranial/intracranial (EC/IC) bypass to prevent stroke. Endarterectomy may be performed when stenosis from plaque and ulceration could lead to further TIAs or stroke. Bypass is performed when endarterectomy is inappropriate, as in complete carotid occlusion or intracranial carotid stenosis.

Surgical intervention in cerebral aneurysm usually involves clipping to prevent rebleeding. Arteriovenous malformation may be excised (preferred treatment) or, if inaccessible, embolized to prevent further bleeding.

Surgical intervention in large intracerebral or subarachnoid hemorrhage (usually cerebellar or lateral basal ganglion hemorrhage) involves evacuation of the clot, if accessible, to prevent herniation.

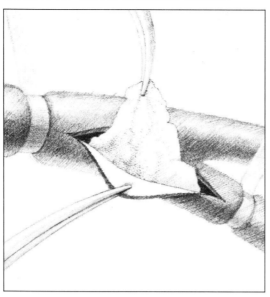

Carotid endarterectomy
Surgical excision removes atherosclerotic plaques from the inner arterial wall, most commonly at carotid arterial bifurcations.

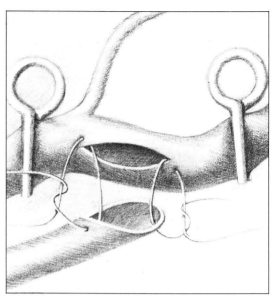

Extracranial/intracranial bypass
Splicing an extracranial artery (such as the superficial temporal artery) to an intracranial artery (such as the middle cerebral artery) bypasses an occlusion.

chance of stroke, ask women about recent pregnancy.

Has the patient recently taken anticoagulants or other drugs that increase susceptibility to hemorrhagic stroke? Does he have a history of blood dyscrasia?

Determine the family history for diabetes, heart disease, stroke, and congenital abnormalities such as AVMs. Because these conditions may be hereditary, a positive family history itself raises the risk of stroke.

Assess weight and alcohol and drug use. Dietary habits, especially heavy use of salt and saturated fats, and drug abuse may contribute to stroke.

Evaluate psychosocial aspects
Because cerebrovascular disease compromises physical, mental, and emotional function, determine the patient's prior activity level and life-style.

Psychosocial history. Was he physically independent before this illness? Will disabling arthritis, amputation, or another disease limit his adaptation to this illness?

Assess the reliability and availability of family and neighbors for physical and emotional support. Evaluate the patient's home; is it on one level or two? With stairs? If an apartment building, are elevators available?

If the patient was employed, will he be able to resume the same work?

Assess previous coping mechanisms. Has

he undergone any major life crisis, such as the death of a spouse, divorce, or job loss, in the past 6 months? How did he adjust? Does he currently suffer from depression, insomnia, anorexia, restlessness, or inability to concentrate? If necessary, muster the help of social service staff and outside support agencies.

Assessment to localize deficits
Of course, you'll assess the patient's condition when you see him, but this may be well after he experiences a stroke or TIA. If you happen to witness a stroke, reassess the patient's condition shortly after onset and then again at regular intervals to note changes. Whenever you perform an assessment, record your findings in detail since they'll serve as the baseline for later evaluation of improvement or deterioration.

Check for cortical involvement. Determining the extent of brain involvement can help you anticipate the total neurologic deficit and improve your care plan. During your initial assessment, evaluate any neurologic deficits and try to establish which brain area is affected—either cerebral hemisphere (anterior circulation) or brain stem and cerebellum (posterior circulation). (See *Sites and signs of neurologic deficits,* page 155.)

Check cardiovascular status. Note the rate, rhythm, and quality of heartbeat. Listen especially for dysrhythmias. Identify murmurs indicating valve insufficiency or stenosis,

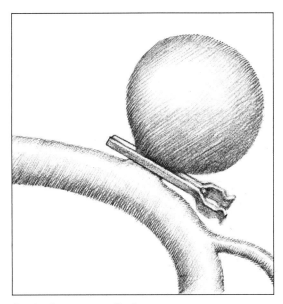

Cerebral aneurysm clipping
Clamping with a metal spring clip isolates an aneurysm.
If clipping is impossible, wrapping an aneurysm with
biologic or synthetic material supports the arterial wall.

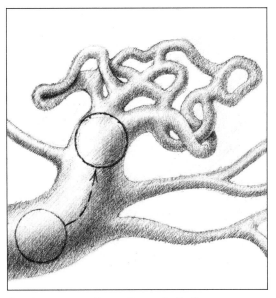

Arteriovenous malformation embolization
Small Silastic beads, placed in the carotid artery with a
catheter, seek out, thrombose, and destroy the malformation.

which may be associated with embolic stroke.
Auscultate the neck for bruits of either carotid
artery; the sound of turbulent blood flow
through narrowed vessels may signal cerebrovascular disease.

Take vital signs to assess ICP. Increased
systolic blood pressure with widening pulse
pressure and decreasing pulse indicates rising
ICP. Blood pressure level may also indicate
hyper- or hypotension, both significant in cerebrovascular disease. Compare blood pressure readings in both arms; in some patients,
subclavian artery blockage may cause a
marked difference.

Evaluate level of consciousness. Use the
Glasgow coma scale to record your findings. A
decreased level usually appears in strokes in
which large areas of the cerebral hemispheres
have been affected by edema, mass effect, or
increased ICP; or in small strokes, when bilateral or in the brain stem. Assess the patient's
awareness of time, place, and person, using
simple sentences that require only yes or no
answers.

Check pupil size and response to light. Dilated, fixed pupils, especially unilaterally, may
be a sign of increased ICP.

Assess higher functions. If the patient is
alert, observe the higher cortical functions,
including speech.

Aphasia, a loss of language function, is associated with stroke in the dominant cerebral
hemisphere, usually the left. The patient may
have trouble understanding spoken words (receptive aphasia) or speaking words correctly
(expressive aphasia), corresponding to damage in Wernicke's area or Broca's speech area,
respectively. Or both areas may be damaged
(global aphasia). Ask the patient if he has
difficulty understanding other people, radio
programs, or television or if he has trouble
speaking or making himself understood. Since
he may be unaware of his speech deficit, listen for errors in his conversation. Consider,
however, that skill dissociation may allow good
repetition of speech in a patient with poor
comprehension. To test receptive language,
ask the patient to follow a few simple commands, such as "Shut your eyes" or "Point to
the door." Ask him to repeat a few simple
words and sentences. Then point to objects
and ask him to name them; sometimes a patient recognizes the object but cannot retrieve
its name.

Watch for dysarthria, which is sometimes
confused with expressive aphasia. With this
deficit in articulation, the cortical ability to
speak and understand language remains intact, but one of the motor components
involved in speech, such as tongue and lip
movement or breath control, is impaired. Dysarthria frequently accompanies aphasia, particularly in the patient with facial weakness.
To assess for it, ask the patient to produce
a few simple sounds and words, such as "ba,"
"sh," and "cat."

Classifying subarachnoid hemorrhage
(Hunt's classification)

Grade I (minimal bleed)
Alert, minimal headache, nuchal rigidity, no neurologic deficit
Grade II (mild bleed)
Alert, mild-to-severe headache, nuchal rigidity, possible cranial nerve (CN) III palsy
Grade III (moderate bleed)
Drowsiness, confusion, headache, nuchal rigidity, possible focal neurologic deficit
Grade IV (moderate-to-severe bleed)
Stupor, nuchal rigidity, mild-to-severe hemiparesis
Grade V (severe bleed)
Coma, decerebrate posturing

Also check for writing disability (agraphia) and lack of reading comprehension (alexia). Assess for them by asking the patient to write his name and a short dictated sentence. If he can't write the sentence, write it for him and ask him to read it.

Watch for neglect syndrome. A patient with cortical involvement of the nondominant hemisphere (usually right) may deny his impairment. He typically ignores half of his body or denies that he has a limb weakness or paralysis. This behavior usually appears in the acute stage of illness but often resolves spontaneously.

Test for motor-sensory impairment. Test for loss of muscle strength and tone, ranging from mild impairment (paresis) to complete paralysis. Gauge muscle strength by asking the patient to move his arms and legs against resistance. Using a 5-point grading system (see Chapter 2), compare strength on both sides. Also test facial movement. If the patient cannot cooperate or has decreased consciousness, approximate muscle strength by observing for spontaneous movement and positioning of the patient's legs (a paralyzed leg tends to rotate outward when the patient's prone). Test muscle tone by gauging resistance when you move a patient's resting joint, such as the wrist or knee. Ordinarily after a stroke, the patient first shows flaccidity, which later changes to spasticity.

Check coordination. Watch the patient walk and then ask him to tap his foot rapidly or pat his knees while you observe for slowness, irregularity, and awkwardness. If a stroke originates in the cerebellum or affects tracts that originate there, disturbances of coordination or voluntary movement may result. The patient may have an ataxic walking gait, unsteady and staggering. Motor weakness may prevent the smooth performance of rapid movements.

Assess cranial nerve function. Seek deficits that imply posterior cerebrovascular disease or brain stem lesions.

Check vision for gaze palsies and double vision (diplopia), which occur with damage to cranial nerves (CN) III, IV, and VI. Look for a field deficit (homonymous hemianopsia), which may occur in both anterior and posterior strokes. (See *Testing for visual field deficits.*) Assess the patient's ability to swallow and to handle oral secretions since dysphagia may result from damage to CN IX and X.

Test for sensory deficit on the same side as motor weakness and on the opposite side; it

may range from slight numbness or a "pins and needles" sensation to complete absence of sensation. Compare the patient's ability to feel a light touch or pinprick at various sites and to feel the identical sensation at contralateral sites. Check if he can distinguish sharp and dull ends of a pin. If the patient's level of consciousness or ability to communicate is diminished, measure sensory perceptions by watching his facial reaction or attempts to move away from the stimulus.

Be alert for apraxia, the inability to complete a deliberate act when no motor or sensory impairment exists. Apraxia represents a cortical motor-planning breakdown involving speech or motor function, not a muscle or nerve deficit. It may occur in isolation or in conjunction with other neurologic deficits such as aphasia. Assess apraxia by observing for consistent ability to perform tasks, such as picking up a cup spontaneously and on demand. An apraxic patient may be inconsistent in his performance, frequently groping for or grossly missing the target.

Once you've established a complete baseline for neurologic deficit, check specific problem areas frequently and note how they're changing. For instance, if a patient has right arm and leg hemiplegia, periodically check the right side to see when movement begins to return. Record your observations with an actual description of the patient's ability, such as "able to shrug right shoulder and move right hip slightly."

Nursing diagnoses shape interventions

With the nursing history and physical assessment as your data base, you can now develop a care plan to fit your patient's specific physical deficits and emotional needs. Typically, your plan for the stroke patient will include the following nursing diagnoses and appropriate interventions.

Ineffective airway clearance related to altered level of consciousness and inability to cough. Prepare to maintain adequate oxygenation to all body tissues and prevent aspiration pneumonia. Begin by keeping an artificial airway at the patient's bedside and an Ambu bag on the unit. Frequently assess respiration rate and rhythm. If irregular respirations occur, record the length and frequency of apnea and notify the doctor since this development may signal intracranial hypertension or extension of a brain stem stroke. Be ready to send arterial blood gases to the laboratory, as ordered.

If the patient is intubated, suction sparingly. A patient with a large hemorrhagic stroke may be hyperventilated to maintain a PCO_2 level below 30 to avoid cerebral vasodilation, which would raise ICP. Suction only when the patient has unclear breath sounds, and limit suction to less than 15 seconds to minimize CO_2 buildup. Hyperventilate with 100% oxygen before and after suctioning.

Turn the patient frequently, elevate the head of the bed if the patient isn't hypotensive, and position his head to the side to help maintain an open airway, prevent aspiration of secretions, and avoid pooling of secretions in the lungs. Clear secretions from his mouth frequently with hard plastic tonsil-tip suction. Give humidified oxygen or room air to prevent thickened secretions that are difficult to remove. Begin to teach coughing and deep breathing when appropriate.

You've met respiratory goals if the patient shows no signs of respiratory distress, hypoventilation, hypoxia, or aspiration pneumonia.

Potential for injury related to unstable cerebrovascular status, immobility, or visual field deficit. To prevent increased ICP, rebleeding from an SAH, falls and injuries from motor deficits and seizures, and complications of bed rest, begin by assessing the patient's neurologic status initially every 2 hours. Include level of consciousness, pupil response, vital signs, and bilateral motor and sensory function. Immediately report changes that signal rising ICP (see *Signs of increased intracranial pressure,* page 162).

After cerebral hemorrhage, use intracranial monitoring, if ordered, to detect ICP changes before they cause clinical signs and to allow prompt intervention to avert permanent damage (see Chapter 6).

In SAH caused by a ruptured aneurysm, maintain a nonstressful environment to prevent rebleeding and further neurologic damage from increased ICP. Place an "aneurysm precaution" sign on the patient's door. Provide a quiet, darkened room, bed rest with minimal activity, and analgesics and sedatives, as ordered. Restrict visitors, phone calls, radio, television, and reading. Elevate the head of the bed 30° to 45° to promote cerebral venous drainage. Caution the patient against coughing or any straining, such as during a bowel movement, because either may increase ICP. Establish a bowel movement regimen to avoid constipation and straining. Take oral or axillary temperatures since rectal temperatures may cause vagal stimulation that raises ICP.

Testing for visual field deficits

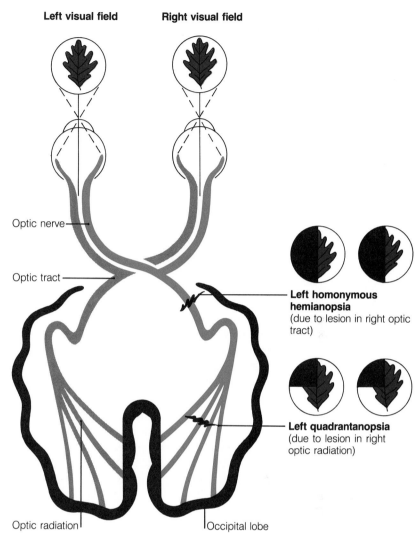

Strokes that involve portions of the visual pathway can cause visual field deficits like those shown above. Here's how to test for them. Stand directly in front of the patient, about 2 feet away from his face, and have him cover one of his eyes. Instruct him to look straight ahead during the test. Now, bring a finger or a pencil from the periphery into his field of vision and have him indicate when he sees the object. Repeat the action moving toward his eyes from each quadrant. Watch his head for gross movements as he becomes aware of the field deficit and begins to compensate for it.

Follow seizure precautions for a patient with intracranial hemorrhage: Tape an oral or nasal airway to the head of the bed, keep padded side rails raised, and have suction equipment ready at bedside. Never allow an unsteady patient to remain out of bed and unattended. Keep the ambulatory patient's environment free of obstacles and clutter. Teach the patient correct techniques for bearing weight, pivoting, and using such devices as wheelchairs, canes, and walkers. Teach the patient with cerebellar involvement that even though he is

Signs of increased intracranial pressure

Deteriorating level of consciousness

Pupillary dilation (especially unilateral)

Decreased pupillary light reflex

Loss of motor function

Sensory deterioration

Rising systolic blood pressure

Widening pulse pressure

Bradycardia

Respiratory pattern changes

Papilledema

Headache

Vomiting

not seriously weakened, ataxia may cause him to lose balance easily and fall. Teach family members about proper body mechanics and alignment and how to assist the patient at home.

If the patient is immobile, guard against complications of bed rest, such as thrombophlebitis and skin breakdown. Apply elastic stockings, and remove them only once a day to wash the legs and check for skin breakdown. Perform frequent range-of-motion exercises on the legs to stimulate peripheral circulation and to prevent venous stasis, which leads to clot formation and pulmonary embolism. If thrombophlebitis does develop, as indicated by redness, swelling, warmth, and streaking of the area and vessel involved, avoid massaging the leg, which can dislodge the clot.

To prevent skin breakdown, turn the patient every 2 hours, pad bony prominences, and supply a foam mattress. Allow him to lie on the paralyzed side only 20 minutes at a time because of increased susceptibility to tissue edema and injury. Elevate his affected arms and legs at intervals to promote reabsorption of dependent edema. Keep the patient's back and perineum clear of perspiration, urine, and feces. Intervene promptly when you see signs of redness, irritation, or skin breakdown.

Help the patient with a visual field deficit by positioning his bed in the room so that his intact side faces the door, if possible. Thus, he won't be surprised by people entering the room. Approach the patient from his intact side, and place objects such as his food tray within his field of vision. Keep the room uncluttered. Teach him to scan his surroundings to avoid obstacles and help judge distances. Caution him to move slowly to compensate for altered depth perception. If double vision is present, try patching the affected eye. If the patient has lost oculomotor nerve control and cannot close his eyelid, protect the cornea by instilling artificial tears every 3 to 4 hours and possibly taping the eyelid closed.

You've met your goals if ICP remains within safe limits and cerebral aneurysm doesn't rebleed and if the patient suffers no falls or seizure-related injuries, shows no signs of thrombophlebitis or decubitus ulcers, and moves about his environment with minimal difficulty.

Alteration in hydration and nutrition related to multiple neurologic deficits. To prevent dehydration and negative nitrogen balance, give fluids intravenously at first. Avoid rapid infusion of fluids, which may raise ICP. Monitor urine output and skin turgor for dehydration. Order tube feedings until swallowing and gag reflexes return. Elevate the head of the bed during and after meals to prevent regurgitation and aspiration. Dilute feedings with water to prevent the osmotic diarrhea that often follows feedings with high solute loads. Before beginning oral feeding, test the patient's swallowing reflex cautiously with a small amount of water; keep the patient upright and have suction equipment handy. When the patient can swallow, begin oral feeding with soft foods, which are easier to swallow than liquids. Because of decreased sensation in the patient's buccal membranes, pretest food and fluids to prevent burns. Encourage self-feeding as much as possible, even though it may prolong mealtimes and require rewarming of food. If necessary, provide several smaller meals a day to maintain adequate intake and prevent starvation and negative nitrogen balance.

You've met your goals if the patient receives adequate fluid and nutritional intake, maintains an appropriate weight, and feeds himself.

Alteration in elimination related to multiple neurologic deficits. To help the patient regain urinary bladder control, first consider the reason for his incontinence. In the acute phase of stroke, incontinence may result from an altered level of consciousness or from bilateral frontal or brain stem lesions. Unless it's vital for monitoring fluid balance, avoid placing an indwelling catheter because of the risk of infection. If you must use a catheter, remove it as soon as the patient's condition stabilizes. In a male, use an external urinary draining device. Before attributing incontinence to neurologic causes, assess the patient's ability to communicate his need to void and his ability to reach a bedpan or urinal. To combat incontinence, offer the bedpan every 2 hours and follow the guidelines for bladder retraining (see Chapter 10). Most patients can regain independent control of this function.

To restore bowel regularity, determine the patient's normal bowel routine and record his bowel movements. Caution against straining during a bowel movement because it raises ICP and risks rebleeding in hemorrhagic stroke. Use suppositories or stool softeners for constipation, particularly if the patient has limited mobility, but avoid enemas because they cause vagal stimulation, which raises ICP. As soon as possible, reestablish a diet with adequate fluid and bulk. Let the able patient use a bedside commode to increase his sense of control.

You've met your goals if the patient maintains urinary continence within his limitations, suffers no urinary infection, and regains independent control of urinary function and if he reestablishes a bowel movement routine and avoids constipation and straining.

Impaired communication related to aphasia and dysarthria. To achieve effective alternative means of communication among patient, staff, and family and to meet the patient's needs, tailor your approach to his disorder.

If the patient has receptive aphasia, keep sentences simple, speak slowly, and repeat directions, using supplementary gestures or pictures.

If the patient has a visual field deficit, stand where he can see you as you talk to him.

Give the patient with expressive aphasia and dysarthria ample time to speak, and supply a letter board, magic slate, or "needs" list to help him communicate.

Reassure the patient and his family that his difficulty with speech relates to the stroke, not to intelligence, and that he's likely to improve in a few months, although recovery may continue for up to 2 years. Encourage the family to speak to the patient in a normal tone. Explain that the patient hears and understands, so they don't need to shout. Warn them that frustration may cause the patient to utter obscenities clearly as a form of automatic speech. Teach the family to support the patient's efforts to speak and to continue speech therapy at home.

You've met your goals if the patient communicates willingly with staff and family, if his frustration seems minimal, and if his needs are being met.

Self-care deficit related to multiple neurologic deficits. To help the patient wash and dress himself and acknowledge his impairment, encourage independence to boost self-esteem. Remind the patient with neglect syndrome to wash and dress all body areas. Make the patient aware of the neglected body parts by sensory stimulation to the affected areas or by assisting with exercises that bring the affected limbs across midline. Advise him to dress the affected side first and undress it last for easier handling of clothes. Suggest clothing with easy, front fastenings.

You've met your goals if the patient handles personal hygiene and grooming well without neglecting impaired body parts.

Alteration in emotional state related to le-sions in specific brain locations and reaction to illness.** To foster appropriate coping mechanisms, make the patient and his family aware that emotional disorders may follow a stroke. After a stroke in the right hemisphere, the patient may appear apathetic or unduly cheerful, tending to minimize or deny his illness. After a stroke in the left hemisphere, especially the left frontal quadrant, the patient often suffers depression. Inappropriate or exaggerated mood swings accompany bilateral frontal damage and pseudobulbar conditions. Ask the patient during a crying or laughing spell if he feels particularly sad or happy; usually, his feelings won't justify the intensity of his external signs of emotion. Help him by identifying inappropriate behavior, praising appropriate behavior, and assisting in setting realistic goals for recovery.

Depression may not always be evident. Once the patient's fully alert, watch for signs of depression, such as sleep disturbances with early morning awakening, loss of appetite and weight, loss of interest and concentration, sadness, anxiety, social withdrawal, brooding, irritability, tearfulness, pessimistic attitude toward the future, and thoughts of death and suicide. Ask his family if they notice a change in the patient since he may express his feelings more openly to them. Encourage the patient to express his feelings, although this may be a difficult task for the patient with aphasia or dysarthria.

Tell the family that the patient's depression could worsen after discharge when he's no longer buoyed by staff attention. The family can help by sympathetically but firmly encouraging rehabilitation. Suggest that the patient seek support through a club of former stroke victims, a church group, or a community program. Persistent depression that interferes with rehabilitation may require mood-elevating drugs or psychiatric consultation.

You've met your goals if the patient and his family accept and expect emotional changes in the patient and if they express their feelings about the disability and define realistic goals.

A rewarding task

Caring for patients with cerebrovascular disease is characteristically arduous and challenging. But it's always worth doing with all the skill you can muster. Giving such competent care can be rewarding when a patient devastated by this disease again becomes a functioning individual through your interventions and encouragement.

Points to remember

- Cerebrovascular disease may be ischemic or hemorrhagic. Its causes include atherosclerotic thrombus, embolus, hypertensive intracerebral hemorrhage, and ruptured cerebral aneurysm.
- Brain cells depend on oxygen and glucose to function. A few minutes of interrupted blood flow causes involved tissue to undergo necrotic changes.
- Deficit severity, type of functional loss or disorder, and prognosis all depend on the specific cerebral focus and extent of ischemia or hemorrhage.
- Computerized tomography scan helps differentiate hemorrhage from infarct. Other tests help locate cause and focus and help guide interventions.
- Medical treatment may include respiratory support; dehydrating agents, anticoagulants, or antihypertensives; and preventive or restorative surgery.
- Emotional support and encouragement can help the patient cope with physical impairments and work harder to regain maximum function.

13 CORRECTING HYDROCEPHALUS

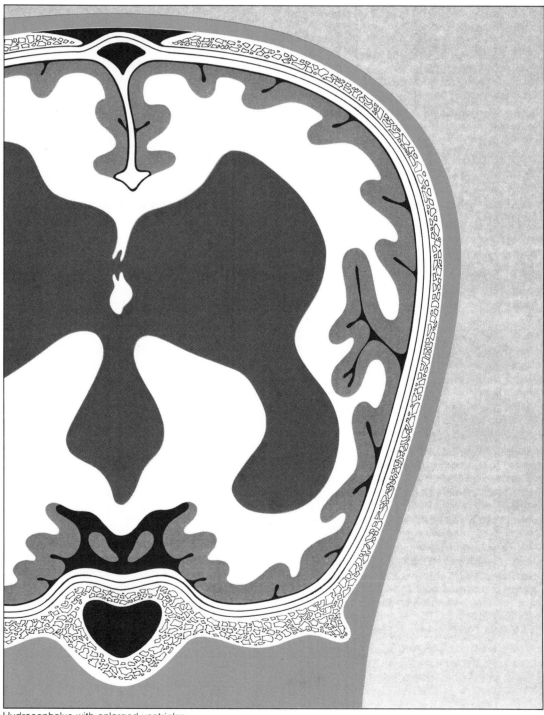

Hydrocephalus with enlarged ventricles

H ydrocephalus. If you think immediately of an infant with a disproportionately large head, that's usually right—head enlargement *is* the unmistakable sign of hydrocephalus in infants. But there's more to this syndrome than meets the eye. For example, did you know that hydrocephalus isn't limited to infants? That head size may remain normal in some patients with hydrocephalus? That hydrocephalus is often confused with other neurologic disorders? And that surgery can sometimes produce dramatic improvement?

Even so, there are no "miracle" cures for hydrocephalus. After surgery, mental and physical impairment often persists. But early detection *can* improve prognosis, so the more you know about this syndrome, the more you can help the patient—and his family.

This chapter will give you the information you need to accurately assess the patient with hydrocephalus and to care for him effectively and compassionately.

What is hydrocephalus?

You've often heard hydrocephalus referred to as "water on the brain." Although simplistic, this colloquial phrase does, in fact, describe the fundamental problem of this syndrome: the presence of too much fluid within the cranial vault. To be exact, hydrocephalus is the excessive accumulation of cerebrospinal fluid (CSF) within the ventricular system, causing dilation of the ventricles. It results from an imbalance between production and reabsorption of CSF.

Although hydrocephalus may be acquired as a result of injury or disease, it's most often congenital. Congenital hydrocephalus, occurring in approximately 1 of every 1,000 births, may be nongenetic—from intracranial hemorrhage or intrauterine infection, for example—or genetic, from stenosis of an aqueduct inherited as an X-linked, recessive trait. This X-linked pattern of inheritance is the cause of hydrocephalus in an estimated 2% of all patients.

Regardless of the cause, the prognosis in hydrocephalus is uniformly poor if the condition remains untreated. Without surgery, hydrocephalus leads to increased intracranial pressure (ICP), which is potentially fatal in patients of all ages; in infants, the associated infection and malnutrition can also have serious consequences. In all patients, the prognosis depends on the underlying cause, its severity, and the effectiveness of treatment.

PATHOPHYSIOLOGY

Hydrocephalus may result from obstruction in CSF flow (noncommunicating hydrocephalus), or from defective reabsorption or (rarely) increased production of CSF (communicating hydrocephalus, including normal-pressure hydrocephalus).

Causes of hydrocephalus

A look at each of these types of hydrocephalus reveals what triggers CSF accumulation.

Noncommunicating hydrocephalus. This hydrocephalus may result from *congenital* stenosis at the aqueduct of Sylvius, between the third and fourth ventricles; at the foramina of Luschka and/or Magendie, the outlets of the fourth ventricle (Dandy-Walker syndrome); or, rarely, at the foramina of Monro, passages of the lateral ventricles to the third ventricle. Such obstruction may be due to genetic or acquired disorders, such as encephalocele, Arnold-Chiari deformity (see *Understanding Arnold-Chiari syndrome,* page 166), tumor, cyst, vascular malformation, or intrauterine infection or hemorrhage.

Acquired stenosis of an aqueduct may result from fibrous adhesions, tumor, blood clot, or inflammatory scarring due to meningitis.

Communicating hydrocephalus. This hydrocephalus also has *congenital* and *acquired* causes. Congenital causes include leptomeningeal inflammation, which may lead to noncommunicating hydrocephalus if scar tissue forms an obstruction. Leptomeningeal inflammation may also be *acquired* from infection, hemorrhage, or particulate matter in CSF, all of which can occlude arachnoid villi, impairing CSF reabsorption.

Communicating hydrocephalus may also result from overproduction of CSF, usually caused by hypertrophy or tumor of the choroid plexus. But since CSF can be reabsorbed three to four times as fast as it's formed, this cause is rare.

Normal-pressure hydrocephalus. Normal-pressure hydrocephalus is a type of communicating hydrocephalus most often seen in adults. In this hydrocephalus, ICP remains normal despite an increase in CSF that causes ventricular enlargement. Conditions that may lead to normal-pressure hydrocephalus include subarachnoid hemorrhage from a bleeding aneurysm, arteriovenous malformation, or head trauma; thrombosis of the superior sagittal sinus; scarring of the basal cistern, usually secondary to head trauma or surgery; and bacterial meningitis. However, in some elderly patients, no cause can be found.

Understanding Arnold-Chiari syndrome
Cross-sectional view

Enlarged ventricles

Pons

Medulla oblongata
Cerebellar elongation

Syringomyelia

Arnold-Chiari syndrome is a congenital malformation of the cervicomedullary function, which often accompanies spina bifida and syringomyelia. It causes hydrocephalus, especially when a myelomeningocele is also present. In this syndrome, the cerebellum and medulla extend down through the foramen magnum into the cervical portion of the spinal canal, impairing drainage of cerebrospinal fluid by compressing the fourth ventricle and closing the foramina of Luschka and Magendie.

Infants with this syndrome exhibit signs and symptoms of both hydrocephalus and meningeal irritation. Treatment requires surgery to insert a ventricular shunt and possible decompression of the cerebellar tonsils.

Ventricular dilation characteristic
Although their causes vary, noncommunicating and communicating hydrocephalus both lead to excessive accumulation of CSF, resulting in ventricular dilation. (See *Ventricular dilation: Hallmark of hydrocephalus.*)

Pattern of onset varies, depending on the location and severity of CSF obstruction. In acute obstruction, dilation may develop rapidly, stretching the ventricular ependyma and disrupting the tight junctions between cells. In partial obstruction or defective reabsorption of CSF, the ventricles enlarge more slowly.

The pattern of ventricular dilation varies as well. Obstruction at the aqueduct of Sylvius usually causes symmetrical dilation of the lateral and third ventricles. Obstruction at the foramina of Magendie and Luschka causes symmetrical dilation of the lateral, third, and fourth ventricles. Since the hypothalamus lies in the floor and lateral walls of the third ventricle, increased pressure due to dilation may impair its function. Obstruction from inflammatory exudate in meningitis may block

the subarachnoid space, dilating the entire ventricular system.

Severity of dilation also varies. In newborns and infants whose cranial sutures haven't fused, the ventricles may reach enormous size if dilation progresses slowly. In older patients, ventricular enlargement is less dramatic because the cranium has a fixed capacity.

Effects of ventricular dilation
Ventricular dilation triggers various compensatory mechanisms that aim to regulate ICP by controlling fluid volume within the cranial vault. Cerebral blood vessels narrow, decreasing cerebral blood flow and increasing cerebral venous pressure. Disruption of the ventricles' ependymal lining allows transventricular reabsorption of some CSF. In infants, expansion of the skull also accommodates increased CSF. When compensatory mechanisms are exhausted, ICP rises. Critically high pressure may increase CSF reabsorption tenfold and may slow its production.

Ventricular dilation exacts the greatest toll on the cortical white matter, which becomes compressed and may eventually atrophy. Its effect on the gray matter is less dramatic: the cerebral cortex may be selectively spared.

Clinical clues to hydrocephalus
Signs and symptoms vary, depending on the patient's age and the type of hydrocephalus. In infants, dramatic enlargement of the head is the definitive sign of hydrocephalus, although initially the head may be normal in size with bulging of the fontanels. Other signs include thin, fragile, and shiny-looking scalp skin; weak, underdeveloped neck muscles; and poor sucking reflex. In severe hydrocephalus, the roof of the orbits is depressed, the eyes are displaced downward, and the scleras are prominent ("setting-sun eyes"). Increased ICP causes listlessness, irritability, vomiting, anorexia, and a high-pitched, shrill cry.

In older children and adults with hydrocephalus, headache, nausea and/or vomiting, and diplopia are common early signs, reflecting increased ICP; later, irritability, restlessness, personality changes, incontinence, and difficulty in walking may also occur.

Cardinal signs of normal-pressure hydrocephalus include impaired mental function, gait disturbances, and urinary incontinence. Forgetfulness and difficulty in participating in conversation are typical early signs of impaired mental function. Later, judgment and analysis also falter, perhaps jeopardizing the patient's safety. Such signs commonly develop over weeks or months and in elderly patients are often mistaken for the results of aging.

Gait disturbance often begins as a slowed pace with wide, zig-zag steps, which makes the patient susceptible to falls and eventually makes independent walking impossible.

Urinary incontinence typically follows the onset of gait disturbance and dementia and probably results from compression of nerve tracts that innervate the bladder.

In addition, tendon reflexes increase, especially in the legs. In advanced stages, the patient may demonstrate Babinski's, grasp, and suck reflexes; hypertension; widening pulse pressure; diminished pulse and respirations; and seizures.

MEDICAL MANAGEMENT

Diagnosis of hydrocephalus can be surprisingly elusive. Normal-pressure hydrocephalus develops so insidiously that telltale signs are easily overlooked. Even in hydrocephalic infants, an abnormally large head isn't conclusive evidence. Subdural hematoma, porencephaly, hydranencephaly, prosencephaly (rare), and achondroplasia can also cause head enlargement; so can a growth spurt after adequate feeding of a malnourished infant. Accurate diagnosis, of course, requires a thorough history and physical examination, but special tests provide the most reliable data.

What diagnostic tests reveal

The following tests are typically part of the diagnostic workup for hydrocephalus:

Computerized tomography (CT) scan. This test reveals ventricular enlargement in hydrocephalus and helps locate the site of CSF obstruction. It also identifies intracranial lesions and shows cortical size and thickness. Serial CT scans monitor the progression of hydrocephalus and its response to treatment.

Pneumoencephalogram. A possible adjunct to the CT scan, this test pinpoints the site of CSF obstruction and shows ventricular enlargement. In normal-pressure hydrocephalus, the injected air readily fills the ventricles. However, since CSF reabsorption is impeded, movement of air into the cerebral subarachnoid space is slight.

Isotope cisternogram (flow study). This test also pinpoints CSF obstruction and evaluates the rate of CSF reabsorption, helping to distinguish noncommunicating from communicating (particularly normal-pressure)

Ventricular dilation: Hallmark of hydrocephalus

Normal
Medial view

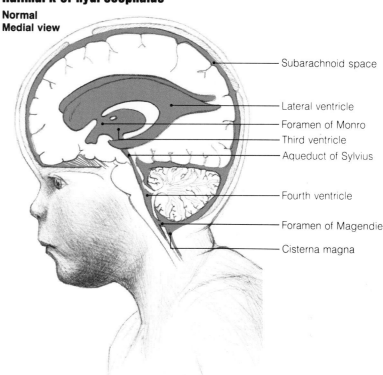

- Subarachnoid space
- Lateral ventricle
- Foramen of Monro
- Third ventricle
- Aqueduct of Sylvius
- Fourth ventricle
- Foramen of Magendie
- Cisterna magna

Hydrocephalus

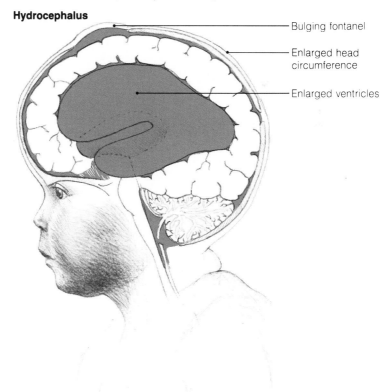

- Bulging fontanel
- Enlarged head circumference
- Enlarged ventricles

Hydrocephalus results from impaired circulation, defective reabsorption, or (rarely) increased production of cerebrospinal fluid (CSF). Subsequent CSF accumulation causes ventricular dilation, which compresses brain tissue and hinders cerebral blood flow. In a child, ventricular dilation swells the still-developing cranium; in an adult, a rigid cranium confines the swelling.

Draining CSF through a surgical shunt

Ventriculoperitoneal shunt

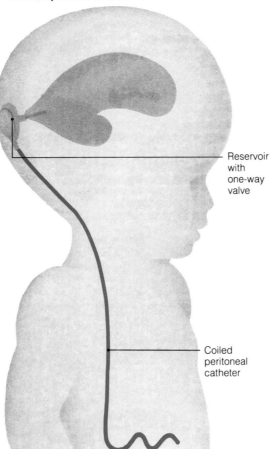

Reservoir
with
one-way
valve

Coiled
peritoneal
catheter

Ventriculoatrial shunt

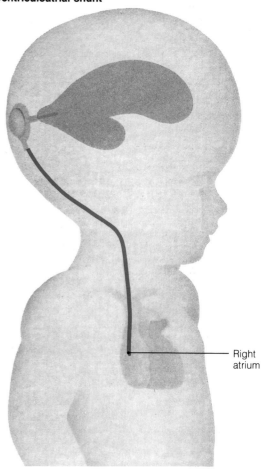

Right
atrium

Surgery for hydrocephalus usually involves insertion of a ventriculoperitoneal shunt, which transports excess cerebrospinal fluid (CSF) from the lateral ventricle into the peritoneal cavity. This shunt is preferred for infants and young children. An overlong catheter can be coiled in the peritoneum; it will uncoil automatically as the child grows. Nevertheless, the catheter must be periodically replaced with a longer one until growth is complete.

A less common procedure is insertion of a ventriculoatrial shunt, which transports excess CSF from the lateral ventricle into the right atrium of the heart, where the fluid enters the venous circulation. This shunt is usually preferred for adults or older children who've completed rapid growth.

With either type of shunt, the system typically consists of a primary catheter, a reservoir, a one-way valve, and a terminal catheter. The primary catheter is inserted in a lateral ventricle and channels CSF from there into a reservoir under the scalp. The one-way valve within the reservoir opens when intracranial pressure (ICP) reaches a certain level, allowing CSF to exit through the terminal catheter. This system prevents a dangerous increase in ICP and backflow of fluid into the ventricles. Note that low-pressure valves are used in normal-pressure hydrocephalus.

hydrocephalus. In normal-pressure hydrocephalus, the injected isotope concentrates in the CSF system and fails to clear within about 48 hours.

Lumbar puncture. Useful for measuring ICP, this test also allows sampling of CSF for laboratory analysis. Elevated CSF protein levels may indicate tumor or infection. Lumbar puncture, however, should be preceded by CT scan in the patient with suspected increased

ICP to detect a possible ventricular shift or brain herniation, and then should be performed with extreme caution to avoid precipitating herniation.

Skull X-rays. These films—now largely replaced by the CT scan—may show thinning of the skull with separation of the sutures and widening of the fontanels in infants. X-rays also show bony erosion and air in the ventricles (from direct intracranial penetration of

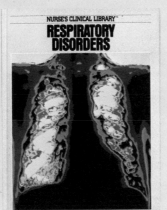
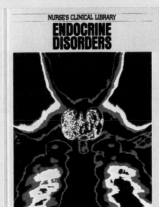
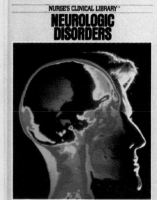
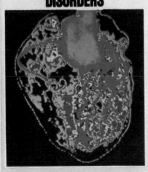
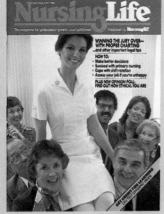

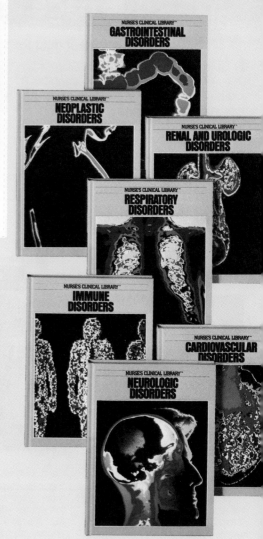

Introduce yourself to the new NURSE'S CLINICAL LIBRARY™ series.

A comprehensive book for each specific body system disorder. That's what makes this set of books so valuable to nurses. No longer will you have to go to one book for drug information, then another for pathophysiology, and still another for diagnostics. Each book in the NURSE'S CLINICAL LIBRARY is a complete source for each body system disorder. And as a subscriber to the series, you save $3.00 off the single-copy price of each book. Act now. Send the postage-paid card above today!

© 1984 Springhouse Corporation

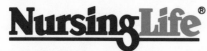
Mail the card at left to get your trial copy of *NursingLife.*

Send no money now. Just mail the card at left and we'll send you a trial copy of *NursingLife,* the fastest growing nursing journal in the world. You'll discover how to avoid malpractice suits, answer touchy ethical questions, get along better with doctors and other nurses, work better under pressure, and much more. Send for yours today!

the dura by facial bone or foreign object).

Other tests. Transillumination of an infant's skull reveals fluid accumulation, and ultrasonography (particularly helpful in children with open fontanels) detects ventricular enlargement. Cerebral arteriography may be done in infants or adults to show ventricular enlargement and associated vascular lesions as demonstrated by displacement of cerebral vessels.

Surgical shunt: Only effective treatment
Surgical shunting transports excess CSF from the enlarged ventricles to an area where it can be reabsorbed or excreted. A ventriculocisternal (Torkildsen) shunt transports CSF from a lateral ventricle to the cisterna magna for reabsorption into the venous sinuses. A ventriculoperitoneal shunt diverts fluid to the peritoneal cavity; a ventriculoatrial shunt, to the right atrium (see *Draining CSF through a surgical shunt*).

Timing has much to do with the outcome of surgery. Shunting obviously can't correct excessive, irreversible brain tissue damage due to ventricular dilation. Since head enlargement may precede brain compression in infants, diagnosis is possible before such damage occurs. Clinical studies in adults with normal-pressure hydrocephalus indicate a better outcome when surgery is performed within 6 months of the onset of symptoms.

Of course, complications can also influence surgical outcome. The shunt's catheter can become kinked or plugged with a blood clot, exudate, brain tissue, or CSF protein. Contamination of the catheter is also fairly common, resulting in meningitis, peritonitis, or septicemia. In addition, the catheter can shift or become dislodged and, rarely, perforate the viscera. (See *Recognize signs of shunt failure*.)

If shunt malfunction or central nervous system (CNS) infection develops, ventriculostomy may be a useful temporary treatment for hydrocephalus. It's also useful for monitoring ICP, sampling CSF, or instilling dyes for diagnostic tests, and it aids in determining the need for a permanent shunt following surgery, such as for SAH or head trauma. In this procedure, a catheter inserted in a lateral ventricle allows drainage of CSF to control ICP. However, too rapid drainage of CSF from the ventricular system can release the tamponade effect created on cortical bridging veins by ventricular dilation and can stretch and rupture those veins, resulting in subdural hematoma. Antisiphon valves help prevent this complication as does postoperative bed rest in a supine position.

A successful shunting procedure often dramatically improves mental status in normal-pressure hydrocephalus, but it may not correct gait disturbance. In all types of hydrocephalus, prognosis varies for infants, but mental retardation and motor and visual deficits may persist.

Recognize that shunting isn't the only surgical treatment for hydrocephalus. Surgical widening of the foramen magnum sometimes achieves decompression in Arnold-Chiari deformity. Or surgical excision of a tumor, cyst, or mass lesion may correct CSF flow in non-communicating hydrocephalus.

Experimental drug therapy to inhibit production of CSF or to increase its reabsorption has been unsuccessful.

NURSING MANAGEMENT
Although the patient's prognosis often depends on a successful shunting procedure, your participation in establishing accurate diagnosis, providing appropriate treatment, and ensuring recovery is very important. Since you'll be spending more time than the doctor with the patient and his family, they'll probably feel more comfortable with you. Hence, your patient history might well reveal much more than the doctor's. Establishing a first-rate history provides a firm basis for your nursing-care plan.

A first-rate patient history
Since the patient will likely be an infant or an adult with impaired mental function, expect to rely on parents or other family members for much of the history. If the patient is an infant, be sure to include a detailed history of the pregnancy, covering any infections incurred and the drugs prescribed during the first two trimesters, and a complete perinatal history. Also, since genetically linked disorders are common causes of neonatal and childhood hydrocephalus, keep in mind that taking a family history for similar or other neurologic disorders is essential.

First, determine the reason for hospitalization. Then explore the patient's symptoms and determine when they were first noticed. Ask the parents if their infant has been irritable, eating poorly, or vomiting frequently. Does holding or rocking make the infant more irritable? Does the infant have a high-pitched, shrill cry? Also find out if they've noticed delayed motor skills. If the patient's an older child or an adult, ask about signs of increas-

Recognize signs of shunt failure

In infants
Tense, bulging fontanels
Abnormal increase in head circumference
Vomiting
Poor feeding
Irritability
Excessive sleepiness

In older children and adults
Headache
Nausea and/or projectile vomiting
"Setting-sun eyes" or paralysis of upward gaze
Lethargy
Irritability
Behavior changes

Measuring head circumference

Routinely measure head circumference in infants and children up to age 3. Using a nonstretchable tape, measure at the greatest circumference— just above the eyebrows and ears and around the occipital prominence at the back of the skull. Suspect hydrocephalus if the measurement exceeds the age-adjusted norm by ½″ (1.3 cm).

After hydrocephalus is diagnosed, take daily measurements pre- and postoperatively. To ensure that all measurements are taken at precisely the same site, draw a picture on the patient's chart showing where to measure the head, or mark the forehead with ink.

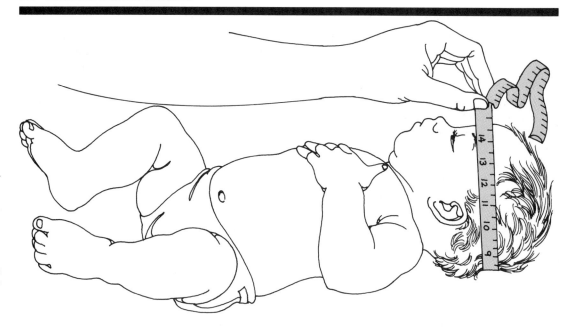

ing ICP—headache, double vision, nausea, vomiting, irritability, urinary incontinence. Does the patient have difficulty walking, remembering things, or paying attention to conversations? Remember that dementia, ataxic gait, and urinary incontinence characterize normal-pressure hydrocephalus.

Also inquire about past treatment for hydrocephalus or a history of other disorders that may produce similar symptoms.

Because hydrocephalus can significantly disrupt family life, try to determine its impact during the history. Keep the following questions in mind.

How do individual family members react to the disease? Has it affected the patient's occupation, schooling, or social life? Determine what physical and social activities the patient can still enjoy. Do other people seem to shun him? Explore the family's emotional and financial resources. Do supportive friends and relatives live nearby? Can the family afford hospitalization and subsequent care?

Physical examination: What meets the eye—and more

Begin the physical examination by evaluating the patient's overall appearance and behavior. If the patient's an infant, measure his head first (see *Measuring head circumference*). Then examine the head for thin, shiny-looking skin; distended scalp veins; and bulging fontanels. Check for a "cracked pot" sound on percussion and a momentary give to the underlying bone, possibly resulting from a prolonged increase in ICP, which may occur with hydrocephalus.

Next, examine the eyes. Are they displaced

downward with the whites prominent? Is nystagmus present? Listen to the child's cry; is it shrill and high-pitched? Note dehydration from poor eating and vomiting, and note lethargy or irritability. Check for poor grasp reflexes, increased muscle tone, and poor motor development.

In older children and adults, check for decreased level of consciousness, an early sign of increased ICP. Look also for later signs, such as motor and pupillary changes, widening pulse pressure, and bradycardia. Examine the eyes for papilledema and nystagmus. Note the presence of Babinski's reflex and an unsteady, uncoordinated gait. Also watch for signs of dementia, such as personality changes, disorientation, and poor judgment.

Nursing diagnoses: The framework of your care plan

Once you complete assessment, you're ready to formulate nursing diagnoses with related goals and interventions. The following diagnoses will probably help shape your care plan:

Potential for increased ICP related to the disease process or to shunt malfunction. To maintain ICP within normal limits, monitor the patient's neurologic status frequently, as appropriate to the patient's status. Also measure and record head circumference daily in infants, and watch for bulging or tender fontanels. In older children and adults, watch for diminished level of consciousness, motor and pupillary changes, altered heart rate or blood pressure, and seizures. Recognize that rising ICP may require prompt decompression to avoid permanent brain damage or death.

After insertion of a shunt, position the patient on the side opposite the operative site, lying flat or with his head slightly elevated, unless the doctor's orders specify otherwise. Frequently check vital signs, level of consciousness, pupil reflex, motor function, and orientation to time, place, and person. Also watch for increased ICP, a possible sign of shunt malfunction. Monitor intake and output and restrict fluids, as ordered. Help the patient regain mobility gradually, but avoid severe neck flexion or head rotation at first.

Potential for infection related to surgical shunting procedure. Meningitis, peritonitis, and septicemia are all possible complications of this procedure. To prevent such infections, maintain the ventriculostomy as a closed system, using strict aseptic technique for dressing changes and fluid withdrawal. Check your hospital's infection-control policy for the recommended maximum length of use. After insertion of a ventriculoperitoneal or ventriculoatrial shunt, watch for signs of CNS infection—change in level of consciousness, nuchal rigidity, Kernig's and Brudzinski's signs (see Chapter 6), fever, headache, and photophobia. Send CSF samples to the laboratory for culture and sensitivity tests, as ordered. With a ventriculoperitoneal shunt, also watch for signs of peritonitis—abdominal tenderness and rigidity, diminished bowel sounds, general lethargy, and fever.

To help prevent infection, be sure to keep wound sites clean and dry. Administer prophylactic antibiotics, as ordered. Check wound sites for redness, swelling, tenderness, and drainage. Notify the doctor immediately if signs of infection develop. Replacement of the shunt may be necessary.

Potential for injury related to neurologic deficits. To avoid injury, take precautions to prevent aspiration, skin breakdown, neck injury, and falls. Assess the hydrocephalic patient's gag and swallow reflexes before feeding him. Offer food slowly in small amounts. After feeding, position the patient on his side to prevent aspiration. Also keep suction equipment nearby. To prevent skin breakdown, turn the patient every 2 hours and place sheepskin under his head. To reduce strain on the neck when turning the infant, move the head, neck, and shoulders with the body. To prevent falls in the ambulatory patient with motor weakness and gait disturbance, keep his room clutter-free, and help his family identify safety risks at home. Reorient the confused or demented patient, as necessary, and supervise his daily activities.

Impaired parent-infant bonding related to prolonged illness and hospitalization. To promote bonding, encourage the parents to spend as much time as possible with their infant. Arrange for liberal visiting hours, if possible. Allow the parents privacy with their infant, and encourage them to participate in his care after appropriate instruction. Also encourage them to stroke and cuddle their infant and to speak soothingly to him. Help them verbalize any feelings of guilt, sorrow, or fear to promote effective coping.

Knowledge deficit regarding hydrocephalus. Educating the patient and his family about hydrocephalus ranks among your most important nursing goals for this disorder. After all, better understanding promotes better compliance with therapy and care. Begin by explaining how hydrocephalus develops and the changes it produces in appearance and behavior. Be sure to consider the family's capacity to understand—based on education and familiarity with medicine. Allow them time to ask questions. Describe necessary diagnostic tests and explain test results as soon as they're available. Also provide routine pre- and postoperative teaching, including specific information about the shunt procedure and the tubes and incisions to expect after surgery. Help the family set realistic goals for rehabilitation, and stress the importance of follow-up care. Be sure to teach parents the signs of shunt failure and of infection, and tell them to notify the doctor immediately if such signs develop.

A successful care plan
Was your care plan a success? Consider it effective if:
• the patient's ICP remains below 15 mm Hg and his neurologic status improves
• the patient remains free of infection
• the patient suffers no injury—such as aspiration, skin breakdown, or falls—due to neurologic deficit
• the patient and his family can verbalize understanding of hydrocephalus and its treatment, when possible, and show no unreasonable fear of hospitalization or surgery
• the family shows the patient affection and acceptance, including normal parent-infant bonding.

Whether the hydrocephalic patient's an infant, child, or adult, your efforts to teach, assist, and encourage the patient and his family can do much toward helping them cope in a positive and realistic way.

Points to remember

• Although most common in newborns, hydrocephalus can also occur in children and adults as a result of injury or disease.
• Dilation of the ventricular system in hydrocephalus compresses the cortical white matter and may cause atrophy.
• Nursing assessment in adults should focus on the following triad of symptoms in normal-pressure hydrocephalus: dementia, incontinence, and gait disturbance.
• Surgery, the only effective treatment for hydrocephalus, involves creating an artificial shunt to drain cerebrospinal fluid from the ventricles to the subarachnoid space, peritoneal cavity, or cardiac chambers.
• Postoperative nursing care emphasizes close monitoring for infection and shunt malfunction.

14 REMOVING TOXINS AND ABNORMAL METABOLITES

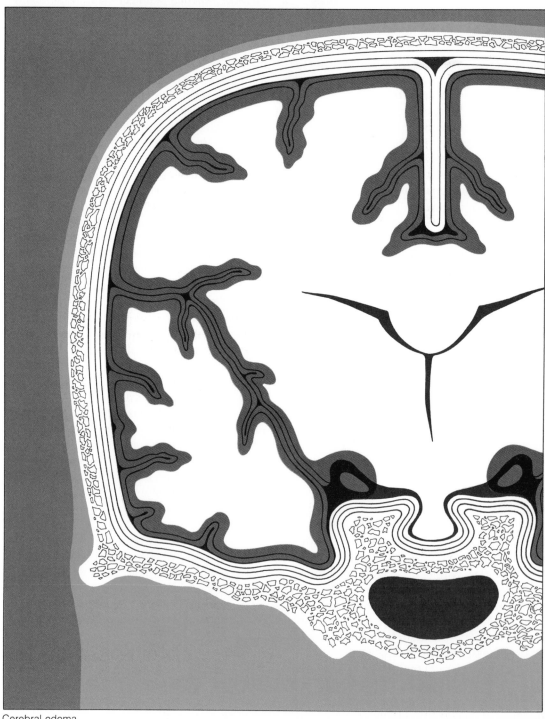

Cerebral edema

Metabolic and toxic disorders affect the nervous system in various, sometimes disastrous, ways. Each year in the United States about 45,000 people die of metabolic disorders, such as hepatic encephalopathy and Reye's syndrome. Each year more than 1 million people suffer the effects of toxins in the home or workplace. Of these, at least 5,000 die of those effects. Others, though they survive, experience permanent neurologic deficits.

Whether you meet such patients in an acute-care or a long-term facility, the challenges they offer may be monumental and many-faceted—ranging from helping them through the acute phase of their disorders to promoting necessary life-style changes; from educating patients and the community to the dangers of environmental toxins to supporting health and safety legislation. To meet these many challenges, you'll need to be thoroughly familiar with the insidious, widespread effects of metabolic and toxic disorders.

PATHOPHYSIOLOGY
Metabolic and environmental toxins interfere with neurologic function by altering cerebral metabolism, resulting in an altered level of consciousness. Pathogenic mechanisms for this alteration include hypoxia, hypoglycemia, metabolic dysfunction, and impaired neurotransmission. (See *Understanding metabolic and toxic disorders,* pages 174 and 175.)

Hypoxia: Three types
Cerebral hypoxia usually results from a larger oxygen supply problem—because ambient gas pressure falls or systemic abnormalities in ventilation, gas transport, or gas exchange interrupt oxygen delivery to the tissues.

Oxygen supply disturbances may be classified as hypoxic hypoxia, anemic hypoxia, or stagnant (ischemic) hypoxia. In hypoxic hypoxia, insufficient oxygen reaches the blood, so that arterial oxygen content and tension diminish. In anemic hypoxia, sufficient oxygen reaches the blood, but hemoglobin is unavailable to bind and transport it. In carbon monoxide poisoning, for example, hemoglobin binds with carbon monoxide much more readily than with oxygen, thereby reducing blood oxygen content. In stagnant hypoxia, circulatory failure renders cerebral blood flow inadequate to supply cerebral tissues.

Cerebral capillaries respond to oxygen deprivation by increasing permeability, which leads to cerebral edema. Aerobic cellular metabolism reverts to anaerobic, which continues for only 3 to 5 minutes before accumulating levels of lactic acid and toxic wastes block circulation, aggravating cerebral edema and causing neuronal death and necrosis.

Hypoxic effects range from transient incoordination and mental dullness to total loss of consciousness and all brain stem reflexes.

Hypoglycemia: Deficient nutrients
Reduced serum glucose levels result from various conditions that disrupt carbohydrate metabolism, such as dietary deficiencies, Reye's syndrome, and some heavy metal poisonings. Glucose metabolism requires certain substances to catalyze molecular changes; for example, thiamine acts as a coenzyme in the Krebs cycle. Dietary deficiency or toxic blockage of these substances ultimately deprives the brain of glucose. For example, heavy metal poisoning disrupts the sulfhydryl compounds essential to form enzymes for glucose metabolism.

Under normal conditions, the brain must rely almost solely on glucose for its energy needs. Because glucose is not stored in the brain in sufficient amounts, the brain must depend on glucose supplied by the blood. When serum glucose levels decline, resultant systemic gluconeogenesis may not compensate for the effects of catabolic waste buildup, cerebral edema, parenchymal damage, and cortical nerve degeneration and gliosis.

Signs of hypoglycemia may progress from confusion and convulsions (associated with reduced levels of gamma-aminobutyric acid, an inhibitory neurotransmitter normally synthesized from glucose by the brain) to stupor and coma. Common effects include cerebral edema (especially with lead poisoning), cerebral hemorrhage (lead and arsenic poisoning), peripheral neuropathy, and neuronal loss and gliosis (manganese and mercury poisoning).

Metabolic dysfunction
Uremic and hepatic encephalopathy and Reye's syndrome impair neurologic function by producing metabolic toxins. In uremic encephalopathy, nitrogenous wastes and other metabolic end products are believed to act as nerve irritants. Peripheral neuropathy may result, with axonal degeneration, segmental demyelination, and cell body chromatolysis of peripheral nerves leading to progressive sensorimotor impairment of lower and then upper *(continued on page 176)*

Understanding metabolic and toxic disorders

Metabolic disorders	Causes	Pathophysiologic mechanisms	Signs and symptoms
Hypoxic encephalopathy	Carbon monoxide poisoning, congestive heart failure, coronary artery disease, suffocation, respiratory failure	Hypoxia causes cessation of aerobic metabolism, which sustains Krebs cycle and electron transport. Neurons catabolize to compensate for loss of their intrinsic energy source but undergo irreversible damage. Accumulated catabolic products fill interstitial tissue, leading to parenchymal damage.	Confusion, stupor, or coma
Hepatic encephalopathy	Hepatitis, cirrhosis, portal-systemic shunt	Ammonia, formed in the bowel, fails to be converted to urea in the liver. It enters systemic circulation, reaches the brain, and interferes with cerebral metabolism.	*Prodromal stage:* disorientation, forgetfulness, slurred speech, slight tremor. *Impending stage:* tremor, asterixis, lethargy, apraxia. *Stuporous stage:* hyperventilation, agitation. *Comatose stage:* hyperactive reflexes, positive Babinski's sign, fetor hepaticus, coma
Uremic encephalopathy	Acute and chronic renal failure, dialysis, renal transplantation	Excretion of nitrogenous wastes and fluid and electrolyte balance are disrupted. Metabolic acidosis, hypocalcemia, hyperphosphatemia, hypernatremia, hyperkalemia, and increased blood urea nitrogen (BUN) and creatinine levels cause CNS and peripheral nerve irritation.	Apathy, fatigue, inattention, irritability, clouded sensorium, hallucinations, muscle twitching, seizures, Kussmaul's and Cheyne-Stokes respirations, coma
Reye's syndrome	Cause unknown but follows acute viral infection, such as influenza type B and varicella, in children and adolescents	Disruption of urea cycle causes hyperammonemia, hypoglycemia, and increased serum fatty acids with subsequent alteration in cerebral metabolism. Fatty infiltration of renal tubules and liver occurs. Encephalopathy results from massive cerebral edema and hepatic dysfunction.	*Stage I:* vomiting, lethargy, hepatic dysfunction. *Stage II:* disorientation, delirium, agitation, hyperventilation, hyperactive reflexes, hepatic dysfunction. *Stage III:* coma, decorticate posturing, hepatic dysfunction. *Stage IV:* deepening coma, decerebrate rigidity, loss of vestibuloocular reflexes, large fixed pupils, increasing hepatic dysfunction. *Stage V:* seizures, absent deep tendon reflexes, respiratory arrest, flaccidity
Toxic disorders			
Alcoholism	Exact cause unknown, but family background apparently contributes	Alcohol depresses subcortical structures that normally regulate cerebro-cortical activity, producing initial excitability of cerebral cortex. Spinal motor neurons initially escape inhibition from higher centers, causing hyperactive tendon reflexes. With increasing amounts of alcohol, depressant action spreads to cerebral cortex, brain stem, and spinal neurons.	*Intoxication:* confusion, stupor, inattentiveness, memory lapses, aggressive behavior. *After abstinence:* nervousness, irritability, diaphoresis, nausea, vomiting; all temporarily relieved by drinking alcohol. Abrupt withdrawal after prolonged or massive use causes delirium tremens (DTs)
Wernicke-Korsakoff syndrome	Thiamine deficiency usually stemming from chronic alcohol abuse	Thiamine deficiency impairs production of coenzymes necessary for CNS energy production. Necrosis and vascular changes occur in the hypothalamus, thalamus, and brain stem. Cerebellar atrophy also results.	Confusion, apathy, listlessness, memory loss, inattentiveness, ocular nerve paralysis, ataxia
Narcotic analgesic abuse	Exact cause unknown, but inability to cope with stress and frustration, desire for immediate gratification, insecurity, and low self-esteem contribute	Analgesics bind with opiate receptors at many CNS sites, altering release of acetylcholine, norepinephrine, substance P, and dopamine—thereby inhibiting neurotransmission. Physical and psychological dependence occur.	*Acute:* hypotension, bradycardia, pinpoint pupils, coma, respiratory depression. *Withdrawal:* diaphoresis, nausea, vomiting, diarrhea, insomnia, dilated pupils, runny nose and tearing eyes, anorexia, chills, fever, persistent back and abdominal pain, tachycardia, increased blood pressure and respiratory rate, spontaneous orgasm

Understanding metabolic and toxic disorders (continued)

Toxic disorders	Causes	Pathophysiologic mechanisms	Signs and symptoms
Barbiturate abuse	Exact cause unknown, but inability to cope with stress and frustration, desire for immediate gratification, insecurity, and low self-esteem contribute	Barbiturates cause CNS depression by decreasing excitability of nerve cells, possibly through increased postsynaptic inhibition of neurotransmission. Physical and psychological dependence can occur.	*Acute:* progressive CNS and respiratory depression. *Chronic:* slurred speech, poor coordination, decreased mental alertness, memory loss, depressed pulse rate and deep tendon reflexes, nystagmus, diplopia, hypotension, dehydration. *Withdrawal:* nervousness, seizures, irritability, orthostatic hypotension, tachycardia, hallucinations, insomnia
Amphetamine abuse	Exact cause unknown, but inability to cope with stress and frustration, desire for immediate gratification, insecurity, and low self-esteem contribute	Amphetamines facilitate CNS neurotransmission by increasing the release of the neurotransmitters dopamine, epinephrine, and 5-HT from storage sites in the nerve terminals. Neurologic and metabolic stimulation and appetite depression result. Psychological dependence can occur.	*Acute:* anxiety, hyperactivity, irritability, insomnia, muscle tension, aggressive or violent behavior, paranoia, psychosis, fever, palpitations, hypertension or hypotension, tachycardia, convulsions, abdominal pain. *Withdrawal:* depression, overwhelming fatigue
Lead poisoning	Ingestion of lead-based paint chips or inhalation of lead-containing dust or fumes. More common in children than adults	Accumulation of lead in the brain causes massive swelling and herniation of cerebellum and temporal lobes, hemorrhage and ischemia in cerebrum and cerebellum, and deposits of protein and mononuclear inflammatory cells around many small blood vessels.	Vomiting, behavior changes, and, at times, seizures, mental deterioration, irritability, and coma
Arsenic poisoning	Inhalation of arsenic-containing insecticides or paint, metal, or enamel fumes	Arsenic forms bonds with sulfhydryl radicals, which appear in peripheral nerve axons and capillary endothelial cells in cerebral tissue and are necessary for cellular metabolism. It causes polyneuropathy and hemorrhagic leukoencephalopathy.	Headache, drowsiness, confusion, delirium, seizures, and, in chronic poisoning, weakness, muscle aches, chills, fever, mucosal irritation
Mercury poisoning	Chronic inhalation or ingestion of mercury-containing compounds found in work environment or contaminated water or food	Mercury inactivates sulfhydryl enzymes and interferes with cellular metabolism. It causes neuronal loss and gliosis of the calcarine cortex and marked degeneration of the granular layer of the cerebellar cortex.	Weakness, fatigue, depression, lethargy, irritability, confusion, ataxia, dysarthria, and tremors of the extremities, tongue, and lips
Manganese poisoning	Chronic inhalation or ingestion of manganese particles during ore mining or processing	Chronic poisoning interferes with neurobiochemical pathways to cause neuronal loss and gliosis of the basal ganglia, resulting in extrapyramidal-like symptoms.	Progressive weakness, fatigue, confusion, hallucinations, drooling, hand tremors, limb stiffness, faint and dysarthric speech, gross rhythmic movement of trunk and head, retropulsive and propulsive gait
Tetanus	Contamination of wound or burn by soil, dust, or animal excreta containing *Clostridium tetani*	Tetanus exotoxin is thought to suppress spinal and brain stem neurons by blocking postsynaptic inhibition, thereby allowing afferent stimuli to produce an exaggerated response. Reciprocal innervation is also abolished, producing muscle spasm.	*Localized:* spasm, increased muscle tone near wound. *Systemic:* marked muscle hypertonicity, hyperactive deep tendon reflexes, tachycardia, diaphoresis, low-grade fever, painful and involuntary muscle contractions, trismus (lockjaw), risus sardonicus
Botulism	Ingestion of food contaminated by *Clostridium botulinum*	Botulism exotoxin affects the presynaptic endings of the neuromuscular junction, interfering with release of acetylcholine, thus disturbing muscle innervation.	Blurred vision, dysarthria, dysphagia, and other cranial nerve impairment followed by descending weakness or paralysis in extremities and trunk, dyspnea and respiratory arrest
Diphtheria	Inhalation or cutaneous contact with *Corynebacterium diphtheriae*	Formation and absorption of an exotoxin causes cranial nerve and peripheral paralysis by disrupting protein synthesis.	Fever, dyspnea, nasal voice, dysphagia, blurred vision, ascending paralysis, respiratory failure, cardiomyopathy

Effects of toxins on neurotransmission

Toxins interfere with neurotransmission by mimicking the actions of neurotransmitter chemicals or by competing with these chemicals for binding sites on the cell membrane.

Impaired acetylcholine release

Normally, the neuron releases the neurotransmitter acetylcholine into the synaptic cleft to complete transmission of a nerve impulse. However, the botulism toxin blocks the release of acetylcholine from the synaptic vesicles (color).

Impaired acetylcholine binding

To accomplish cell depolarization, receptor sites on the muscle membrane take up acetylcholine. However, the neuromuscular blocking agent curare and its medicinal forms, such as pancuronium, compete with acetylcholine for receptor sites (color), blocking depolarization.

Postsynaptic inhibition

In normal postsynaptic inhibition, the activation of inhibitory fibers diminishes the excitatory response of the neuron. However, the tetanus toxin blocks these inhibitory fibers (color), causing hyperexcitability of the neuron.

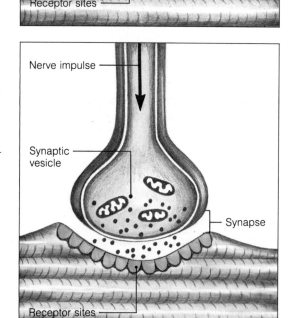

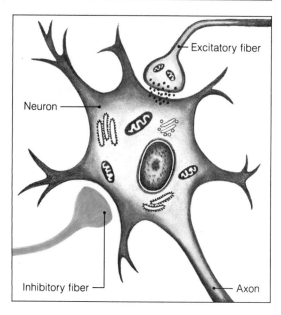

extremities. Central nervous system (CNS) involvement may also occur, with cerebral edema producing stupor and coma.

In hepatic encephalopathy and Reye's syndrome, the liver fails to convert ammonia to urea for excretion, and ammonia builds up to toxic levels. This buildup may overload cerebral metabolic pathways, depleting alpha-ketoglutarate, necessary for production of high-energy phosphate compounds, or it may directly inhibit cerebral neurotransmission.

Impaired neurotransmission

Many toxic substances can disrupt neurotransmission. (See *Effects of toxins on neurotransmission*.) *Alcohol* initially inhibits higher regulatory centers in the brain and then proceeds to block cerebrocortical, brain stem, and spinal cord pathways.

Narcotics alter release of various neurotransmitters, thereby blocking the pain pathway. Brain stem depression may lead to cardiorespiratory arrest; respiratory depression (CO_2 retention), to cerebrovascular dilation and increased intracranial pressure (ICP).

Barbiturates inhibit transmission of stimuli along CNS pathways by decreasing neuron excitability. They may affect all areas of the nervous system but most profoundly affect the reticular formation of the sensitive thalamus and midbrain. High doses lead quickly to loss of consciousness but do not usually cause cerebral edema and ischemia, because these drugs reduce oxygen consumption and increase supplies of glucose and high-energy phosphate compounds in brain tissue.

Amphetamines affect neurotransmission by promoting release of dopamine and other excitatory chemicals from their storage sites. Although these drugs usually do not cause pathologic lesions, excessive use may lead to toxic cardiovascular effects and psychotic behavior.

Bacterial toxins also affect neurotransmission. *Tetanus toxin* suppresses spinal and brain stem inhibitory neuron control, thereby interfering with the reflex arc. It also alters neurotransmission directly at skeletal muscles and, possibly, in the cerebral cortex and hypothalamus. Blockage of postsynaptic inhibition produces neuronal excitation that leads to sustained muscle spasm and severe sympathetic effects.

Diphtheria toxin inhibits protein synthesis in the neuron, which causes Schwann's cell damage and subsequent cranial nerve impairment and delayed peripheral neuropathy. *Bot-*

ulism toxin interferes with release of acetylcholine in presynaptic terminals at the myoneural junction, causing cranial nerve impairment and descending muscle paralysis.

MEDICAL MANAGEMENT
Diagnosis of metabolic and toxic disorders relies heavily on the patient history and physical examination. However, it frequently requires confirming laboratory tests (see *Testing for metabolic and toxic disorders*). After diagnosis, treatment aims to support vital functions and to remove the toxic agent or compensate for its effects.

Varied treatment
In *hypoxic encephalopathy,* treatment includes oxygen administration and, if necessary, cardiopulmonary resuscitation. Dexamethasone and an osmotic diuretic, such as mannitol, help reduce cerebral edema. Hypothermia may reduce hypoxic effects by lowering the cerebral metabolic rate. Mild hyperventilation promotes cerebral vasoconstriction and may help reduce ICP.

In *hepatic encephalopathy,* treatment requires elimination of ammonigenic material from the GI tract by decreased dietary intake of protein (because normal bacterial degradation of amino acids in the gut produces ammonia); catharsis (using sorbitol) to produce osmotic diarrhea and prevent accumulation of ammonigenic blood proteins and nitrogenous body wastes; neomycin and kanamycin to suppress bacterial flora, preventing them from converting amino acids into ammonia; and lactulose to increase colonic acidity, prevent bacterial growth, and promote excretion of ammonia. Occasionally, hemodialysis can temporarily clear some toxins from the blood. Similarly, exchange transfusions may provide dramatic but temporary relief.

In *Reye's syndrome,* treatment depends on the stage of the illness. In stage I, it includes monitoring vital signs and level of consciousness, giving vitamin K to help correct hypoprothrombinemia, and using diet, fluids, and drugs to keep glucose levels high, ammonia levels low, and plasma osmolality normal. In stage II, baseline treatment continues and administration of phenytoin prevents seizures. In stage III, baseline and seizure treatment continues. In addition, endotracheal intubation and mechanical ventilation control PCO_2 levels, and administration of mannitol counteracts rising ICP and rising serum osmolality. ICP monitoring helps detect intracranial

hypertension. In stage IV, all previous care measures continue and barbiturate coma, decompressive craniotomy, hypothermia, exchange transfusion, and hemodialysis may be attempted to prevent fatal complications.

In *uremic encephalopathy,* hemodialysis is the primary treatment.

Prevention after emergency care
Almost all toxic disorders may require emergency care to prevent fatal complications. (See *Treating toxic disorders,* pages 178 and 179.) After emergency care, subsequent care measures aim to prevent recurrence of the disorder. Tetanus and diphtheria, for example, require immunization to prevent subsequent infection. Occupational exposure to heavy metals may require use of masks and protective clothing on the job or even a change of profession to avoid further toxicity.

Obviously, the most prevalent sources of recurring toxicity are alcoholism and drug dependence. Treating them requires abstinence, significant life-style changes, and, at times, psychological counseling to determine and correct the underlying cause for dependence.

Alcoholism. In alcoholism, two forms of treatment promote abstinence: aversion therapy and supportive counseling. Aversion therapy uses a daily dose of disulfiram, which interferes with alcohol metabolism and causes toxic blood levels of acetaldehyde if the patient drinks alcohol within 12 hours of taking the drug. This distressing reaction includes headache, dyspnea, nausea, vomiting, diaphoresis, facial flushing, chest pain, tachycardia, and hypotension and may last up to 3 hours. Severe reactions can cause death.

Supportive counseling may improve the alcoholic patient's ability to deal with anxiety, stress, and frustration and may allow him to gain insight into the personal conflicts that led him to alcoholism. Self-help groups, such as Alcoholics Anonymous (AA), provide peer support. Halfway houses, job training programs, and sheltered workshops offer rehabilitation for the patient who's lost contact with his family and friends, has a long history of unemployment, or has had trouble with the law. Counseling of family members may also help eliminate destructive interactions.

If the alcoholic patient also suffers from Wernicke-Korsakoff syndrome, treatment includes administration of thiamine, to help reverse neurologic symptoms, and maintenance of nutrition and hydration.

Testing for metabolic and toxic disorders

Metabolic disorders
Blood tests
• Detect rising levels of liver enzymes and ammonia in hepatic encephalopathy and Reye's syndrome.
• Detect rising blood urea nitrogen and creatinine levels in uremic encephalopathy.
• Show depressed oxyhemoglobin levels and increased carboxyhemoglobin saturation in carbon monoxide poisoning.
Radiologic tests
• Skull X-rays and CT scan can demonstrate small or "absent" ventricles caused by cerebral edema in Reye's syndrome or other conditions such as hepatic or uremic encephalopathy. CT scan also demonstrates cerebral atrophy and helps rule out other conditions.
Electroencephalography
• Reveals a slow pattern in hypoxic, hepatic, and uremic encephalopathy and may indicate a seizure tendency.

Toxic disorders
Blood and urine screening
• Acidification and illumination of a urine sample detects coproporphyrin, a product of poor heme synthesis in lead poisoning.
• Urinalysis can detect all narcotics and can quantify arsenic, mercury, amphetamines, and most narcotics.
• Serum analysis can detect barbiturates, alcohol (ethanol), and manganese.
Special tests
• Skeletal X-rays reveal lead lines in long bones of children, helping confirm chronic lead poisoning.
• CT scan may detect degenerative or hemorrhagic cerebral lesions in heavy metal poisoning, alcoholism, and Wernicke-Korsakoff syndrome.
• EEG reveals a slow pattern in heavy metal poisoning and in barbiturate and narcotic abuse.
• In botulism, EMG shows diminished muscle action potential after one supramaximal nerve stimulus.

Treating toxic disorders

Many toxic disorders require prompt, aggressive treatment to support vital functions, to prevent potentially fatal complications, and, if appropriate, to remove the toxin or diminish its effect.

Alcohol withdrawal syndrome

Initial treatment of acute withdrawal aims to protect the patient from injury, to relieve his symptoms, and to correct associated disorders. If the patient's combative or disoriented, apply restraints and give tranquilizers. Administer I.V. glucose to correct hypoglycemia and I.V. fluids containing thiamine and other B complex vitamins to correct nutritional deficiencies and to help metabolize glucose. Monitor I.V. therapy carefully to prevent congestive heart failure. If symptoms develop, prepare to administer I.V. furosemide.

If withdrawal symptoms are severe, monitor the patient's mental status, heart rate, breath sounds, blood pressure, and rectal temperature every 4 to 6 hours. Orient the patient to his surroundings, since he may experience terrifying tactile or visual hallucinations.

Drug abuse

Treatment, of course, varies according to the drug abused. For *narcotic analgesics*, assist with gastric lavage or, if the patient is alert, induce vomiting to stop further drug absorption. Maintain respirations by endotracheal intubation and me-

chanical ventilation. As ordered, give oxygen to correct hypoxemia and naloxone to reverse the narcotic effect.

For *barbiturate abuse*, maintain respiration by endotracheal intubation. Give diuretics and I.V. fluids to promote diuresis and I.V. sodium bicarbonate to alkalize blood pH, thereby promoting drug excretion. If ordered, prepare for hemodialysis.

For *amphetamine abuse*, give an alpha-adrenergic blocking agent, as ordered, to inhibit life-threatening autonomic effects, such as hypertensive crisis and dysrhythmia. Also give ammonium chloride to acidify urine and to promote amphetamine excretion, and haloperidol, chlorpromazine, or other antipsychotic drugs to control amphetamine-induced psychosis. If necessary, administer I.V. fluids to curb dehydration, and insert an endotracheal tube to support respirations.

Heavy metal poisoning

Lead poisoning requires prompt treatment during acute symptomatic episodes to prevent chronic, irreversible effects, such as cognitive deficits in children. First, establish the adequacy of urine output. Then give I.M. dimercaprol (BAL) and calcium disodium edetate (EDTA), as ordered. Also give mannitol and prednisolone to relieve cerebral edema and diazepam to control seizures. Reduce fever with cooling blankets, and maintain urine output

with I.V. fluids. Be sure to restrict oral fluids for 3 days.

To treat *arsenic poisoning*, assist with gastric lavage or promote emesis. Give I.M. dimercaprol, as ordered. Also give I.V. fluids and, if necessary, vasopressors to maintain blood pressure. Provide pain medication for polyneuropathy and muscle ache.

To treat *mercury poisoning*, assist with gastric lavage or promote emesis. Give dimercaprol and penicillamine I.M., as ordered, and prepare to assist with hemodialysis to promote removal of the mercury-dimercaprol complex. Give I.V. fluids and watch for signs of GI perforation, such as hematemesis and bloody stool.

To treat *manganese poisoning*, provide supportive care. Place the patient in bed, and raise the side rails to prevent falls. If ordered, administer levodopa, which acts as an inhibitory neurotransmitter to reverse neurologic symptoms.

Bacterial toxins

To treat *tetanus*, thoroughly debride and cleanse the wound, and obtain an accurate history of allergies to immunizations or penicillin. If ordered, give tetanus immune human globulin or tetanus antitoxin, to confer temporary immunization, and high-dose antibiotics. If symptoms develop despite treatment, maintain an adequate airway and ventilation to prevent pneumonia and atelectasis. Suction

Drug dependence. In drug dependence, treatment includes psychological counseling and rehabilitative services. For heroin dependence, it also includes substituting the drug methadone. In barbiturate dependence, withdrawal requires stabilization doses of short- or long-acting barbiturates followed by progressively reduced doses until completion of withdrawal. In amphetamine dependence, progressively reduced doses of amphetamine and administration of antipsychotics or antidepressants counteract withdrawal symptoms.

NURSING MANAGEMENT

In metabolic and toxic disorders, nursing management aims to monitor the patient's progress, to detect potentially life-threatening changes in his condition, to evaluate the disorder's effect on the patient's life-style, and to promote the goals of rehabilitation.

Patient history: Address key areas

Note the primary reason for the patient's hospitalization, and ask the patient about current symptoms. Next, consider his age. Reye's syn-

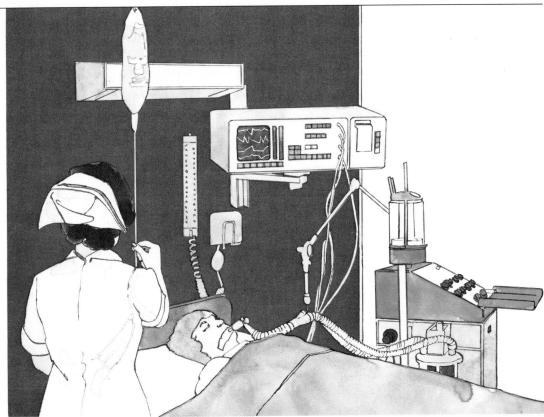

often and be alert for signs of respiratory distress.

If necessary, insert an artificial airway to prevent tongue injury and to maintain respirations during spasms. Keep tracheostomy equipment readily available. Give muscle relaxants and sedatives, as ordered. Keep the patient's room dark and quiet because even minimal stimulation can provoke muscle spasms. Monitor the EKG frequently for dysrhythmias. Accurately record intake and output. If urinary retention develops, insert an indwelling (Foley) catheter. Lastly, turn the patient frequently to prevent decubiti and pulmonary stasis.

To treat *botulism*, first obtain an accurate patient history of allergies (especially to horse serum), and perform a skin test to determine sensitivity to the botulism antitoxin. If ordered, give antitoxin to neutralize any circulating toxin. Keep epinephrine and resuscitation equipment readily available, and watch for signs of anaphylaxis. Monitor cardiac and respiratory function, and assess reflexes and movement of extremities. Administer I.V. fluids, turn the patient frequently, and promote deep-breathing exercises.

To treat *diphtheria*, enforce strict isolation to prevent transmission of the disease. Obtain a patient history of allergies, and perform a skin test. If ordered, administer diphtheria antitoxin. Keep epinephrine and resuscitation equipment readily available, and watch for signs of anaphylaxis. Give antibiotics to eliminate *Corynebacterium diphtheriae* from the upper respiratory tract and to terminate the carrier state. Monitor respirations carefully, and watch for signs of airway obstruction. Be alert for signs of myocarditis, such as heart murmurs and EKG changes. Also watch for signs of shock, which can develop suddenly. If neuritis develops, tell the patient it's usually transient.

drome, for example, rarely occurs in patients over age 20. Alcoholic encephalopathy, in contrast, tends to appear in older adults after many years of alcohol abuse.

Ask about the onset of the patient's symptoms. Acute onset may indicate tetanus, botulism, or Reye's syndrome; gradual onset may indicate lead poisoning.

Ask about predisposing or contributing factors, such as alcohol and drug use or unusual food cravings (pica in children). Investigate the influence of the patient's work or home environment. Does he work with toxic chemicals, live in an old building (lead poisoning), or have frequent exposures to fuel exhaust fumes (carbon monoxide poisoning)?

Examine the patient's medical history. A contaminated puncture wound may implicate tetanus. A history of eating questionably preserved food may implicate botulism. Hypertension, renal failure, congestive heart failure, liver disease, or recent viral illness may worsen or even cause toxic effects.

Assess the psychosocial effects. Metabolic

Recognizing alcohol withdrawal syndrome

The most acute complication of alcohol abuse, alcohol withdrawal syndrome (delirium tremens) follows abrupt withdrawal after prolonged or massive use. It usually begins 12 to 36 hours after cessation of drinking. Its earliest signs include coarse tremors, depression, disorientation, and shortened attention span. Later signs include anorexia, insomnia, diaphoresis, fever, tachycardia, tachypnea, and seizures. This syndrome also produces bizarre tactile and visual hallucinations. If untreated, it carries a 15% to 20% mortality.

disorders, for example, alter frontal lobe and limbic system function, resulting in emotional lability. Alcoholism and drug dependence adversely affect family life, friendships, and job or scholastic performance.

Examine all body systems

Begin your examination by assessing the patient's neurologic status, especially his level of consciousness. In tetanus, botulism, and heavy metal poisoning, the patient may appear alert or mildly drowsy. In the prodromal stages of Reye's syndrome and hepatic encephalopathy, he may appear disoriented and lethargic. In alcohol withdrawal syndrome, he may appear disoriented and speak incoherently. (See *Recognizing alcohol withdrawal syndrome*.)

Next, assess the cranial nerves, which can be damaged by diphtheria or botulism exotoxins or thiamine deficiency. Be alert for dysarthria, dysphagia, visual disturbances, and extraocular muscle palsies.

Assess the musculoskeletal system. Evaluate the patient's muscle strength—symmetrical weakness, especially during exertion, that's accompanied by tingling in the hands and feet commonly occurs in heavy metal poisoning, botulism, and nutritional deficiencies. Check for asterixis, a flapping tremor of the outstretched hand that's typical in hepatic encephalopathy and may occur in uremic or hypoxic encephalopathy. Also check for muscle twitching, which occurs especially in uremic encephalopathy. Check for characteristic signs of tetanus—risus sardonicus, a grin caused by facial muscle spasm; a rigid, boardlike abdomen; and rigidly extended legs.

Assess the respiratory system. Begin by checking respiratory rate and pattern. Hypoventilation may result from abuse of alcohol or CNS-depressing drugs. Kussmaul's respiration may compensate for metabolic acidosis caused by uremic encephalopathy. Respiratory depression may occur in tetanus, diphtheria, and botulism.

Check for unusual breath odor. An odor of ammonia or a musty, sweet breath odor (fetor hepaticus) occurs in hepatic encephalopathy. A fruity odor (acetone breath) results from metabolic acidosis in alcohol-related nutritional deficiencies.

Assess the cardiovascular system. Check blood pressure and pulse. Elevated systolic pressure and widening pulse pressure may indicate rising ICP. Hypotension may signal seriously deteriorating neurologic status. Signs of heart failure may result from chronic alco-

holism and hepatic encephalopathy; dysrhythmia, from accumulation of metabolic toxins.

Assess the skin. Check skin color. Cherry-red skin, for example, indicates carbon monoxide poisoning. Uremic frost—a fine, white coating covering the entire skin—characterizes uremic encephalopathy. Dark lines at the gingival margins indicate lead poisoning. Be sure to check for signs of drug abuse—needle tracks on the arms and legs, between the fingers and toes, and even under the tongue. Also check for infected wounds, which can indicate tetanus.

Formulate nursing diagnoses

In metabolic and toxic disorders, nursing diagnoses typically address the patient's physical, emotional, and cognitive problems revealed by your history and examination.

Potential for injury related to neurologic deficits. To prevent patient injury, position the patient comfortably, place the bed in a low position, raise the side rails, and, if appropriate, apply restraints. Observe the patient frequently, orient him to reality, and, if ordered, administer tranquilizers. Don't allow the patient to walk without help. In metabolic disorders, alcohol withdrawal syndrome, tetanus, or lead poisoning, tape an oral airway to the head of the bed for emergency use in seizures.

To prevent skin breakdown and other complications of prolonged bed rest, turn the patient every 2 hours; massage his back, arms, and legs to stimulate circulation; and cushion pressure points. Encourage active range-of-motion (ROM) exercises or perform passive ROM exercises to prevent muscle atrophy and contractures.

Consider your interventions successful if the patient remains free of injury and shows no signs of skin breakdown or other complications of immobility.

Fluid and electrolyte imbalance related to reduced oral intake and vomiting. To maintain balanced intake and output and normal serum electrolyte levels, to promote elimination of the toxin or help reduce its effect, and to prevent elevated ICP and cerebral edema, assess the patient for edema and signs of dehydration—poor skin turgor, fever, and low urine output. If ordered, give I.V. replacement and monitor urine output. If output falls below 20 ml/hour, notify the doctor and prepare to administer an osmotic diuretic or furosemide I.V. Monitor electrolyte balance concomitantly, because diuretics can easily alter levels, particularly of potassium. Be alert for signs of rising ICP—altered level of consciousness, widening pulse pressure, and bradycardia.

In heavy metal toxicity, give chelating agents, as ordered, to promote elimination of the toxin. If necessary, prepare for dialysis or for exchange transfusion.

In hepatic encephalopathy, give lactulose as ordered to acidify the colon and to promote elimination of ammonia in the stool. Because lactulose causes diarrhea, assist the patient in using the bedpan or bathroom, keep the perineum clean and dry, and monitor serum electrolyte and ammonia levels. For excessive vomiting, give an antiemetic and monitor serum electrolytes.

Your interventions have been effective if urine output is at least 20 ml/hour and the patient shows no signs of dehydration, increased ICP, or electrolyte imbalance.

Nutritional deficiency related to anorexia, nausea, vomiting, and decreased level of consciousness. To meet the patient's nutritional requirements and prevent weight loss, give nasogastric feedings or intravenous hyperalimentation (IVH), as ordered. With nasogastric feedings, be sure to use a soft, plastic, flexible tube to prevent irritation of the gastric mucosa. Elevate the patient's head to avoid aspiration of vomitus, and frequently check the patency, position, and residual volume of the feeding tube. With IVH, be alert for complications, such as hyperglycemia and fluid and electrolyte imbalance. Prevent infection by meticulous I.V. dressing changes, and monitor routine lab studies to allow appropriate changes in the composition of the infused solution. Weigh the patient daily, and report any loss to the doctor and dietitian. In the alcoholic patient, be sure to provide supplementary thiamine.

Your interventions were successful if the patient's nutritional requirements are met, his weight remains stable, and he incurs no complications from nasogastric or IVH feedings.

Ineffective coping related to chronic alcohol or drug abuse. To help the patient comply with treatment and develop effective coping mechanisms, provide a firm but supportive environment, and set limits on the patient's behavior. Work closely with the doctor, counselor, and other staff to help the patient understand and accept the prescribed treatment plan. Warn the patient receiving disulfiram about the effects of ingesting anything that contains alcohol in any form, including most mouthwashes, cough syrups, liquid vitamins, and cold remedies. Encourage him to join a

support group, such as AA, and, if appropriate, encourage family involvement in rehabilitation programs.

Help the drug-abusing patient to understand the reasons for his dependence, and encourage him to seek counseling.

Consider your interventions successful if the patient understands and accepts the prescribed treatment programs and seeks counseling or joins a support group.

Knowledge deficit about prevention or recurrence of toxic disorders. Teach the patient or his parents the signs and causes of the disorder and preventive measures. In lead poisoning of a child, tell parents that toxicity usually results from ingestion of lead-based paint chips from toys, furniture, or peeling walls. Initial toxic signs develop over 3 to 6 weeks and include decreased appetite, lethargy, and irritability. Later, vomiting, abdominal pain, and faulty coordination appear, followed by stupor, seizures, and coma.

Tell the patient with tetanus, or his parents, that prevention depends solely on immunization. Encourage compliance with the prescribed immunization schedule and reinforcement with a booster every 10 years.

Tell the patient with botulism that it results from faulty food preservation or processing. Advise him to avoid even tasting food from a bulging or malodorous can and to boil any utensil that touches such food.

Teach the patient who works in an industrial setting that headache, fainting, dizziness, drowsiness, or other neurologic symptoms that appear at work but subside at home indicate chronic exposure to toxins. Advise him to report his symptoms to his employer, and be sure that you inform public health officials.

Consider your interventions successful if the patient or his parents recognize the causes of toxic disorders and understand preventive measures.

The nursing challenge
Caring for patients with metabolic or toxic disorders becomes an often prolonged and sometimes frustrating commitment. The mainstay in managing toxic disorders is deceptively simple: avoidance of further exposure. Alcohol and drug abusers, however, have such deep-seated psychological and social problems that noncompliance with treatment is common. Still, for these patients and for others whose prognosis is somewhat brighter, your supportive nursing care can make the difference between relapse and recovery.

 Points to remember

- Metabolic and toxic disorders interfere with neurologic function by causing hypoxia, hypoglycemia, metabolic alterations, or impaired neurotransmission.
- The cause of Reye's syndrome is unknown, but acute viral infection commonly precedes it.
- Detection of metabolic and toxic disorders depends on a careful patient history and physical examination. Diagnostic tests, especially blood and urine studies, help confirm diagnosis.
- Almost all toxic disorders may require emergency care to prevent fatal complications.

APPENDIX

Neurologic drugs

Anticonvulsants

Drug, dose, and route	Interactions	Side effects	Special considerations
acetazolamide 375 mg to 1 g P.O. daily in divided doses	*Ephedrine, pseudoephedrine:* increased CNS stimulation. *Lithium:* decreased therapeutic effects. *Methenamine:* antagonized methenamine effect.	Aplastic anemia, hyperchloremic acidosis	Obtain CBC and serum electrolytes every 3 months. Also, drug is usually given with other anticonvulsants. Monitor for hyperglycemia in prediabetics or diabetics on insulin or oral drugs.
carbamazepine 800 mg to 1.2 g P.O. daily in divided doses	*Nicotinic acid:* may decrease carbamazepine levels. Monitor for lack of therapeutic effect. *Propoxyphene:* may increase carbamazepine levels. Use another analgesic. *Troleandomycin, erythromycin, isoniazid:* may increase carbamazepine blood levels. Use together cautiously.	Blood dyscrasias, dizziness, drowsiness, ataxia, nausea, stomatitis, dry mouth	May cause mild-to-moderate dizziness when first taken. Effect usually disappears within 4 days. Obtain CBC and platelet counts weekly for first 3 months, then monthly. Tell patient to notify doctor immediately if fever, sore throat, mouth ulcers, or easy bruising occurs. When used for trigeminal neuralgia, an attempt should be made every 3 months to decrease dose or to stop drug.
clonazepam 0.5 to 2 mg P.O. t.i.d.	None significant.	Drowsiness, ataxia, increased salivation	Warn patient to avoid activities that require alertness and good psychomotor coordination until CNS response to drug has been determined. Never withdraw drug suddenly. Tell patient to report side effects immediately. Also monitor patient for oversedation.
diazepam *For status epilepticus:* 5 to 20 mg by slow I.V. push; may repeat q 5 to 10 minutes to maximum dose of 60 mg	None significant.	Cardiovascular collapse, drowsiness, ataxia, pain at injection site, thrombophlebitis	Don't mix with other drugs or I.V. fluids. Avoid storing in plastic syringe or infusing through plastic tubing. Infuse at rate not exceeding 5 mg/minute and preferably at 2 mg/minute to decrease risk of respiratory depression and hypotension. Monitor respirations every 5 to 15 minutes and before each repeated dose. Have emergency resuscitative equipment and oxygen at bedside. Also watch for phlebitis at injection site.
ethosuximide 20 mg/kg P.O. in divided doses; maximum dose—1.5 g daily	None significant.	Nausea, vomiting, anorexia, epigastric distress, drowsiness, euphoria, dizziness, blood dyscrasias	Warn patient to avoid activities that require alertness and good psychomotor coordination until CNS response to drug has been determined. Obtain CBC every 3 months. Never withdraw drug suddenly.
ethotoin 2 to 3 g P.O. daily in divided doses	*Alcohol, folic acid, loxapine:* decreased ethotoin activity. *Oral anticoagulants, antihistamines, chloramphenicol, diazepam, diazoxide, disulfiram, isoniazid, phenylbutazone, salicylates, valproate:* increased ethotoin activity and toxicity.	Nausea, vomiting, diarrhea, lymphadenopathy	Give after meals. Schedule doses as evenly as possible over 24 hours. Stop drug at once if lymphadenopathy or lupus-like syndrome develops. Hydantoin derivative of choice in young adults who are prone to gingival hyperplasia caused by phenytoin. Otherwise, it's infrequently used for treating epilepsy.
mephenytoin 200 to 600 mg P.O. daily in three divided doses	*Alcohol, folic acid, loxapine:* decreased mephenytoin activity. *Oral anticoagulants, antihistamines, chloramphenicol, diazepam, diazoxide, disulfiram, isoniazid, phenylbutazone, salicylates, valproate:* increased mephenytoin activity and toxicity.	Drowsiness, blood dyscrasias, skin rash, exfoliative dermatitis	Tell patient to notify doctor if fever, sore throat, bleeding, or skin rash occurs. These signs may indicate serious blood dyscrasias. Check CBC and platelet count initially and every 2 weeks thereafter, up to 2 weeks after full dose attained; then monthly. Stop drug if neutrophil count falls below 1,600/mm³.
mephobarbital 400 to 600 mg P.O. daily in single or divided doses	*MAO inhibitors:* potentiates barbiturate effect. *Oral anticoagulants:* possible decreased anticoagulant effect. *Rifampin:* may decrease barbiturate levels. Monitor for decreased effect.	Dizziness, drowsiness, lethargy, skin eruptions	Warn patient to avoid activities that require alertness and good psychomotor coordination until CNS response to drug has been determined. Store drug in light-resistant container. In adults, give total or largest dose at night if seizures occur then. Warn patient to use drug cautiously with alcohol, narcotics, or other CNS depressant.
paraldehyde *For status epilepticus:* 5 to 10 ml I.M.; 0.2 to 0.4 ml/kg in 0.9% saline by I.V. injection	*Alcohol:* increased CNS depression. Use together cautiously. *Disulfiram:* increased paraldehyde blood levels; possible toxic disulfiram reaction. Use together cautiously.	Pulmonary edema or hemorrhage, circulatory collapse (from I.V. use), foul breath odor, skin rash	Divide 10 ml I.M. dose into two injections. Inject deeply, away from nerve trunks, and massage injection site. Use glass syringe and bottle for parenteral dose since drug reacts with plastic. Don't use if solution is brown or has a vinegary odor, or if container has been open longer than 24 hours.
paramethadione 0.9 to 2.4 g P.O. daily in three or four divided doses	None significant.	Blood dyscrasias, drowsiness, exfoliative dermatitis, skin rash, photophobia	Tell patient to immediately report sore throat, fever, malaise, bruises, petechiae, or epistaxis. Advise him to wear dark glasses if photophobia occurs.

Anticonvulsants (continued)

Drug, dose, and route	Interactions	Side effects	Special considerations
phenobarbital *For status epilepticus:* 10 mg/kg by I.V. infusion no faster than 50 mg/minute; maximum dose—20 mg/kg *For epilepsy:* usual maintenance dose—100 to 200 mg P.O. daily in single or divided doses	*Alcohol and other CNS depressants, including narcotic analgesics:* excessive CNS depression. *MAO inhibitors:* potentiated barbiturate effect. *Oral anticoagulants:* possible decreased anticoagulant effect. *Rifampin:* may decrease barbiturate levels. Monitor for decreased effect.	Lethargy, drowsiness, hangover, skin eruptions	Reserve I.V. injection for emergency treatment, and give slowly under close supervision. Monitor respirations carefully. Watch for signs of barbiturate toxicity: asthmatic breathing, cyanosis, clammy skin, hypotension, coma. Overdose can be fatal. Don't use injection solution if it contains a precipitate.
phensuximide 500 mg to 1 g P.O. b.i.d. or t.i.d.	None significant.	Nausea, vomiting, drowsiness, dizziness	Never withdraw drug suddenly to avoid petit mal seizures. Report side effects immediately. Drug may cause pink, red, or reddish-brown urine.
phenytoin *For status epilepticus:* 500 mg to 1 g I.V. at 50 mg/minute. *For epilepsy:* maintenance dose—300 to 600 mg P.O. daily or in divided doses	*Alcohol, folic acid, loxapine:* decreased phenytoin activity. *Oral anticoagulants, antihistamines, chloramphenicol, cimetidine, diazepam, diazoxide, disulfiram, isoniazid, phenylbutazone, salicylates, thioridazine, valproate:* phenytoin toxicity risk.	Nausea, vomiting, gingival hyperplasia, blood dyscrasias, rash, exfoliative dermatitis, hirsutism, nystagmus, diplopia, blurred vision, drowsiness, dizziness, confusion, hallucinations, slurred speech	Give divided doses with or after meals to decrease GI side effects. Stop drug if skin rash appears. If rash is scarlet or measles-like, resume drug after rash clears. If rash reappears, stop drug. If rash is exfoliative, purpuric, or bullous, don't resume drug. Provide patient with instructions (see below). Use only clear solution for injection. Consider slight yellowing acceptable. Don't refrigerate drug.
primidone 250 mg P.O. t.i.d. or q.i.d.	*Carbamazepine:* increased primidone levels. Observe for toxicity. *Phenytoin:* stimulates conversion of primidone to phenobarbital. Observe for increased phenobarbital effect.	Drowsiness, diplopia, lethargy, nausea, vomiting	Warn patient to avoid activities that require alertness and good psychomotor coordination until CNS response to drug has been determined. Drug is partially converted to phenobarbital by body metabolism. Shake liquid suspension well.
valproic acid **valproate sodium** 15 to 30 mg/kg daily, usually in divided doses	*Antacids, aspirin:* may cause valproic acid toxicity. Use together cautiously and monitor blood levels.	Nausea, vomiting, indigestion, thrombocytopenia, hepatotoxicity	Obtain liver function studies, platelet counts, and prothrombin time before starting drug and every month thereafter. Nonspecific symptoms, such as fever and lethargy, may signal severe hepatotoxicity.

PATIENT-TEACHING AID

Controlling seizures with phenytoin

Dear Patient,

Your doctor has prescribed phenytoin (Dilantin) to help you control seizures. Remember:
• Carry identification saying that you use this drug. Report its use before any surgery or emergency treatment.
• Take phenytoin exactly as your doctor orders, preferably at the same time(s) each day.
• Tell your doctor immediately if you're pregnant, nursing, or planning a pregnancy; if you have or develop any other medical conditions; or if you're taking any other prescription or nonprescription drugs.
• Don't start or stop taking any other drugs without first asking your doctor. Any change may alter phenytoin's effectiveness.
• If you're taking *liquid phenytoin,* shake the bottle well and use a medical measuring spoon to ensure correct dosage. If

you're taking *phenytoin tablets,* chew or crush them. If you're taking *capsules,* swallow them whole.
• If phenytoin upsets your stomach, ask your doctor about taking it with food or milk. Also ask about use of alcohol, which may alter the drug's effectiveness.
• Miss a dose? *If you normally take one dose a day,* take the missed dose immediately, then resume your normal schedule. However, if you don't remember the missed dose until the next day, don't take it and don't double your daily dose; just resume your normal schedule. *If you normally take several doses a day,* take the missed dose immediately (unless your next scheduled dose is within 4 hours), then resume your normal schedule. Don't double-dose. *If you miss doses for 2 or more days,* call your doctor.
• See your doctor regularly,

especially at first, since your dosage may need adjusting.
• Don't stop taking this drug without first asking your doctor. Abrupt withdrawal may cause adverse reactions.
• Call your doctor immediately if you develop involuntary eye movements, blurred or double vision, skin rash, drowsiness, dizziness, confusion, hallucinations, slurred speech, or other adverse reactions.
• Don't be alarmed if phenytoin causes gray stool and pink to reddish-brown urine.
• Because phenytoin may cause gum tenderness, swelling, or bleeding, brush and floss carefully and see your dentist regularly.
• When refilling your prescription, don't change brands or dosage forms or allow generic substitutions without first asking your doctor. Phenytoin comes in several forms, and each acts differently in the body.

Anti-infectives

Drug, dose, and route	Interactions	Side effects	Special considerations
cefotaxime 1 g I.V. or I.M. q 6 to 8 hours; maximum dose—12 g daily in life-threatening infections	*Probenecid:* may inhibit excretion and increase blood levels of cefotaxime.	Diarrhea, pseudomembranous colitis, rash, urticaria, pain at injection site, thrombophlebitis (with I.V. administration)	Give drug I.V. rather than I.M. in life-threatening infection. When administering I.M., inject deep into a large muscle mass, such as the gluteus or lateral aspect of thigh.
chloramphenicol 50 to 100 mg/kg P.O. or I.V. daily in divided doses q 6 hours; maximum dose—100 mg/kg daily	*Acetaminophen:* elevated chloramphenicol levels. *Oral anticoagulants:* possible bleeding. *Penicillins:* antagonized antibacterial effect. Give penicillin at least 1 hour before. *Sulfonylureas:* increased hypoglycemia.	Aplastic anemia, granulocytopenia, dose-related anemia	Monitor CBC, platelet and reticulocyte counts, and serum iron levels before and every 2 days during therapy. Stop drug immediately if anemia, reticulocytopenia, leukopenia, or thrombocytopenia develops.
moxalactam 2 to 6 g I.V. or I.M. daily in divided doses q 8 hours; maximum dose—12 g daily in life-threatening infections	*Ethyl alcohol:* may cause disulfiram-like reaction. Warn patient not to drink alcohol for several days after discontinuing moxalactam.	Hypoprothrombinemia with possible severe bleeding, diarrhea, pseudomembranous colitis, rash, urticaria, pain at injection site, thrombophlebitis	When administering I.M., inject deep into a large muscle mass, such as the gluteus or lateral aspect of thigh. If severe bleeding occurs after high doses, promptly give vitamin K.
nafcillin 2 to 12 g I.V. or I.M. daily in divided doses q 4 to 6 hours	*Aminoglycoside antibiotics:* separate I.V. nafcillin dose by at least 1 hour. Don't mix together in same I.V. container. *Chloramphenicol, erythromycin, tetracyclines:* antibiotic antagonism. Give nafcillin at least 1 hour before. *Probenecid:* increased blood levels of nafcillin. (Probenecid is often used for this purpose.)	Hypersensitivity, skin rash, thrombophlebitis	Before giving nafcillin, ask patient if he's had any allergic reactions to penicillin. Check drug's expiration date. Give intermittently I.V. to prevent vein irritation. Also change site every 48 hours.
penicillin G 1.2 to 24 million units I.M. or I.V. daily in divided doses q 4 hours	*Aminoglycoside antibiotics:* separate I.V. penicillin dose by at least 1 hour. Don't mix together in same I.V. container. *Chloramphenicol, erythromycin, tetracyclines:* antibiotic antagonism. Give penicillin at least 1 hour before bacteriostatic antibiotics. *Probenecid:* increased blood levels of penicillin. (Probenecid is often used for this purpose.)	Hypersensitivity, skin rash, thrombophlebitis	Before giving penicillin, ask the patient if he's had any allergic reactions to this drug. Check drug's expiration date. Give intermittently I.V. to prevent vein irritation. Also change site every 48 hours. Superinfection may occur with prolonged therapy, especially in elderly and debilitated patients.
vidarabine 15 mg/kg daily for 10 days; give by slow I.V. infusion over 12 to 24 hours	*Allopurinol:* increased incidence of CNS side effects.	Anorexia, nausea, tremor, dizziness, confusion	Don't give I.M. or S.C. because of low solubility and poor absorption. Administer with an in-line I.V. filter 0.45 μm or smaller. CNS side effects must be distinguished from symptoms of encephalitis.

Antimyasthenics

Drug, dose, and route	Interactions	Side effects	Special considerations
neostigmine 15 to 30 mg P.O. t.i.d.; 0.5 to 2 mg I.M. or I.V. q 1 to 3 hours, as needed	*Procainamide, aminoglycoside antibiotics, quinidine:* may reverse cholinergic effect on muscle. Observe for lack of therapeutic effect. *Succinylcholine:* prolonged respiratory depression and possible apnea.	Nausea, vomiting, diarrhea, muscle cramps, respiratory depression	Monitor vital signs frequently, especially respirations. Keep atropine injection available to treat serious side effects. Give drug with milk or food to reduce GI side effects. Document patient's response after each dose. Show patient how to observe and record variations in muscle strength.
pyridostigmine 60 to 180 mg P.O. b.i.d. or q.i.d. with maximum dose of 1,500 mg; 2 mg I.M. or very slow I.V. injection q 3 hours	*Procainamide, aminoglycoside antibiotics, quinidine:* may reverse cholinergic effect on muscle. Observe for lack of therapeutic effect. *Succinylcholine:* prolonged respiratory depression and possible apnea.	Nausea, vomiting, diarrhea, headache	Parenteral dose is ⅓₀ of oral dose. Double-check all orders for I.M. or I.V. administration. Adjust dose depending on patient response.

Antineoplastics

Drug, dose, and route	Interactions	Side effects	Special considerations
carmustine (BCNU) 100 mg/m² by slow I.V. infusion daily for 2 days; repeat dose q 6 weeks if platelets above 100,000/mm³ and WBC above 4,000/mm³	*Cimetidine:* increased bone marrow suppression. Avoid use if possible.	Bone marrow suppression, including leukopenia and thrombocytopenia; nausea; vomiting; pain at infusion site; pulmonary fibrosis	Warn patient to watch for signs of infection and bone marrow suppression, such as fever, sore throat, anemia, fatigue, easy bruising, nose or gum bleeds, and tarry stools. Take temperature daily. To reduce pain on infusion, dilute drug further or slow the infusion rate. Avoid contact with skin, as carmustine causes a brown stain. If drug comes into contact with skin, wash off thoroughly. Solution is unstable in plastic I.V. bags. Administer only in glass containers.

Antineoplastics (continued)

Drug, dose, and route	Interactions	Side effects	Special considerations
lomustine (CCNU) 130 mg/m² P.O. in a single dose q 6 weeks; give only if platelets above 100,000/mm³ and WBC above 4,000/mm³	None significant.	Bone marrow suppression, including leukopenia and thrombocytopenia; nausea; vomiting	Give drug 2 to 4 hours after meals. To avoid nausea, give antiemetic before administering. Monitor blood counts weekly. Don't give more often than every 7 weeks; bone marrow suppression is cumulative and delayed.

Antiparkinson drugs

Drug, dose, and route	Interactions	Side effects	Special considerations
levodopa 0.5 to 1 g P.O. daily b.i.d., t.i.d., or q.i.d. Increase dose by 0.75 g every 3 to 7 days; maximum dose—8 g daily	*Antacids:* may increase levodopa effect. *Anticholinergic drugs, tricyclic antidepressants, benzodiazepines, clonidine, papaverine, phenothiazines and other antipsychotics, phenytoin:* decreased levodopa effect. *Pyridoxine:* decreased levodopa effect. Check vitamin preparations and nutritional supplements for content of vitamin B₆ (pyridoxine).	Choreiform, dystonic and dyskinetic movements; involuntary grimacing; myoclonic body jerks; psychiatric disturbances; nausea; vomiting; anorexia; orthostatic hypotension	Adjust dose according to patient's response. Monitor vital signs, especially while adjusting dose. Warn patient and family not to increase drug dose without the doctor's orders. Warn patient of possible dizziness and orthostatic hypotension, especially at start of therapy. Inform patient and family that multivitamin preparations, fortified cereals, and certain over-the-counter drugs may contain pyridoxine (vitamin B₆), which can reverse the effects of levodopa.
levodopa-carbidopa 3 to 6 tablets of 25 mg carbidopa/250 mg levodopa P.O. daily in divided doses; maximum dose—8 tablets daily	*Papaverine, diazepam, clonidine, phenothiazines and other antipsychotics:* may antagonize parkinsonian actions. Use together cautiously.	Choreiform, dystonic, and dyskinetic movements; involuntary grimacing; myoclonic body jerks; orthostatic hypotension	Adjust dose according to patient's response. Drug effects occur more rapidly with levodopa-carbidopa than with levodopa alone. Monitor vital signs, especially while adjusting dose. If patient is receiving levodopa, discontinue this drug for at least 8 hours before starting levodopa-carbidopa.

Antithrombotics

Drug, dose, and route	Interactions	Side effects	Special considerations
aspirin 1,300 mg P.O. daily	*Ammonium chloride (and other urine acidifiers):* increased aspirin levels. Monitor for aspirin toxicity. *Antacids in high doses (and other urine alkalinizers), corticosteroids:* decreased aspirin effect. *Oral anticoagulants and heparin:* increased risk of bleeding.	Prolonged bleeding time, nausea, vomiting, GI distress, and occult bleeding	Advise patients receiving large doses of aspirin for an extended period to watch for petechiae, bleeding gums, and GI bleeding, and to maintain adequate fluid intake. Give with food, milk, antacid, or water to reduce GI side effects. Obtain hemoglobin levels and prothrombin time periodically.
dipyridamole *For transient ischemic attacks:* 400 to 800 mg P.O. daily in divided doses	None significant.	Headache, dizziness, hypotension, nausea	Give 1 hour before meals. Monitor blood pressure and observe for side effects, especially with large doses. Also watch for signs of bleeding and for prolonged bleeding time.
heparin 7,500 to 10,000 units by I.V. bolus, then 1,000 units hourly by I.V. infusion	*Aspirin:* may increase bleeding risk. Don't use together.	Hemorrhage and excessive bleeding, thrombocytopenia	Measure partial thromboplastin time (PTT) carefully and regularly. Anticoagulation exists when PTT values are 1.5 to 2 times control values. When intermittent I.V. therapy is used, always draw blood 30 minutes before next scheduled dose to avoid spuriously elevated PTT. Avoid excessive I.M. injections of other drugs to prevent or minimize hematomas.
sulfinpyrazone *For transient ischemic attacks:* 600 to 800 mg P.O. daily in divided doses	*Oral anticoagulants:* possible bleeding. *Probenecid:* inhibited renal excretion of sulfinpyrazone. Use together cautiously.	Nausea, dyspepsia, epigastric pain	Give with milk, food, or antacid to reduce GI side effects.
warfarin maintenance dose—2 to 10 mg daily P.O.	*Allopurinol, chloramphenicol, danazol, cloifibrate, diflunisal, dextrothyroxine, thyroid drugs, heparin, anabolic steroids, cimetidine, disulfiram, glucagon, inhalation anesthetics, metronidazole, quinidine, influenza vaccine, sulindac, sulfonamides:* increased prothrombin time. Monitor for bleeding. *Ethacrynic acid, indomethacin, mefenamic acid, oxyphenbutazone, phenylbutazone, salicylates:* increased prothrombin time; ulcerogenic effects. *Griseofulvin, haloperidol, carbamazepine, paraldehyde, rifampin:* reduced anticoagulant effect. *Glutethimide, chloral hydrate, sulfinpyrazone, triclofos sodium:* increased or decreased prothrombin time.	Hemorrhage and excessive bleeding, dermatitis, skin rash, fever	Regularly measure prothrombin time (PT) to monitor anticoagulant effect. PT should be 1.5 to 2 times normal. When PT exceeds 2.5 times control value, bleeding risk is high. Give drug at the same time daily. Stress importance of complying with recommended dose and keeping follow-up appointments. Advise patient to carry a card that identifies him as a potential bleeder. Also suggest that he use an electric razor when shaving to avoid scratching skin and to brush his teeth with a soft toothbrush. Tell female patient to report unusually heavy menses. The dose may need to be adjusted. Fever and skin rash signal severe complications. Elderly patients and those with renal or hepatic failure are especially sensitive to warfarin effect.

Heavy metal antagonists

Drug, dose, and route	Interactions	Side effects	Special considerations
dimercaprol 2 to 5 mg/kg by deep I.M. injection daily to q.i.d.	^{131}I *uptake thyroid tests:* decreased iodine uptake. Don't schedule patient for this test during course of dimercaprol therapy. *Iron:* formed toxic metal complex. Don't use together.	Transient hypertension, tachycardia, nausea, vomiting, renal damage	Give only by deep I.M. route, and massage injection site after giving drug. Drug has an unpleasant, garlicky odor. Keep urine alkaline to prevent renal damage. Oral $NaHCO_3$ may be ordered.
edetate calcium disodium 1 g in 500 ml of 5% dextrose or 0.9% sodium chloride by I.V. infusion; 1 g I.M.	None significant.	Nephrotoxicity with acute tubular necrosis, fever, and chills 4 to 8 hours after infusion	Encourage fluids to promote excretion of edetate-metal complex (except in lead poisoning, since excess fluid may raise ICP). Monitor intake and output, urinalysis, BUN, and EKGs. To avoid toxicity, use drug with dimercaprol. Procaine HCl may be added to I.M. solutions to minimize pain. Avoid rapid I.V. infusions, and watch for local reactions afterward.

Miscellaneous

Drug, dose, and route	Interactions	Side effects	Special considerations
dexamethasone *For cerebral edema:* 10 mg I.V., then 4 to 6 mg I.M. q 6 hours for 2 to 4 days; then decrease dose over 5 to 7 days	*Indomethacin, aspirin:* increased risk of GI distress and bleeding. Use together cautiously.	Atrophy at I.M. injection sites, euphoria, insomnia, peptic ulcer	Give I.M. injection deep into gluteal muscle. Avoid S.C. injections, which may result in atrophy and sterile abscesses. When possible, replace I.M. with P.O. route.
disulfiram *For chronic alcoholism:* 125 to 500 mg P.O. daily	*Alcohol:* disulfiram reaction (blurred vision, confusion, dyspnea, tachycardia, hypotension, flushing, nausea, vomiting, sweating, thirst, vertigo). *Isoniazid (INH):* ataxia or marked change in behavior. Avoid use. *Metronidazole:* psychotic reaction. Don't use together. *Paraldehyde:* toxic levels of the acetaldehyde. Don't use together.	Drowsiness, headache, garlic-like taste, peripheral neuritis	Warn patient to avoid all alcohol, including that found in foods, medications like cough syrup and liniments, and toiletries like shaving lotion. Tell him that disulfiram reaction may occur as long as 2 weeks after single dose of disulfiram. The longer patient remains on drug, the more sensitive he becomes to alcohol. Blood alcohol level of 5 to 10 mg/dl may trigger a mild reaction; a level of 50 mg/dl a severe reaction; unconsciousness usually occurs at level of 125 to 150 ml/dl. Reaction may last ½ hour to several hours, or as long as alcohol remains in blood. Reassure patient that most side effects subside after 2 weeks of therapy.
ergotamine *For migraine headache:* 2 mg P.O. or S.L., then 1 to 2 mg P.O. hourly or S.L. q ½ hour. Maximum dose—6 mg daily	*Beta-adrenergic blockers:* possible increased vasoconstriction.	Numbness and tingling in fingers and toes, muscle pains	Most effective when used during prodromal stage of headache or as soon as possible after onset. Sublingual tablet is preferred during early stage of attack because of its rapid absorption. Prolonged exposure to cold weather should be avoided whenever possible. Cold may increase many of the side effects. Avoid prolonged administration and don't exceed recommended dosage.
lactulose *For hepatic coma:* 20 to 30 g (30 to 45 ml) P.O. t.i.d. or q.i.d. until patient has two or three soft stools daily	None significant.	Cramps, belching, flatulence, diarrhea, hypernatremia	If desired, minimize drug's sweet taste by diluting with water or fruit juice or giving with food. Reduce dosage if diarrhea occurs. Replace fluid loss. Monitor serum sodium for possible hypernatremia, especially with high doses.
methysergide *For migraine headache prophylaxis:* 2 to 4 mg P.O. b.i.d. with meals	None significant.	Retroperitoneal and pulmonary fibrosis, vertigo, euphoria	Stop drug every 6 months; then restart after at least 3 or 4 weeks. Tell patient not to stop drug abruptly; may cause rebound headaches. Stop gradually over 2 to 3 weeks. Not for treatment of migraine or vascular headache in progress or for treatment of tension (muscle contraction) headaches.
neomycin *For hepatic coma:* 1 to 3 g P.O. q.i.d. for 5 to 6 days	*Dimenhydrinate:* may mask symptoms of ototoxicity. *Ethacrynic acid, furosemide:* increased ototoxicity. *Other aminoglycosides, methoxyflurane:* increase ototoxicity and nephrotoxicity.	Ototoxicity, nephrotoxicity	Drug isn't absorbed at recommended dosage. However, more than 4 g of neomycin daily may be systemically absorbed and may lead to nephrotoxicity. Monitor renal function (urine output, specific gravity, BUN and creatinine levels, and creatinine clearance). Notify doctor of signs of decreasing renal function.
propranolol *For migraine headache prophylaxis:* 160 to 240 mg P.O. daily in divided doses or once daily as sustained-release capsule	*Barbiturates, rifampin:* decreased effect of propranolol. *Chlorpromazine, cimetidine:* increased effect of propranolol. *Insulin, oral hypoglycemics:* monitor patient for altered dosage requirements.	Fatigue, lethargy, bradycardia, heart failure, heart block, hypotension	Monitor blood pressure for hypotension due to propranolol's beta-blocking action. To improve poor compliance with therapy, change dosage schedule to once or twice daily. Recognize that drug masks common signs of shock and hypoglycemia. Drug is for prophylaxis only; it won't effectively treat migraine already in progress.

Selected References and Acknowledgments

Selected References

Adams, R.D., and Victor, M. *Principles of Neurology*, 2nd ed. New York: McGraw-Hill Book Co., 1981.

◆

Ambielli, M. "Migraine Headache: Current Therapy," *Journal of Neurosurgical Nursing* 14:203-6, August 1982.

◆

Barrett-Griesemer, Patricia. "A Guide to Headaches—and How to Relieve Their Pain," *Nursing81* 11:50-7, April 1981.

◆

Bowers, S.A., and Marshall, L.F. "Severe Head Injury: Current Treatment and Research," *Journal of Neurosurgical Nursing* 14(5):210-9, October 1982.

◆

Bresler, David E., and Trubo, Richard. *Free Yourself from Pain*. New York: Simon & Schuster, 1979.

◆

Collins, R. Douglas. *Illustrated Manual of Neurologic Diagnosis*, 2nd ed. Philadelphia: J.B. Lippincott Co., 1982.

◆

Conway-Rutkowski, Barbara Lang. *Carini and Owens' Neurological and Neurosurgical Nursing*, 8th ed. St. Louis: C.V. Mosby Co., 1982.

◆

Ducker, Thomas. "The Surgical Treatment of Stroke," in *Neurological Emergencies: Recognition and Management*. Edited by Michael Salcman. New York: Raven Press Pubs., 1980.

◆

Edelson, Edward. "Scanning the Body Magnetic," *Science*, July/August 1983.

◆

Fleischer, Alan, and Barrow, Daniel. "Axioms on Head Injury," *Hospital Medicine*, March 1982.

◆

Gilroy, John, and Meyer, John S. *Medical Neurology*, 3rd ed. New York: Macmillan Pub. Co., 1979.

◆

Griswold, Kim, et al. "An Approach to the Care of the Patient with Guillain-Barre Syndrome," *Heart & Lung* 13:66-72, January 1984.

◆

Hausman, K.A. "Nursing Care of the Patient with Hydrocephalus," *Journal of Neurosurgical Nursing* 13:326-32, December 1981.

◆

Hickey, Joanne V.X. *The Clinical Practice of Neurological and Neurosurgical Nursing*. Philadelphia: J.B. Lippincott Co., 1981.

Holland, Nancy J., et al. "Overview of Multiple Sclerosis and Nursing Care of the MS Patient," *Journal of Neurosurgical Nursing* 13:28-33, February 1981.

◆

Litel, Gerald R. *Neurosurgery and the Clinical Team: A Guide for Nurses, Technicians, and Students*. New York: Springer Publishing Co., 1980.

◆

McQuat, F. "The Insidious Spinal Cord Tumor," *Journal of Neurosurgical Nursing* 13:18-22, February 1981.

◆

Martin, Nancy, et al. *Comprehensive Rehabilitation Nursing*. New York: McGraw-Hill Book Co., 1980.

◆

Meinhart, Noreen T., and McCaffery, Margo. *Pain, A Nursing Approach to Assessment and Analysis*. Norwalk, Conn.: Appleton-Century-Crofts, 1983.

◆

Melzack, Ronald, and Wall, Patrick D. *The Challenge of Pain*. New York: Basic Books, 1983.

◆

Moore, D.E., and Blacker, H.M. "How Effective Is TENS for Chronic Pain?" *American Journal of Nursing* 83(8):1175-7, August 1983.

◆

Nikas, Diana L. *The Critically Ill Neurosurgical Patient*. (Contemporary Issues in Critical Care Nursing Series.) New York: Churchill Livingstone, 1982.

◆

Norman, Susan E., et al. "Seizure Disorders," *American Journal of Nursing* 81:983-1000, May 1981.

◆

Pansky, Ben, and Allen, Delmas J. *Review of Neuroscience*. New York: Macmillan Publishing Co., 1980.

◆

Plum, Fred, and Posner, Jerome. *The Diagnosis of Stupor and Coma*, 3rd ed. Philadelphia: F.A. Davis Co., 1980.

◆

Professional Information Committee of the National Medical Advisory Board. *Myasthenia Gravis: A Manual for Nurses*. New York: Myasthenia Gravis Foundation, 1981.

◆

Pryse-Phillips, William, and Murray, T.J. *Concise Textbook—Essential Neurology*, 2nd ed. New Hyde Park, N.Y.: Medical Examination Publishing Co., 1982.

Rimel, R.W. "A Prospective Study of Patients with Central Nervous System Trauma," *Journal of Neurosurgical Nursing* 13:132-41, June 1981.

◆

Robinson, Robert, and Price, Thomas. "Post-Stroke Depressive Disorders: A Follow-up Study of 103 Patients," *Stroke* 13(1982):635-41.

◆

Snyder, Mariah, and Jackle, Mary. *Neurologic Problems: A Critical Care Nursing Focus*. Bowie, Md.: Robert J. Brady Co., 1981.

◆

Speers, I. "Cerebral Edema," *Journal of Neurosurgical Nursing* 13:102-15, April 1981.

◆

Wallace, Kathleen G., and Hays, Judith. "Nursing Management of Chronic Pain," *Journal of Neurosurgical Nursing* 14(4):185-91, August 1982.

◆

Wiley, Loy, ed. "Muscular Dystrophy—A Nursing Point of View. Nursing Grand Rounds," *Nursing80* 10:45-9, January 1980.

Acknowledgments

◆ p. 40: Photo courtesy of Thomas J. Brady, MD, Assoc. Professor of Radiology, Harvard Univ. Medical School, and Asst. Radiologist, Massachusetts General Hospital, Boston.
◆ p. 41 top: Photo courtesy of Abass Alavi, MD, Professor of Radiology and Neurology, and Chief, Division of Nuclear Medicine, Hospital of the University of Pennsylvania, Philadelphia.
◆ p. 41 middle: Photo courtesy of Marc S. Lapayowker, MD, Chairman, Department of Radiology, Abington (Pa.) Memorial Hospital.
◆ p. 41 bottom: Photo courtesy of S. Warren Gross, MD, Chairman, Department of Radiology, Warminster (Pa.) General Hospital.
◆ p. 103 top: Photo reprinted from Donald L. Schotland, MD, *Muscular Dystrophy*, Medcom, Inc., 1971, and used with permission.
◆ p. 103 bottom: Photo courtesy of Lucy Rorke, MD, Neuropathology Department, Children's Hospital of Philadelphia.
◆ p. 114: Illustration adapted from Gail Solomon and Fred Plum, *Clinical Management of Seizures* (Philadelphia: W.B. Saunders, 1976), and used with permission.
◆ p. 156: Chart adapted from Mary T. O'Brien and Phyllis J. Pallett, *Total Care of the Stroke Patient* (Boston: Little, Brown & Co., 1978), and used with permission.

INDEX

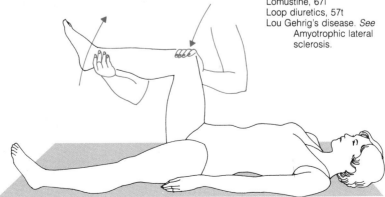

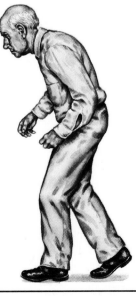

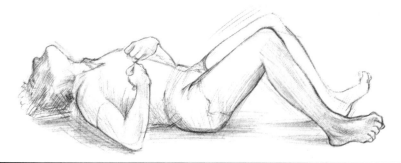

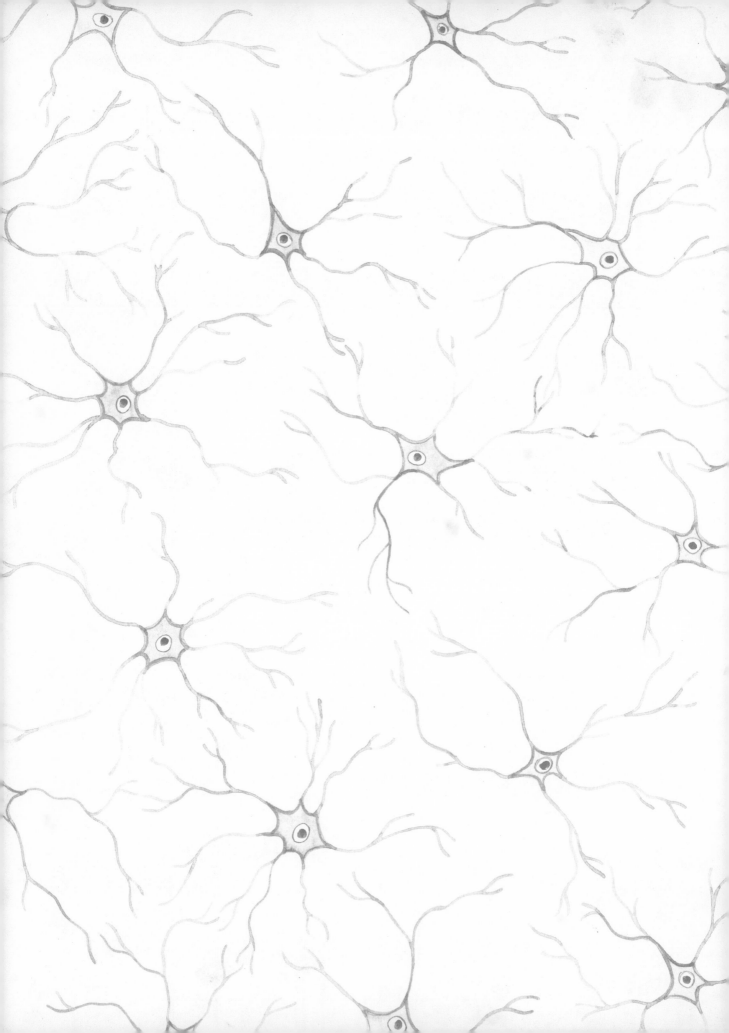